Cognitive-Behavioural Therapy

Research and practice in
health and social care

Second edition

Brian Sheldon

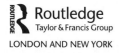
Routledge
Taylor & Francis Group

LONDON AND NEW YORK

First edition published
by Routledge 1995

This edition published 2011
by Routledge
2 Park Square, Milton Park, Abingdon, Oxon OX14 4RN

Simultaneously published in the USA and Canada
by Routledge
270 Madison Avenue, New York, NY 10016

Routledge is an imprint of the Taylor & Francis Group, an informa business

© 1995, 2011 Brian Sheldon

Typeset in Baskerville by
Keystroke, Station Road, Codsall, Wolverhampton
Printed and bound in Great Britain by
TJ International Ltd, Padstow, Cornwall

British Library Cataloguing in Publication Data
A catalogue record for this book is available from the British Library

Library of Congress Cataloging in Publication Data
Sheldon, Brian.
    Cognitive-behavioural therapy : research and practice in health and social care /
    Brian Sheldon. — 2nd ed.
        p. cm.
    Includes bibliographical references and index.
    1. Social case work—Great Britain. 2. Social case work—Moral and ethical aspects.
    3. Behavior modification. 4. Behaviorism (Psychology) 5. Cognitive therapy.
    6. Behavior therapy. I. Title. II. Title: Cognitive behavioral therapy.
    [DNLM: 1. Cognitive Therapy. 2. Ethics, Professional. 3. Social Work. WM
    425.5.C6]
    HV245.S47 2011
    361.3′20941—dc22   2010027991

ISBN13: 978–0–415–56436–6 (hbk)
ISBN13: 978–0–415–56435–9 (pbk)
ISBN13: 978–0–203–83371–1 (ebk)

For my grandsons Sonny and Cassius Ashcroft,
with abiding love.

Contents

Illustrations

Figures

Tables

About the author

Brian Sheldon is Emeritus Professor of Applied Social Research at the University of Exeter (UK). Before that he was Director of the Centre for Evidence-Based Social Services (a collaboration with twenty Local Authorities and Health Departments and the Department of Health) charged with research, development and dissemination functions. He holds qualifications in nursing, psychiatric social work and a PhD in psychology – which accounts for the multi-disciplinary nature of this book. He is the author of five books, many chapters in edited collections, and many research papers, mainly on the theme of developing evidence-based policy and practice in social care, health and throughout the helping professions. He is an ex-president of the British Association for Behavioural and Cognitive Psychotherapies, and throughout his academic career has continued to practise. He is an enthusiastic teacher of evidence-based approaches in general, and cognitive-behavioural therapy (CBT) in particular, both at home (387 conference presentations in ten years) and abroad, in the US, China and Scandinavia.

Brian Sheldon (who wrote his first paper on this subject in 1978) has campaigned steadily for the adoption of CBT approaches into mainstream practice. It now looks to be happening, so *sometimes* rationality wins out over fashion and vested interests. The task now is to ensure that the most needy gain ready access to this most scientifically validated and applicable of psychological treatments.

Preface

This book is intended as a comprehensive guide to cognitive-behavioural approaches particularly in the fields of health and social care. One can readily think of a range of helping professionals who may find it useful – social workers, psychiatric nurses, occupational therapists – but a new body of specialist, cognitive-behavioural therapists is emerging who see this as their main job, not as a subsidiary part of their professional duties, and it is intended for them too.

Although it started out as a second edition of *Cognitive-Behavioural Therapy* (Sheldon 1995), that book was aimed mainly at social workers who were then dragging their feet a little as to whether they could build CBT approaches into their practice (I confess some considerable loyalty to them but I'm now advocating a coalition). For now, when health and social care professionals are in ever closer cooperation, and the 'tribal customs' seem less worth defending than before, we have a chance to integrate services as never before, with considerable backing from research, and not just out of political convenience.

Dedicated graduate and postgraduate courses are now taking off at last, and this volume may be of some use to them and to psychologists whose courses have not always contained very much of this material. There may be a few GPs who would like to know more about what they are hoping to prescribe against the bureaucratic odds, and recently two of them plus a consultant anaesthetist attended my multi-disciplinary course in CBT, something to be celebrated I think.

The precepts which have informed me in writing this book are as follows: (1) that there is too much of a divide between academic research on the effectiveness of approaches, and routine clinical practice – with all its compromises and distractions. Therefore I have tried to write a 'real-world' text with real case examples; (2) much CBT practice (particularly when privately funded or on a contract) is carried out in consulting rooms and is, effectively, cognitive therapy with a 'homework' assignment or two. On the research evidence, and given the history of psychotherapy, this is a mistake. That a 'cognitive revolution' has occurred is without doubt, but less talked about is the 'behavioural revolution' which has influenced cognitive therapy. This book takes an integrated approach to human experience, both regarding what has gone wrong, and the prospects for recovery and rehabilitation. Thus, thinking, emotion and behaviour should never be artificially separated, or one or other element privileged over the others; (3) nor should helping professionals with an interest in these techniques, nor free-standing CBT professionals, ever allow themselves to be classified as 'psychological technicians'. They need to know about how this amalgam was developed; how well its approaches stand up to experimental scrutiny and to systematic reviews; what they are clearly good for, and what they *might* be good for if sympathetically adapted in the future.

This book looks at the historic development of this discipline, at the philosophical under-pinnings of it, and at the ethical considerations which sometimes come into play. It also looks at process factors, the *how* of helping as well as the *what*.

Acknowledgements

I would like to extend my gratitude to Rachael Macdonald, B.Sc. Cantab., Keith Walters, Dr Stephanie Tierney, Maggie Scoble, Sandra and Keith Andrews, Lindsay Andrews, the Routledge staff and Jodie Tierney for their invaluable assistance in the production of this book. My thanks also to the Centre for Evidence-Based Social Services team as abiding conditioned reinforcers, and to my co-author and friend, Professor Geraldine Macdonald of Queens University, Belfast who is always in my head when I write something.

Equal with colleagues in a ring
I sit on each calm evening,
  Enchanted as the flowers
The opening light draws out of hiding
From leaves with all its dove-like pleading
  Its logic and its powers.

That later we, though parted then
May still recall these evenings when
  Fear gave his watch no look;
The lion griefs loped from the shade
And on our knees their muzzles laid,
  And Death put down his book.
          W.H. Auden, 'A Summer Night'

Part One

History, development and distinctive features of cognitive-behavioural therapy

1 Origins and development of cognitive-behavioural therapy

With a name like yours, you might be any shape almost.

(Lewis Carroll 1872: 192)

Definition

Cognitive-behavioural therapy (CBT) is an evidence-based psychological approach, practised by a range of professionals, for the treatment of mental health and other personal and family problems. It seeks to help clients to analyse and 'reality test' existing patterns of thinking, emotional reactions and behaviour identified via an assessment of current difficulties, and to try out new approaches in a stepwise fashion, monitoring and evaluating effects in all three areas.

This will do for now, since in complex fields (this is one) definitions, though necessary, tend to be either pithy but self-referential (so that one worries about the details left out) or all-encompassing but rather like short essays in themselves. Pity the 2008 Reith Lecturer Daniel Barenboim who had to define *Music*. He came up with 'sonorous air' and then spent five hours on the complications. Adopting this approach, there follows a critical review of the main characteristics of CBT both as a collection of techniques and as a discipline.

The interrelation of thoughts, feelings and behaviour

CBT promotes rational/logical analysis of thoughts, whether in the direction of less pessimistic, less fatalistic appraisals in cases of depression; in the direction of less sanguine estimates of risk in harm reduction approaches to substance misuse or in relapse-prevention programmes in mental health. It also encourages an analysis of emotions, their circumstantial triggers, and the consequences they have for thinking and behaviour. CBT encourages clients empirically to test out their fears or avoidance reactions to see what *actually* happens if they react differently. Next comes a concentration on behaviour linked to problems, or which may even constitute 'the problem' itself. For research has repeatedly told us that the gap between insight, understanding and future action remains the largest, most underestimated obstacle to useful, therapeutically derived change. After all, are we not ourselves (usually the much less up against it) *full* of knowledge about semi-automatic patterns of cognitive appraisal, stereotypes, preferences, prejudices, habits; emotional over- or under-reactions; avoidant or self-defeating actions? But do we not often continue in very similar ways?

Thus the behavioural psychology principles: (1) that no one ever learned to swim through tutorials on the topic; (2) that some clients are simply unequipped by previous learning experiences to behave differently (behavioural deficits); (3) that these gaps need remedial action, and that positive reinforcement for new, trial behaviours must be arranged; (4) that whatever concomitant interpretive cognitions are implicated, when it come to evaluations of therapeutic good intentions, useful change in *behaviour* is the Gold Standard which gives credence to reports of changed mood or more rational patterns of thought.

It is interesting to note in this connection how, over the decades, different schools of psychology have emphasised one or other of these three strands of human experience (see Figure 1.1). Thus, psychoanalysis held/holds that feelings, particularly repressed sexual feelings, trump everything else. The radical behaviourists held that hard- or impossible-to-verify inner experiences such as thoughts and feelings are *concomitants* of interaction with an ambivalent physical and social environment; and were/are a bar to scientific development, suggesting that these probably do not even exist in the forms in which they are popularly conceived (see Chapter 4; Skinner 1953, 1974). Cognitive therapists (see Beck 1976), on the other hand, see thoughts and patterns of inaccurate causal attribution as primary; as more than just the triggers and maintainers of maladaptive emotions and behaviour. Their thinking is that the other two brute elements will fall into line when these cognitions have been clarified. However, some persuasive research suggests that it may just be the other way around, and that they are underestimating the power of emotion (see Le Doux 2003).

Unreconstructed proponents of each of these schools will always react to such summaries as (hurt but coping) victims of stereotyping, but analyses of the psychological knowledge on which their disciplines rest (see Bergin & Garfield 1994; Eysenck 1978, 1985) confirm *just* these emphases; *just* these practices, *just* these priorities, *just* these blindspots. However, when psychoanalysts came to evaluate their work (if they did at all) they could not escape at least glancing at subsequent behavioural change, not just at the 'revealing' content of the therapeutic discourse. Similarly, behaviour therapists have always wielded much of their influence through words, interpretations and plans. The point being that in each case these other considerations were seen as *subsidiary* influences.

The questions for all would-be helpers considering a particular approach are therefore: (1) what are their views of the direction of causality in problems – the key element in aetiology – and (2) what factors are routinely being privileged over others? One can now encounter, oxymoronically, 'brief, psychoanalytical therapy' delivered by therapists who have not themselves been analysed; cognitive therapists who accompany their clients on behavioural expeditions or give 'homework assignments', or behaviourists who devote a considerable portion of their sessions to how clients interpret and selectively perceive stimuli – including environmental feedback from their own behaviour. This does not however alter the point that schools of psychotherapy have tended to carve up human experience to match their embedded theoretical views on the causes of problems and therefore on the priorities for interventions.

I would like to have been able to end this first foray with the sentence, 'By contrast, CBT practitioners . . .' but in all honesty I cannot. So I will say instead that a close reading of the literature of CBT in its academic and practice forms shows a promising trend towards the *integration* of these three elements, both when investigating causes and regarding the priorities of practice (see Lambert 2004: ch. 10).

This *combination* of targets of potential influence, plus the fact that the means by which it is sought derive from rigorous studies, and which are then themselves subjected to evaluation, places CBT in a dominant position. There is simply nothing to compare with this approach elsewhere in the literature on psycho-social interventions (see Lambert 2004; NIHCE 2005a, 2005b, 2007a, 2007b). What could stand in the way of steady consolidation and wider application then? I see two factors which might do so.

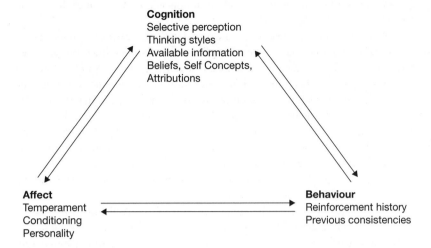

Figure 1.1 Interactions between cognition, behaviour and affect

First, we still tend to undervalue the need for a 'logical fit' between *nature and development of* research, and studies of therapeutic *effects*, even though its presence appears to be the best predictor of positive outcomes. An earlier generation of psychiatrists did just go 'empirical', i.e. they tried out approaches that *seemed* to work in one or another setting then casually extrapolated them to other, quite different ones and just waited to see what happened without too many concerns as to *why* it did. And ourselves?:

> Referring to Cognitive-Behaviour Therapy by its acronym – CBT – gives the appearance of a unitary therapy, but CBT is better seen as an increasingly diverse set of problem-specific interventions. These draw on a common base of behavioural and cognitive models of psychological disorders and utilize a set of overlapping techniques, but show significant variations in the way in which these techniques are applied.
>
> (Roth & Pilling 2008: 129)

CBT is broadening, then; the approach is increasingly in the hands of people from different professional backgrounds who emphasise different features of the model, and, it is strongly implied in the contemporary literature that this augers well for creative diversity. 'Let a hundred flowers bloom, a hundred schools of thought contend' (Mao Tse Tung). So long as they *do* freely and openly contend, that is. Research designs able to prise out worthwhile effect sizes connectable to small behavioural differences and verbal emphases among therapists are notoriously hard to pull off. One such area of 'development' is the increasing tendency for one or other element of the CBT model to receive additional and sometimes exclusive emphasis: most notably the cognitive component. Under the banner of CBT many practitioners have adopted an approach that might more accurately be called Cbt, just as an earlier generation clung to the known effectiveness of what amounted to cBt. We also, with the rather belated discovery of process factors by clinical psychologists (social workers have been obsessed by them for decades), see forms of attempted engagement with clients that are much closer to the 'humanistic' approaches of Carl Rogers, Beisteck and others (see Lambert *et al.* 2004; Sheldon & Macdonald 2009), cbT as it might be called. The adjectives have started to proliferate and we now have 'ecological', humanistic', 'meta', 'mindfulness' and other forms advertised.

Second, a sense of novelty, and having one's name associated with a new approach can be very reinforcing, but take note that many other disciplines have skipped down the primrose path to sectarian certainty before. Early studies of the effectiveness of social work (see Sheldon 1986) have shown that *process* had become all, but at the expense of outcome research. The results of the early experimental trials were disappointing to say the least (Fischer 1973, 1976; Macdonald & Sheldon 1992). Colleagues in family therapy are only now beginning to talk civilly to each other, having splintered into many different sects (e.g. Milan School, functional, structural, postmodernist), emphasising what to outsiders are not very distinctive aspects of technique, i.e. seeing everybody together. Freud (and he would have known) described similar tendencies in psychoanalysis as due to 'the narcissism of small differences'. We should, perhaps, apply a little learning theory to these tendencies.

What environmental factors shape the behaviour of therapists? Well, the B in CBT is awkward for a start; it takes one out of the controlled conditions of the interview room and into the rain; to the school gates, into homes after 6 p.m., into the hospital, into meetings with employers, *outside* to see for oneself the obstacles to change present in real-life conditions. How much more professionally comfortable and 'efficient' (i.e. convenient) just to talk about and analyse *thoughts* about these contingencies and how best to respond to them. Add to these enticements the preference of modern 'top-down' organisations for 'battery' rather than 'free range' employees – so that staff in the helping professions now struggle to see their clients face to face for more than 20 per cent of the working week – and you have a recipe for 'virtual reality' therapy (see Sheldon & Chilvers 2000; Sheldon & Macdonald 2009).

Please let it be understood that I am arguing here against a *general*, a priori aetiology-squeezing preference; I am in favour of decisions based on a specific history and a formulation regarding *which* psychological and environmental factors probably hold sway in a given case. Indeed, collaboratively adjusting therapeutic content according to the client's history and goals should be a hallmark of CBT. Thus, if a range of problems, from low self-esteem to poor relationships with one's children, are traceable back to sexual abuse in childhood, then the cognitions regarding semi-conscious complicity that might be leading to inappropriate self-attribution and not to the machinations of the perpetrator, might mean that 80 per cent of sessions are sensibly devoted to trying to straighten out such mistaken, self-blaming thoughts. 'I think I was a prostitute at seven' began one client when her childhood history was probed by the present author. (Her stepfather had given her 'pocket money' and treats for 'secret favours' – she blamed herself, not him.) However, in other cases, say, in anxiety-based conditions, it is a failure to experiment with what might *actually* happen if fears are confronted, which might point to a predominantly behavioural approach. 'Horses for courses' then, not semi-automatic pre-selection of favoured emphases, should, if we were to take our own routine advice to clients, guide our practice.

Then there is the 'look-no-hands' effect to consider. In other words, the culturally pre-scribed view that the less directly related, the more distant, the less observable a set of contingencies associated with change, the greater the prestige and perceived expertise accorded to the helper. Which is why a mental health nurse exercising considerable expertise in line with a large body of research, walking a trembling agoraphobic client around a supermarket, is seen as giving technical back-up; but exploring the alleged, dark, visceral psycho-sexual origins of this fear in the consulting room is seen as more skilled. This is so even though the first approach will probably take about six one-hour sessions to complete and be very effective, and the second, three to five years, and probably make little difference other than to the client's bank balance (see Skinner 1974; Rachman & Wilson 1980; Eysenck 1985; Lambert 2004).

We need thus to consider whether the tendency to tinker about with tried-and-trusted treatment protocols and try continually to rebrand them is always a sign of disciplinary confidence and a wish to experiment, or whether it is sometimes closer to intellectual fidgeting or empire building. True experiments to see whether the range of CBT's effectiveness can be extended beyond its established clientele have been undertaken and sometimes the answer has been 'not really', or 'a little' (see Bergin & Garfield 1994; Lambert 2004); but then carefully controlled investigations with disappointing results are very precious so long as methodological standards have not been relaxed in the face of the worthy aspirations and the enthusiasm of participants, and that we take the lessons.

CBT is an evidence-based approach (discuss)

Above all other considerations, CBT claims to be an evidence-informed discipline, and we need to take a look at what this implies – since it must be more than a slogan. It means that practitioners should actively select a given approach because of the quantity and quality of research evidence, and not for any other reason associated with familiarity, occupational congeniality or 'image'.

Evidence-based practice is in fact quite an old idea. Mary Richmond was writing about the obstacles to it on the eve of the Russian Revolution (Richmond 1917); the first controlled experiments on the effects of social work were undertaken in the late 1940s/early 1950s (see Fischer 1976; Sheldon 1986; Sheldon & Macdonald 2009: chs 3–4) – as early as any medical trials, but with poor outcomes. The results now, from a very much larger body of research, are much more positive, due largely to the adoption of behavioural and cognitive behavioural approaches and the principles of task-centred casework (see Reid & Hanrahan 1980; Sheldon & Macdonald 2009: ch.10).

This idea, with its own regularly changing brand names, now appears to have found its time throughout the helping professions, so let us look at the essential factors, beginning with a definition:

> Evidence-Based practice is the conscientious, explicit and judicious use of current best evidence in making decisions about the future well-being of clients.
>
> (adapted from Sackett *et al.* 1996)

How does this definition, adapted from the field of evidence-based medicine, translate to psycho-social approaches? The word *conscientious* surely reminds us of the need to give practical expression to hovering codes of ethics, particularly regarding the validity and reliability of recipes from research which we then try out on vulnerable people. There is after all no point in 'happy-clappy' mission statement commitments to provide non-discriminatory, non-postcode lottery-based, speedy access to *ineffective* help.

Hippocrates counselled his student physicians thus: 'First, do no harm.' Can it be said that we in the would-be helping professions, and psychotherapy in particular, do no harm? Sins of omission (e.g. blinkeredly underestimated suicide risks in mental health cases (see Appleby 1997; Parsloe 1999), or of 'commission' (e.g. moral panic attacks following failures of vigilance in child maltreatment cases), or scares about child sexual abuse under the influence of 'recovered memory' doctrines, have all hit the headlines and have led to the development of a 'blame culture' in professional life, which probably increases rather than diminishes risks (see O'Neill 2002; Munro 2006). Any intervention with a capacity for good may well carry a capacity for harm (you can overdose on vitamin C if you try hard enough). But the 'frozen watchfulness' which characterises many services today is not really a valid ethical option. We must instead acknowledge that it is perfectly possible for well-meaning, good-hearted, intelligent, well-qualified, hard-working professionals to do little good at all with a promising approach, or even sometimes to make things worse. This is a fact of professional life about which, pending the delivery to us of the long awaited crystal ball technology with which so far only journalists and politicians have been equipped, we can only acknowledge and take judicious precautions against, i.e.:

1   Outside genuine clinical experiments, we can ensure that the approach we are using has been tried out before and has been subjected to methodically robust studies. In other words we can search the back catalogue for advice on applications and known side-effects. This is easier said than done where clients, having saved up problems with which they have struggled for some time, are anxious to begin doing *something now* about their troubles. Thus there is often a tension between thinking, assessing and doing. If the need for the former is explained to clients – as something that *we* need if we are to help – my experience is that most accept it on the medical analogy that instant diagnosis and treatment in all but dire emergencies would not be reassuring. Evidence-based practice then depends on reading, appraising and tailoring, not on stock responses to predefined problems. The pressure is on for just this, but outcome evidence is clear that 'bespoke' rather than 'off-the-peg' interventions are superior and safer (see Wodarski & Thyer 1998: vol. 2; Sheldon & Macdonald 2009: chs 3, 4 and 10; Gambrill 2010).

2   We should make use of standardised risk assessment tools and diagnostic profiles and look more closely at epidemiological data. For example, even where there is apparent contrition, reviews of cases of violence against women show that 60 per cent of perpetrators do it again anyway. Nothing predicts behaviour like behaviour. The question must be: Does the *present* case have features which place it firmly in the 40 per cent cohort and will it stay there? Thus risk assessments are not one-off exercises (see Chapter 6). Reviews in the light of new information; of progress or lack of it; concerns from third parties and so on are vital. For even in intensive cases, would-be helpers are, inevitably, not *in situ* for much of the time.

3   We can try to avoid falling in love with theories; either those on which interventions are based, or those which try to account for the aetiology of the problems that confront us. This is difficult, because those who make use of applied psychology are required to give something of themselves emotionally and so tend to form other than 'just good friends' attachments to the ideas behind what we do. We are consequently prone to sulk when others criticise our faith in them.

The literature of the helping professions is full of examples where 'commitment to' this or that (one of the commonest phrases in professional references) has overtaken a conscientious mindset and the need for a self-denying ordinance regarding questions of evidence. There is one famous example: three of Freud's cases featuring the 'neuroses' of six women – supposedly exhibiting 'hysterical conversion symptoms' – would today have brought him before the General Medical Council. In the case of one patient (Emma B) being treated for 'hysterical nosebleeds', it later transpired that a ribbon of surgical gauze had been left in one of her nasal cavities during an operation. What was the reaction to the news that this was the case? A letter from Freud to his collaborator Fleiss contains the following views:

She began to feel restless out of unconscious longing and the intention of drawing me to her side. And since I did not come during the night, she renewed the haemorrhage as an unfailing means of reactivating my affections.

(Freud, in Malcolm 1984: 49)

Note the absence of repentance (Think again, Leon Festinger). The preservation of the theory is all, as it was during the infamous Orkney Islands cases of alleged 'satanic abuse' of children there (see Dalrymple 1994; Sheldon & Macdonald 2009: 43). Many children were brought into care in an almost military-style operation, and were interviewed by child therapists about the lurid stories featuring 'infant sacrifices and fiery crosses' that were circulating, but persistent denials from the children that anything of the sort had taken place were always reinterpreted.

To misdiagnose something in a complex case is forgivable providing that counter-information has been attended to, and not zealously explained away. Evidence-based practice is thus an ethical as well as a technical requirement for good practice.

Explicitness is the next keyword in our definition (Latin, *explicitus est liber*, the book is unrolled). However, until recently the very last thing that most users of psychotherapeutic techniques would be guilty of is giving considered, explicit advice. Intendedly helpful relationships were, until the advent of behaviour therapy, characterised by a more tactical, coded form of communication. Client opinion studies of the process of what it was like to receive psychological or social assistance are littered with accounts of confusion about diagnosis; roles; the purpose and direction of interpretations, and complaints about an apparently cool, uncaring demeanour from the would-be helper, resulting in disengagement in many cases (see Strupp *et al.* 1977; Eysenck 1985).

Yet, for reasons already discussed, the edifice which Freud and his followers erected remains prominent in the culture, and failures in outcome experiments and accounts of serious professional misjudgement are set aside. Here is W.H. Auden's forgiving appraisal of the man:

> If often he was wrong and, at times absurd,
> To us he is no more a person
> Now but a whole climate of opinion.
> (Auden 1976: 273–276)

But can you think of any other belief system where adulation, *despite* scientific or practical failures, or adverse reactions would still be merited? (Marxian political theory or 'market capitalism' are – given recent experience – the best candidate answers.)

Let us turn next to the contribution of 'person-centred' 'humanistic' approaches. These doctrines assume two things: (1) that solutions to problems lie inside people and require only release through supportive, confirmatory and clarificatory statements; and (2) that any attempts at advice or an explicit statement of opinion will serve only to weaken an already compromised capacity for self-direction, and may in any case be ignored as externally-imposed when difficulties arise in implementation. This approach too can threaten *genuineness* (see p. 70) in therapeutic encounters (see Truax & Carkhuff 1967; Hill & Lambert 2004), since clients tend to get thoughts and feelings they already know they have relentlessly batted back to them. Just imagine bumping into Carl Rogers on campus, asking the way to the library, and getting back 'I sense that you feel lost'.

The idea central to CBT is that therapeutic relationships should be based on an open, contractual, negotiating style, where the therapist and the client are recognised as bringing two overlapping types of expertise to the encounter: the client's 'insider' knowledge of the details of history and current circumstances, and of the thoughts and feelings which accompany their dilemmas; and that of the therapist, who has knowledge to contribute from research and theory, clinical experience, plus a measure of objectivity. There are provisos though. First, a rather romantic view has grown up, particularly in the mental health field, that clients' views contain a special kind of truth and should always predominate in the design and delivery of services. But then, realistically, it is these very personal but not always accurate certainties that therapists often have to encourage clients to analyse and think about. It is surely the pre-set rules of free discussion, which are more likely to give clients a voice, either individually or collectively. A jump from 'the clinician always knows best' to 'clients always know best' is no solution to power imbalances. Second, what *kind* of research and theory? Over the years we have seen similarly polarised patterns develop in psychotherapeutic practice, from the 'outcome is all' stance of the behaviourists and some modern managers, to the 'process is all' views of Rogers and others (see Sheldon & Macdonald 2009: ch. 6). However, regarding this brand of 'humanistic' psychology we need to remind ourselves that there is nothing particularly 'humanistic' about an approach which does not achieve good results.

What professionals *say* they believe in and hope to achieve, and what they actually *do*, are, research tells us, somewhat different things. Similarly, many previous approaches developed in closely controlled experimental studies do not always 'travel well' to routine practice (see Orlinsky *et al.* 2004; Roth & Pilling 2008).

We also have some relevant evidence from the social work field, since this group once had a dubious reputation for long-term 'supportive' interventions which were not always well focused, but who then eventually decided to do something about the problem. Look at this conclusion from a study of mental health aftercare:

> These examples point to the conclusion that it was not unreasonable for clients to perceive social work as a relatively timeless friendship in which help was available to weather crises rather than to resolve or avoid them.
>
> (Fisher *et al.* 1984: 63; see also Macdonald & Sheldon 1997: ch. 6)

However, just before this confirmation of the staying power of process-dominated approaches, a review appeared containing evidence of useful change attributable to the use of focused, time-limited approaches, largely concerned with the 'here and now'.

> In brief, one is struck by the dominance of structured forms of practice in these experiments – that is, of practice that takes the form of well-explicated, well-organised procedures usually carried out in a stepwise manner and designed to achieve relatively specific goals. The influence of the behavioural movement is quite apparent and pervasive.
>
> (Reid & Hanrahan 1980: 11–12)

At the World Behavioural Therapy Conference in Edinburgh in 1988, I saw a wonderful T-shirt logo: 'Talk Normal' it read, and to this day (readily forgiving the grammatical lapse) I can think of no better advice regarding the technical and ethical usefulness of explicit communication free of 'special voices'.

The next key word in our definition of evidence-based practice is *judicious*, which means '*sensible, prudent; sound in Judgement*' (OED).

This principle presses upon us that not all that *could* be done *should* be done, but also that some interventions which appear expensive in the short term may turn out to be a bargain in the longer term. Preventive work with children and adolescents springs to mind. But not waiting until the next serious crisis grabs our attention before investing in some precautionary involve-ment, though an obvious approach, is threatening to budgetary control staff, and does not reinforce cooperation among politicians elected for a term of four to five years – hence the mess and chronic indecision over the care of elderly people despite a convincing Royal Commission Report; endless research reviews and government reports over the years (see Wanless 2006).

In the NHS and Social Services, managing these pressures reminds one of the tricks perfected by jugglers of keeping two dozen plates spinning on a table at once. They had to develop an acute sense of which plate (or person in our case) is wobbling dangerously and give it/them a quick 'spin'. This situation gives the surface impression of skill and control, but ignores the effectiveness question. Study after study has shown that clients value helpers who are on side with them in a problem-solving, problem-preventing way, and are conscious of a steady, predictable, stepwise process which addresses difficulties until a growing sense of competence begins to appear (see Lambert 2004; Sheldon & Macdonald 2009: Part 1). Such a preventive emphasis (get your car serviced; don't wait until your wobbly tooth drops out before seeing the dentist) needs to be distinguished from (not *always* as judicious as they sound) mass screening programmes. These are often replete with false positives and false negatives, produce increased anxiety, and not always much improved treatment (see Gambrill 2010). The same applies to the modern political obsession for mass databases, which when con-cerned with allegedly foreseeable trouble provide a rich culture medium in which unintended consequences grow and multiply.

A corollary to all this is that each individual therapeutic encounter should ideally be thought about by both parties in the light of what went on in the previous meeting, and that the early stages of each interview should be about agenda-setting. Easy to say, but many studies reveal how the parties bring different expectations with them into the interview room and then fail to notice any discrepancies. Typical of this is the desire of the therapist to get back to the 'forensics' of earlier experiences to make sure that the common origins of difficulties are pinned down, and the client's desire to discuss *current* difficulties (see Mayer & Timms 1970; Salzberger-Wittenberg 1970; Sheldon & Macdonald 2009: ch. 3).

Thus evidence-based practice is about weighing up such tensions, competing claims and differences in understanding, making them explicit, and then choosing an openly negotiated way forward. However, there are many influences in professional life which blow us away from such a sensible course. Pragmatic judgement about the *content* of schemes as well as their names, shape, whether they might deliver credible *numbers*; and clinically and not just *statistically* significant outcomes, has been out of fashion for four decades at least. This impacts distractingly upon day-to-day practice, directing us towards too much concern for the *wants* of the monitoring classes, and too little for the *needs* of clients. These distortions also influence who gets referred in the first place. Clinically depressed elderly people often do not, for example, despite the fact that the outcomes from CBT are as good as with any other age group, and that there are many other collateral benefits from regular contact (to say nothing of a debt of honour to repay).

This brings us to the next key phrase in our definition: *current best evidence*. Let us take 'best' first. This is an awkward idea in some participating disciplines. It implies that some studies, either of the origins of psychological problems or of how best to approach them, are superior to others, and not just 'different'. Look at this frank account about the current standing of the applied social sciences – which overlap considerably with applied psychology:

> Social scientists, like medical scientists, have a vast store of factual information and an arsenal of sophisticated statistical techniques for its analysis. They are intellectually capable.

Many of their leading thinkers will tell you, if asked, that all is well, that the disciplines are on track – sort of, more or less. Still it is obvious to even casual inspection that the efforts of social scientists are snarled by disunity and a failure of vision. And the reasons for the confusion are becoming increasingly clear. Social scientists by and large spurn the idea of the hierarchical ordering of knowledge that unites and drives the natural sciences. Split into independent cadres, they stress precision in words within their speciality, but seldom spread the same technical language from one speciality to the next. A great many even enjoy the resulting overall atmosphere of chaos, mistaking it for creative ferment.

(Wilson and Fairburn 1998: 201)

Francis Bacon (1605) addressed the epistemological difficulties alluded to above succinctly when he declared that '*What is known depends upon how it is known*'. Quite.

Despite the continuing debates on what exactly *is* evidence, sometimes it is hard not to see these as a form of avoidance behaviour (see Chapter 4). For me it is difficult to conceive that any fair-minded surveyor of the field of psychotherapy effectiveness would not conclude – after all the conflicts over the alleged superiority of different methods (see Eysenck 1985); after all the 'pre-emptive disqualification' attempts by psychoanalysts and now the 'postmodernists' (see Sheldon 2001; Webb 2001), after all the methodological wrangling over studies and reviews – that the arguments put forward by Wilson (above) have not settled the matter. In Thomas Kuhn's (1970) terms we have now embarked upon a period of 'normal science'. That is, what the 'game' is has been decided upon; the rules have been written down; anyone can take part if they qualify and abide by these rules; the 'offside' rule has been clarified; you *can* argue with the umpires, providing you do so evidentially and respectfully and it doesn't go on for ever. 'Pitch conditions', and who/what the home team is up against will make a difference, so expectations may need to be considered. The rest is down to score rates, which, given their feedback effects, should rise steadily before they tail off. The staging costs too need to have an eye kept on them, but otherwise these matters have been pretty well sorted. We have a paradigm to work within, and we can tinker with the rules as we go along, so let's get on with it. In other words, for once there *is* a little room for complacency regarding CBT applications.

Table 1.1 gives an explanation of the hierarchy of research and evaluation methods, ordered according to the degree to which they minimise the effects of sources of bias.

As for the need for occasional changes of emphasis in the standard protocol, there are a few remaining problems with some kinds of research and our attitudes to them which still deserve attention.

Research studies are sometimes divided artificially into *qualitative* or *quantative* types. The first description is often accompanied by explanations that the usual methodological rules should be relaxed owing to the worthiness of the endeavour, or because of 'complexity'. If we are seeking to understand what it is like for clients to stay in a psychiatric unit, or how helpful or otherwise they find the local day centre, then we should probably conduct interviews against a pre-piloted schedule, standardised as far as possible in line with existing knowledge, but with scope for capturing outlying opinions and experiences. Qualitative research therefore seeks to answer why? and how? questions and needs to address feelings as well as yes/no/how much? outcomes. However, the rules about sample representativeness and not leading the witnesses, and about not casually extrapolating from one dataset to others, still apply. Similarly, there need to be transparent rules about sample selection and the selection of 'telling' testimony from the welter of 'ordinary' comments. For qualitative, interview-based studies typically generate masses of data – which raises the question, Why was *that* particular comment included in the report and others regarded as 'less relevant'? The answer is usually through pattern-seeking and pattern-making by the researcher. There are now software programmes to help contain these tendencies, but they are not consistently used, and the researchers' a priori views (e.g. 'something is wrong with this service' so scan for negative comments to confirm this) lead often to our overlooking less polarised or less dramatic testimonies. I once worked next door to a qualitative researcher who had the task of reducing hours of tape recordings of service users' comments to summaries suitable for publication. One could hear the constant clunking of the editor's foot pedal, and fast-forward whirring noises, which always raised the question: Why are we going to get to read *that* testimony, and not the rest?

Complex fields and complex interventions research are still worryingly under-represented in the research output on CBT (see Chapter 2). This concerns me because many of our regular areas of operation are with conditions that are bio-psycho-social in nature and require an *array* of services. Nevertheless, these have increased in quantity and quality in recent years (see www.cochrane.org; james.lindlibrary.org; MRC 2003).The fact is that we are rarely, if ever, dealing with single interventions for unidimensional problems, the point being that it takes an awful lot of self-deception or later special pleading to exclude quantitative factors from qualitative research, or qualitative factors from quantitative research. Rather we must look to the concept of *attributive confidence* and issues of validity and rehability whatever the methodology employed. Otherwise mere therapeutic fashion will fill the vacuum.

If you have some sympathy with these precepts, then these words, from arguably our best-ever cultural historian, might resonate:

> Our intellectual history is a succession of periods of inflation and deflation; when the imagination grows too luxuriant at the expense of careful observations and detail there is a salutary reaction towards austerity and the unadorned facts; where the accounts of these grow so colourless, bleak and pessimistic, the public begins to wonders why so dreary an activity, so little connected with human interest, is worth pursuing at all.
>
> (Berlin 1996: 27)

We have intellectual resources as never before to support our discipline, and unprecedented access to these via the internet. However, there are side-effects to contend with. Training courses often move too quickly away from the teaching of basic theory, particularly learning theory, in all its generalisable richness, to specialist work within modules about this or that particular type of case. We often equip students with critical appraisal skills (see Gibbs 1991) much too late in the sequence, when 'internet promiscuity' may already have established itself – i.e. the habit of clicking on supportive studies to back an intervention, or a take on an essay pretty well decided upon already. Systematic reviews, the best remedy for such bad habits, nevertheless need to be to be approached with the same forensic attitudes as experimental studies (see Littell (2008) for an excellent guide to chastity in this regard).

The word 'theory' as used above, evokes mixed feelings in our culture. It means two things at once:

> *Theory:* a plausible or scientifically acceptable general principle or body of knowledge offered to explain phenomena. The analysis of facts is their relation to one another. *Theory*, abstract thought; speculation.
>
> (OED)

In the applied psychology field the British, closely followed by the Americans, but hardly at all by the continental Europeans, have tended towards the vernacular 'it's just theory', so

Table 1.1 Questions of attributive confidence in different types of research

Methodology	Procedure	Attributive confidence
Systematic reviews of randomised controlled trials: These synthesise the evidence from research on the effects of an intervention designed to address an issue for a pre-specified sample/ population. Where possible, effect sizes from comparisons of one approach with another, or with no intervention, are calculated.	Reviews are conducted in line with a pre-specified protocol, in which reviewers make explicit their working assumptions and proposed methodology. Exhaustive searches for relevant studies, an unvarnished presentation of results and implications, plus regular updating, are other hallmarks.	Well-conducted systematic reviews minimise sources of reviewer bias. If well managed, they provide our most secure results. Negative conclusions are also valuable.
Randomised controlled trials in which participants are randomly allocated to an experimental intervention or a control group, and the results compared.	One group (the experimental group) receives as consistent as possible an exposure to the intervention under test. The other receives no service, or management as usual, or non-specific attention (since attention and belief in the expertise of helpers also have strong effects). Rarely, studies have three conditions – no intervention, standard intervention and test intervention – compared. Outcomes are assessed against specific quantitative outcome indicators (e.g. readmission to hospital, recidivism).	Well-conducted trials minimise a number of sources of bias, but each of these needs to be carefully assessed, including confounders such as significant baseline differences across groups (which randomisation may not eliminate); biases in allocation concealment, outcome assessment and differential drop-out rates between the two groups.
Quasi-experimental studies	These are comparison studies in which participants have been matched on variables known to confound results (e.g. race, gender, class).	Useful where different services are routinely introduced in one area but not in another and a good source of hypotheses for more rigorous tests. The absence of random allocation means we can never be sure that we are comparing like with like, given that unknown factors may also influence outcomes.
Narrative reviews: These are not usually as exhaustive as systematic reviews and tend to have less explicit inclusion and exclusion criteria.	Authors draw up a list of topics which they wish to search (e.g. 'social work in general hospitals'; 'supported housing for learning disabled people') and then track down likely sources and look for emergent trends and implications.	They suffer from the problem of 'convenience samples' (i.e. sources readily available to the authors), and from a higher possibility of selective perception than where a very tight, prepublished protocol is in place. Reviewers are more susceptible to privileging evidence that supports their preferred world views. Nevertheless, they are a good starting point in the absence of something more rigorous.

Table 1.1 (continued)

Methodology	Procedure	Attributive confidence
Single group, pre-post tests: Sometimes known as time-series designs, these procedures compare problems and gains on a before-and-after basis in a single sample.	Baseline (i.e. pre-intervention, preferably standardised) measures are taken in key problem areas prior to intervention (see Fischer and Corcoran (2007) for an accessible manual). They are then repeated at the end of the programme for comparison purposes.	Most evaluations in Social Services are post-only (see below) and so it is difficult to calculate the value added. This approach takes 'snapshots' of functions on a before-and-after basis. Nevertheless, it cannot determine the extent to which any improvements that occur are due to the mere passage of time (maturational factors) or to other factors unconnected with the intervention.
Post-test-only measures: This approach reviews outcomes only, without benefit of specific pre-intervention (baseline) measures.	A sample is chosen against criteria of need, type and extent of problem(s). The intervention is made, and then measures of outcomes are implemented.	Since many routine approaches and projects are still not evaluated at all, this may be better than nothing. It can be improved by standardised referral criteria being in place at the outset.
Client-opinion studies: Largely qualitative studies (occasionally with quantitative elements). Usually post-only, but there is no reason why pre-post qualitative measures should not be taken (there are, however, few examples of this happening).	A sample of clients receiving a particular intervention, or those with a particular set of problems, receiving a range of interventions are interviewed for their opinions on the effects of services and, usually, on the way in which services were provided.	These studies are rich in qualitative detail about what it is like to be on the receiving end of services. However, a common problem is representativeness. Do the respondents in the sample reflect the range of service user and problem characteristics? Random sampling of populations helps here. Should be routine in Health and Social Services as part of the service-planning process.
Single case designs: Largely quantitative measures (though there is no reason why standardised qualitative measures should not be included) (see Fischer and Corcoran 2007). Applied to single cases.	Measures are taken on a before-and-after basis (AB design) or before/after/follow-up basis (ABA designs), or even in experimental forms (ABAB designs) where interventions are baselined, the intervention made, then withdrawn, and then reinstated and differences noted. Mainly used in behaviour therapy, though there is no reason why this should be so, providing that case-specific behavioural change in line with the aims of a given approach are prespecified.	Should be more widely used by practitioners whatever the intervention method in use. Enable staff and clients to assess progress and adjust accordingly.

Source: Sheldon & Macdonald (2009: 75–77).

'proper scientific work not yet done' usage of the term. However, the awkward fact about theories and theorising, the process of 'joining up the dots' of observations and of scattered research findings, is that we are psychologically incapable of not having them or of not doing it. This is what we in CBT tell our clients in effect, and we should take the advice ourselves. Scores of studies on perception in all of our five senses and in memory all point to a tendency to see, hear and remember what we expect, and to transform these selections into patterns and predictions. This is particularly so if they are concordant with existing beliefs. Let us look at two examples. First, the assumption that negative, self-blaming thinking plays a major role in cases of clinical depression (it does) but the question is: Is this widely reported association causal or concomitant? In a classic study, Lewinsohn *et al.* (1981) gathered a large community sample of people with no particular clinical history and administered a standardised test of cognitive styles, then waited to see which of the participants acquired a diagnosis of clinical depression, and compared these with the rest. Against expectations, they concluded that:

> Prior to becoming depressed, these future depressives did not subscribe to irrational beliefs, they did not have lower expectations for positive outcomes or higher expectations for negative outcomes, they did not attribute success experiences to external causes and failure experience to internal causes, nor did they perceive themselves as having less control over the events in their lives.
>
> (Lewinsohn *et al.* 1981: 218)

A second example concerns R.D. Laing's proposal that schizophrenia was a product of disordered family communication and family power games. Most clinicians have seen these at work – as they often are in cases of anorexia nervosa. Yet, growing evidence on inherited factors, on brain chemistry differences (see Gottesman 1991; McGuffin *et al.* 2005) cast doubt upon a *causal* rule for such factors. More likely, clinicians were observing the social and psychological fall-out from debilitating illness and, under the influence of *One Flew over the Cuckoo's Nest* cultural influences, mixed the cocktail of 'postmodern' French philosophy (see Foucault 1965, 1987) and home-grown anti-establishment attitudes, that became 'anti-psychiatry'. It fitted the cultural mood of the 1960s and 1970s when psychiatrists of this persuasion began to appear on book jackets wearing kaftans. But with what harm (the theories, not the kaftans)? is the question. For we in the helping professions *try out* approaches, not just consider them.

So, since we cannot be above theorising, what can we do to anchor these propositions in solid, empirical research? Here are some suggestions.

The qualities of theories

We must begin by recognising that theories are not created equal; that many are logically incompatible with each other, and that we should *mind* that this is so and try to achieve a coherent synthesis. How? My first piece of advice is that the philosophy of science has already provided some good guidance (see Popper 1963; Oakley 2000). Here is a list of reasonable tests of beliefs and propositions:

1   In order to check up on the status of a theory at all it must be potentially refutable. This is Karl Popper's demarcation between what counts as scientific knowledge and what does not. Some theories contain inbuilt defences against disbelief (e.g. much of Freud's and

Marx's work; the literature on 'recovered memory' effects in the child abuse field). Although the arguments have great explanatory range (I dearly miss the presence of the occasional 'somewhat' or 'sometimes' in such accounts), they must occupy a lower position in any hierarchy stressing validity and reliability. The personal 'blind spots' of the unanalysed critic on the one hand, or the prejudices of class or gender on the other, withhold 'true understanding'. Daniel Dennett (2006) aptly calls this 'pre-emptive dis-qualification'. New interpretations arise to cope with each successive attack and the theory is in all cases left intact, or, as in debates about religion, there is a general charge of 'disrespect'. This intellectual sleight of hand is also to be found at the level of practice: if the goals of intervention are loosely defined ('flexible goals' as they are euphemistically called; see Chapter 6), then how are we to know with any certainty what has been achieved? Einstein once said of a paper critical of his work that it was 'not even wrong'. Irrefutability, either at the level of theories for practice or practice theory, is not a virtue but a vice.

2 Popper's second criterion of worth is that of 'riskiness of prediction'. The preferable theory is, contra-intuitively, the one that *prohibits* the most. Thus we should learn to prefer those explanations which place themselves at the greatest risk of refutation by predicting what ought *not* to occur. Cognitive-behavioural theories are thus preferable to psycho-dynamic and family therapy theories in this respect since they predict that direct intervention will not produce symptom substitution. If they do (they don't), the theory is endangered. Psychoanalytical concepts and 'humanistic psychology' run no such risks since, if the right degree or direction of behavioural change does not follow, then clients are deemed, retrospectively, not to have attained 'true insight' but are engaging in 'defensive intellectualisation', or to be 'unmotivated' as if their internal springs had wound down.

3 The next point of evaluation concerns testability. The good theory is that which produces relevant and testable hypotheses. Many quite elaborate theories produce very low yields of these operational 'so, on the best current evidence, what we should consider doing is . . .' statements, contrary to what we expect from our medical advisers and gas fitters.

4 Obviously the next point must concern the history of any attempts which have been made to test a theory or concept. Would-be helpers often respond to ideas because they are attractive in themselves; because they find ready support in an established system of values, because they have flattering implications, or because their tutors like them.

5 The next test is concerned with the degree of simplicity in a given theory. This test is called variously 'Occam's Razor' (after the philosopher William of Occam, or Ockham (1285–1349)) or the 'law of parsimony'. It proposes that the more economical the explanation of a given set of factors or events, the more preferable. Thus 'persuasion', or 'selective reinforcement of responses', might be preferable concepts to 'insight' for explaining therapeutically derived changes in clients.

6 Logical consistency comes next: the greater the harmony or internal consistency within a theory, the more preferable. Freud's adaptation of the Oedipus theory to cover little girls, the 'Electra Complex', has been taken up by feminist writers, who have largely ignored the fact that it has problems of internal inconsistency. What Freud predicts should happen is logically at odds with the rest of his theory.

7 Clarity of expression: the less ambiguous the presentation of a theory, the more preferable. This is not simply a reference to style (which can be a problem) but to the quality and clarity of the prescription contained within a statement. Thus, if the phrase 'family homeostasis' is used it must be operationally defined; otherwise potential users of the concept are entitled to ask how they will recognise this phenomenon should they

come across it, or think it absent. Getting the research question and attendant propositions right at the outset is a major precautionary feature of good systematic reviews.

8   In circumstances where no convincing explanation is available, the best that can be done is to attempt to develop what Karl Popper called 'criteria of relative potential satisfactoriness'. That is, we should try to construct the best 'template' possible as a guide to future investigation.

This leaves the word *current* in our definition of evidence-based practice to consider. This word needs to be distinguished from the rest, since not all findings that are recent *replace* earlier findings; in fact, such relegations are rare. More usually, earlier findings are built upon, added to or modified, and practitioners need to keep abreast of these changes. But they also need to remember that reviews and scatters of robust research should not be left unconsidered because of some idiosyncratic 'best before' date, particularly since much contemporary psychological research is more timid than it once was (see Schachter & Singer 1962; Milgram 1974). A good example to follow is that of the *Diagnostic and Statistical Manual* (DSM) with reworkings based on reliability studies and evidence-based revisions appearing every few years. We are now on DSM IV^{TR} (text revision). There are interesting changes to material on personality disorders (once seen as 'a diagnosis hardly worth making'); on the growth in recommendations for the use of CBT; and regarding grey areas on the borderlines of different diagnoses. There are occasions, particularly regarding pharmacological interventions, where major changes are recommended as a matter of urgency, but in complex psycho-social interventions, benign, ratchet-like progress is typified by smaller clicks and slippages. 'Multi-Systemic Therapy' (MST) is a short-term, home- and community-based intervention, and a close cousin of CBT, for social, emotional and/or behavioural problems (see Henggeler *et al.* 1998: ch. 8; Littell 2008; Sheldon & Macdonald 2009). There are thirty-seven reviews in print, but only 60 per cent of these are fully systematic, and questions have been raised about their independence, inclusion/exclusion criteria, and over-optimistic reports of results (confirmation bias). Thus we are in a less confident position than many thought previously regarding this approach, but it develops apace nevertheless (see Littell 2008).

If we wish to develop a knowledge base that is, for now, quite secure, and as free as possible from ideological bewitchment as we can make it, we cannot afford not to look out for and register such new developments – as we all expect to happen in medicine and air traffic control where we have an immediate personal interest. So, we all dislike the image of the ECT-happy psychiatrist – 'I've seen it work for years, we don't know how, but it does' (it does *a bit* in very serious case of depression, but with noteworthy side-effects) and the Prozac-happy GP – 'the answer's Fluoxetine, now what's the problem?' But how often do we ourselves fall into such convenient routines, ignoring effect-size balances and placing failures into a convenient 'nothing works for everyone' category?

A few years ago, to challenge the defensive position that psycho-social interventions are 'just different', and that less onerous rules have to be applied, was to invite derision. I set up a little experiment at a large multi-disciplinary mental health conference (see Sheldon & Chilvers 2000). This concerned 'case-management' – a method of organising contact and planning with clients which owes its origins to attempts to introduce 'business methods' to health and welfare services by Sir Roy Griffiths in 1988. He was the financial head of a large supermarket chain (we leave aside here, with the due humility rarely extended to us by consultants from other fields, the question of what a supermarket organised by members of the helping professions would be like to shop in). The conclusions of a systematic review of the effects of case-management approaches in mental health cases vs. standard clinical and social care (see Marshall *et al.* 1998) were read out, but the name of a mythical, neuroleptic medication, Lususoproxene, was substituted (Lusus is Latin for joke or playfulness). Here is what the audience heard:

> Lususoproxene increased the numbers remaining in contact with services. Lususoproxene doubled the approximate numbers admitted to psychiatric hospital. Except for a positive finding from one study, Lususoproxene showed no significant advantages over standard care on any psychiatric or social variable. Cost data did not favour Lususoproxene but insufficient information was available to permit definitive conclusions.

The audience were then asked what should be done about this medication and were overwhelmingly of the opinion that is should no longer be used. When they were let in on the Lusus, there was much discussion about this being a 'different sort of field' and therefore comparisons were invalid, and since these are matters of 'policy' practitioners can do little to influence them ('learned helplessness'). The consensus was that we might 'use with caution'. When asked 'how *much* caution?' the audience came to no particular conclusions, except for suggesting that guidelines and procedures are one thing and what actually goes on in practice is quite another: the 'Good Soldier Schweik' defence (see Hašek 1923).

The need to preserve a role for *intuition* or practice wisdom is the argument usually put forward to this conundrum of too much to know, too much to appraise and too much to do. The safeguarding of these allegedly valuable commodities is seen by some as the main case against the idea of evidence-based practice. I think that we cannot realistically do without either. Not even in the physical sciences do we proceed inductively until a mass of separate observations suddenly coalese into a pattern that we recognise as truth; they always need an interpreter (see Popper 1963: 53).

Translate this to the assessment process in CBT (see Chapter 6) and it means that (1) we cannot not have hunches, it's just not the way we are built, but (2) we are also built to have awareness of them, and so can turn them into potentially refutable hypotheses, and say to ourselves and our supervisors, 'what would it take for this idea not to be really the case?' We can watch out along the way for contra-evidence as well as psychologically tempting 'confirmations'. Our intuitions are thus only as good as our watchfulness procedures regarding these.

Practice wisdom is in the same territory; experience is valuable if it is valid, applicable experience, is pertinent to a given case and not just deemed to be so since it reminds one of other cases. Intuition is celebrated in our culture. Most cop dramas set a wise, case-hardened pro against a jumped-up superior who 'goes by the book'. Most medical dramas celebrate the 'off-the-wall' diagnosis which is difficult to defend to the style-cramping medical establishment. Entertaining if you are not *actually* being investigated by, or treated by, such people. A sensible compromise is on offer in the following quotation:

> Most contemporary scholarship on judgement concerns itself with how we might counteract biases that intrude on rational decision making by means of rigorous training in (social) statistics and probability theory. This effort is designed to improve our judgement by strengthening our reason. There is much to gain from this endeavour, for intuitive biases are many and their influence in decision making is often pernicious. An education in reason is all for the good. The problem is that this education is generally portrayed as a means of *replacing* intuitions with conscious, rational thought, and that any

such effort will prove counter-productive. The alternative, however, is not simply to give free range to intuitions. The task is to educate them.

(Thiele 2006: 120)

Cognitive-behavioural therapy is a structured, time-limited approach

Research across the helping professions has long shown that there are welcome effects which appear semi-independent of the actual techniques being employed. One such set derives from the *structuring* of encounters, another from process factors or therapist variables (see Chapter 2).

Early findings from outcome studies, and from client opinion and follow-up reports (see Eysenck 1985; Sheldon & Macdonald 2009: ch. 6) regularly reported a sense of vagueness about goals and how exactly they were to be achieved; a tendency to dwell on the long-lost origins of problems rather than deal with them in the here and now; far too much emphasis on 'insight' and too little on producing the behavioural and circumstantial changes that clients usually have their eyes on, and above all worries about sheer length of time that resolutions were expected to take. 'Therapeutic Micawberism.' As Dickens's character might have said, '*Something is definitely going to turn up in this case one of these days.*'

A later concentration on efficiency alongside effectiveness was born of two sets of factors: (1) many of the programmes for psychological and social help were publicly supported, or, in the US, tightly grant-aided (a set of dynamics amusingly characterised as 'Bambi meets Godzilla' by Lambert (2004: ch.1)); (2) the results of long-term interventions were being called increasingly into question by controlled studies (see Eysenck 1960, 1985): not only did these (predominantly psychoanalytic) methods not work, but they took forever not to work; (3) the emergence of behaviour therapy which is by its nature short-term, problem-focused and time-limited (see Wolpe 1958; Eysenck 1960, 1985: ch. 3) promised better, quicker results, without any evidence of the predicted 'symptom substitution' effect which was supposed to be its Achilles heel.

A meta-analysis of outcome studies by Howard *et al.* (1986) brought to our attention buried data on length of contact vs. reported gains (see Figure 1.2).

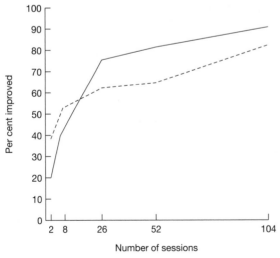

Figure 1.2 Relation of number of sessions and percentage of patients/clients improved

Note
Solid line = client ratings; dotted line = objective ratings (see Howard *et al.* (1986)).

Structured, time-limited approaches cut down on the scope for things clients regularly report that they find unhelpful, but humour in their therapists. That is, getting interminably stuck in histories; forays into 'interesting' side-issues; miscommunications which neither of the parties notice happening. This sort of occurrence is evident from an early study of the effects of counselling for clients from multi-problem families:

> There is almost a Kafkaresque quality about these interactions. To exaggerate only slightly, each of the parties assumed that the other shared certain of his/her underlying conceptions about behaviour and the ways in which it might be altered. Then, unaware of the inappropriateness of their extrapolations, each found special reasons to account for the others conduct.

> (Mayer & Timms 1970: 77)

The effect is still to be had (for an empirical study see Thwaite & Bennett-Levy 2007).

Clients often sign up for help at some personal cost because they want something troubling to stop, or something more fulfilling to begin. Positive and negative reinforcement effects operating in professional encounters are known to be important in recovery, but how are they to be recognised and interpreted unless there is a structure to support evaluation and feedback, i.e. a gentle, progress-chasing style?

Problems can often seem defeating to clients because they always consider them as a whole. Much of the success of behaviour therapy and CBT comes from an approach which breaks down problems into smaller, more manageable pieces. This has both positive and negative reinforcement effects. The rest has not been forgotten, just put on hold for a time – the time frame having been negotiated. There are also the benign effects of positive generalisation to be grateful for.

The question before us is: How much of a 'dose' of CBT is optimal? There are guidelines from BABCP and the American NABCP; there is experimental research, but then there are NHS and Social Services accountants. It is very pleasing to have (at last) effective forms of help for such disabling conditions as clinical depression, phobias, panic attacks or obsessive-compulsive disorder, but such benefits cannot be measured (and funded) as if they were the human equivalents of medications – however administratively convenient the idea. Most studies of the 'dose–effect' relationship show that between eight and ten sessions will give us most of what we want. But clients come in all shapes and sizes; older people may not want something quite so fast-paced; and some clients are far from being the YAVIS type (young, attractive, verbal, intelligent and successful) which featured in early reports of psychotherapy effects. It is tempting too to insert an 'R' for rich into this acronym.

Clients asked for their views on time-limited approaches regularly raise the issue of whether or not a *little* more time might not been enabled them to, as they see it, complete their tasks, rather than just being 'significantly improved' for cost–benefit analysis purposes. In my own practice I have regularly extended therapeutic contact for specific purposes which will not take for ever, and there is empirical support for this, for follow-up appointments, and for 'booster sessions' if problems recur. Clients value a little controlled flexibility in professional dealings, as do we all.

The history of cognitive-behavioural approaches

> Those who know no history are often condemned to relive it.
>
> (Karl Marx, paraphrasing Hegel)

Although there have been some genuinely reciprocal influences, on the whole CBT owes its present shape and scope to the grafting on of cognitive theories to applied behavioural psychology, which already worked well when nothing much else did. The transplant produced little in the way of 'auto-immune' responses, and it will be interesting to look at why, since schools of psychotherapy are often powerfully rejecting of what they see as 'foreign material'. Here is my own account, based on contemporary reports and my own experience as President of the then British Association for Behavioural Psychotherapy, at the time charged with helping to negotiate the terms of a merger so that we could secure government backing for a registration scheme incorporating the 'C' word.

1   Two pioneering sets of studies stand out as being influential. First, Wolpe (1958) through his research and clinical work on the principle of *reciprocal inhibition*, based on the work of Pavlov (1927) and the latter's colleague Cover Jones, who first raised the idea of therapeutic applications; and second, the work of Aaron T. Beck (1964, 1976), who pioneered cognitive therapy for depression and made important contributions to the academic study of the influence of thought patterns on this and other conditions. However the large influence of two other figures cannot be overlooked. Donald Meichenbaum (1977) produced a consolidating textbook full of accounts of clinical applications; and Albert Bandura, who in his *Principles of Behavior Modification* (1969) wrote a scientifically well-grounded account of how cognitively mediated and vicarious factors (modelling) influence learning.

2   Behaviourism, through producing many robust studies testifying to the effectiveness of therapeutic offshoots (see Bergin & Garfield 1971, 1978; Rachman & Wilson 1980), was coming to be seen as a philosophical dead-end (see Ayer 1973 and Chapter 3, this volume). The argument that internal events such as thoughts and all but the strongest of feelings were invisible to external observation and thus beyond the scope of science, and that we must therefore pretend that they don't *really* exist and try (interestingly, but vainly) to substitute behavioural correlates (Skinner 1953, 1974) was counter-cultural; upset most contemporary philosophers, but was reacted to by most informed commentators in 'so much the worse for science then' terms. However, one powerful effect that behaviourism did have was to bind together adherents into a school which defined itself by what it definitely was not: namely wishy-washy, ineffective in application, unscientific, mystical.

Thus, small bands who were Pharisaically 'glad that they were not as other men' tried to hold conversations about their work without mentioning minds, thoughts or attitudes, the point being that in almost all the accounts of the development of CBT, early proponents were *escaping* something, but were not entirely happy with the self-denying ordinance required by behaviourism. Here is Aaron Beck on the issue. Having come across anomalous findings in studies of depression (those of others, and his own) he saw his task as revising psychoanalytical theory so that 'laboratory findings' and clinical theory could be reconciled (fat chance then). He describes this attempt as requiring an 'amazing reappraisal' of his own belief system.

> Concurrently, I became somewhat painfully aware that the early promise of psychoanalysis that I had observed in the early 1950s was not borne out by the middle and late fifties – as my fellow psychoanalytic students and other colleagues entered their sixth and seventh years of psychoanalysis with no striking improvement

in their behaviour or feelings! Furthermore, I noted that many of my depressed patients reacted adversely to therapeutic interventions.

(Beck 1976: 16)

3   One should be careful of the 'great figures' views of history; they undoubtedly play a part, but so also does the climate in which their proposals either find favour or are sidelined. Looking at the assumptions of the major schools of psychology, one can see, as it were, 'sociological receptors' in place (e.g. the influence of 'steam-age' constructs in much of Freud's work, which is full of allusions to 'pressure vessel' dynamics, 'safety valves', etc.). The climate of unstoppable scientific progress in the 1950s certainly influenced the reception of behaviourist ideas – imagine that time, when clean, safe, nuclear science promised to remove the need for electricity bills (ahem) – and reworkings of mental health problems as purely environmental responses made redundant any suspicions that they might contain innate predispositions or have deep, dark psychosexual origins. Here is the philosopher Mary Midgley's reminiscence on the mood of those times:

> Any explanation that evoked culture, however vague, abstract, far-fetched, infertile and implausible, tended to be readily accepted, while any explanation in terms of innate tendencies, however careful, rigorous, well documented, limited and specific, tended to be ignored.

(Midgley 2003: 142–143)

The necessary correctives took a while to emerge in the literature (see Tsuang & Vandermey 1980; Gottesman 1991; Sheldon 1994; Pinker 2004).

4   The invention of the computer and associated interest in the idea of artificial intelligence influenced the development of systems models for thinking. Computer metaphors abound in cognitive therapy circles: 'hardware', 'software', 'information overload', 'download', etc. These analogies are often accompanied by decision trees and input/output flowcharts that resemble circuit diagrams. Whether thinking is not more analogue than digital is a question for later. The point for now is that we have learned much about decision flows and feedback loops from *them* (computers) even though we built them in the first place.

This discipline (cognitive science) has undergone rapid development and the danger now is desiccation, because in defining itself as a field it has come close to separating thinking from emotion. Have these people never been in love? Indeed, in *The Mind's New Science: A History of the Cognitive Revolution*, Howard Gardner (1987) lists its de-emphasis of affect as one of its defining features. This discipline is another example of historical compartmentalisation (see Damassio 1994). However, some modern authors argue for the benefits of *concilience* (see Pinker 2004); that is, that some of the most promising scientific developments occur when investigators hop over disciplinary fences to see what the neighbours are up to. Nevertheless, a defined disciplinary territory, with better than fair results in the outcome-research stakes, did mean that there was a common language within which to discuss the possibilities of a merger. Joseph Le Doux in his influential book *The Emotional Brain* (2003) plots a different course:

> All along some cognitive scientists have recognized that emotion is important. A. I. pioneer Herbert Simon (1962) for example, argued that cognitive models needed to

account for emotions in order to approximate real minds, and around the same time social psychologist Robert Abelson suggested that the field of cognitive psychology needed to lean towards 'hot cognitions' as opposed to the 'cold' logical processes that it had been focusing on.

(Le Doux 2003: 38)

Awkwardly for scientists, in clinical practice the *cases* which come our way require that the ever-present, wired-in interplay between thinking, feeling and behaving *have* to be addressed together, and this recognition is a plausible explanation for the fact that CBT has been practitioner-driven to a surprising degree, sometimes leaving theorists struggling to catch up (see Hollon & Beck 2004). But then Victorian engineers probably spent little time thinking about Boyle's law; they just put together something that worked, and probably had more influence on science than it had on them.

5   Aaron Beck's view on the factors encouraging a merger between cognitive therapy and behaviour therapy is that research into the former's efficacy and range could not be ignored by a discipline which put scientific rigour to the fore in debates about comparative results (see Beck 1976; Rachman & Wilson 1980; Dobson 1989). Standards for systematic reviews and experimental trials are tighter now (see Littell 2008), and results tapered off when cognitive methods were applied in other than cases of depression and panic attacks. Nevertheless, there existed a body of methodologically good-enough research. Here was the home team position in the mid 1990s:

> CT has typically fared well in comparisons with alternative interventions with respect to the reduction of acute distress. Nevertheless it would be premature to conclude that the efficacy of CT has been established or that CT is superior to any other interventions.
>
> (Hollon & Beck 1994: 428)

6   This conclusion was based on the following factors: (a) the comparisons studies did not always reflect fully clinical populations; (b) measurements of changes in beliefs alongside concordant behavioural change were not always well carried out; (c) the adoption of some behavioural add-ons (as they were seen to be), as recommended by Beck and his followers, blur the issue of which influences exactly were responsible for positive changes; (d) *worthwhile* moderations in mood disorders (the majority) are harder to measure than distinct recovery; (e) few placebo-controlled trials existed, unlike in pharmacology. Nevertheless, it is possible to see some promise in the commitment to scientific procedure and undeniable progress in the number and quality of trials, and reviews (see Craighead *et al.* 1994; Lambert 2004: ch. 10).

Thus the groundwork for a more formal consolidation of the overlapping approaches had been done, and a plan was in place (best represented in early textbooks which explained, defined and demonstrated a deliberate combination of techniques such as that of Meichenbaum (1977)).

The transition from 'just good friends' to 'going steady', to formal union was strongly condoned by the interest of government in starting to encourage but control and regulate the burgeoning private psychotherapy market. In Britain the clear message in the late 1980s and 1990s was that they were not interested in internecine squabbles: 'physicians heal thyselves' sums up the mood, and that they would be legislating anyway. That questions of evidence regarding comparative efficacy were recognised, but beyond the principle of *caveat emptor*, then general consumer protection measures; the increased availability of training; a code of ethics; independent oversight; evidence of competence rather than of allegiance or reputation, would for registration purposes handle the matter.

Although many behaviour therapists didn't like the 'psycho', in behavioural psycho-therapy, negotiators were aware of the 'cognitive revolution' claims and decided to pool their case for official recognition so as jointly to see off attempts by the psychoanalysts to have self-serving requirements such as extended personal experience of the therapeutic method being employed written into the rules. Thus a 'see your long apprenticeship model, and raise you a scientific proof of efficacy test' is the Poker image that comes to mind regarding these negotiations. Ironically then, a merger was effected by a simple, governmental behaviour-modification scheme; it didn't hurt that much, and so far there have been no major side-effects (see www.BABCP.org).

7   One of the most powerful motivations for the changes described above, and certainly regarding their consolidation, is more psychological than historical. Behaviour therapists have always suffered from an image that their discipline implies a 'narrow', mechanistic view of the human condition. The early reaction to this was to form square and defend. In my book *Cognitive-Behavioural Therapy* (Sheldon 1995), the forerunner to this one, Chapter 1 was entitled 'Behaviour therapy in a cold climate' and began with these words:

> During twenty years as a behaviour therapist and teacher of behavioural psychol-ogy, the prospect that this well-researched and broadly applicable approach might leap to prominence has always seemed tantalizingly close. However, the plain fact is that although each generation of students produces a handful of enthusiasts and the journals and publication lists now contain much more of this work than hitherto, these methods are not as widely used by professionals as empirical research suggests they should be. We are still a school.
>
> (Sheldon 1995: 4)

Happily we are no longer just a school. I am not in the advertising business, but the mere insertion of the word *cognitive* in front of *behavioural* has, in Pavlovian fashion, produced quite a different emotional reaction in professionals, clients, critics and the general public. A less defensive attitude has resulted in a wider inclusion of cognitive factors and an unprecedented surge of scholarly publications and experimental research. Type *cognitive-behavioural therapy* into a search engine today, and stand back; there are *thousands* of studies (see Chapter 2). Intellectually justified optimism for this merger has also been accompanied by an increase in positive self-regard among staff in the NHS and Social Services who incorporate CBT approaches into their practice. In addition, we now have graduate and professional courses in CBT itself, not just as an adjunct to other professional training. Something very useful has been achieved, and rather against the odds.

2 Research on the effectiveness of cognitive-behavioural therapy

Science is organized doubt.

(Sir Martin Rees FRS, Astronomer Royal)

Suppose we were to apply the various tests of attributive confidence (laid out in Chapter 1, pp. 14–15) to the research and theory underpinning CBT, how well would it fare in comparison with other methods, or compared to no intervention at all? What works? Although politicians and research funders like the simplicity of this phrase, and though it has performed a useful function in cutting through academic obfuscation (cf. Macdonald & Roberts 1995) it is too simple for its own good. What we should be asking instead is more complicated: (1) What exactly *is* the 'what'? (2) *How* does it produce its effects? How is '*works*' assessed? Is it measured against tangible behavioural change and standardised psychological measures, or more subjectively? (3) Can we be reasonably sure that any apparently useful results are attributable to the method(s) and not to collateral factors? (4) What are the essential ingredients of the intervention and what forgo-able add-ons? (5) How long do any beneficial effects last in comparison with other interventions? (6) For what conditions, and against what diagnostic criteria have methods been used and to what differential effects? (7) How much does it cost in relation to other approaches? (8) Who gets what is claimed to work and who doesn't? (9) Are there any side-effects; how foreseeable are they, and how remediable are they?

We have got much better in recent years in both experimental studies and systematic reviews of these questions in determining effects and staying power and linking these to diagnostic criteria (see Lambert *et al.* 2004). However, we have made less good progress in standardising the main ingredients of the CBT 'recipe' and how well it cooks up under different conditions. Even the 'Bible' of psychotherapeutic practice (see Bergin & Garfield 1971, 1994; Lambert 2004) still often separates cognitive and behavioural components in a bid to tease out what exactly clients are being exposed to, with what differential effects. Such 'the medium is a large part of the message' factors hardly trouble pharmacological investigations once the experimental 'blinding' procedures are in place – not that these are ever perfect – but are an ever-present influence in psycho-social research.

The next point of concern is whether therapeutic procedures are delivered as per the recipe and by people expert at using them. In the past 'qualified or not?' was about the best we could do. There is now an increasing use of treatment protocols and routine audio and CCTV recordings' key competencies have been approved and deployed (see Bennett-Levy *et al.* 2009). The charge here is that the demands of the evaluation and what is convenient for *it* take over and make untypically rigid the approach under study. The awkward trade-off is that if methods of helping are to be properly evaluated, we need to be sure that we know what clients are actually getting, rather than just what label it has been given; but then helpers need to feel free to, say, sit there and listen rather than administer cognitive challenges when the former seems appropriate in an individual case without worrying too much about protocol compliance scores. Blind inter-rater reliability scores from transcripts of about 80 per cent-plus are probably as close as we shall ever get, or clinically *can afford* to get, to the standardised procedures of drug trials. Processes and substances are different things. We must keep an eye on these issues, but resist fussing over them: in horse-riding terms, 'methodological dressage', for we are more typically engaged in 'point-to-point' gallops across rough country.

The main message of this large, robust research literature is that there is something in the CBT recipe that transcends such questions about the precise mix of ingredients, exact culinary technique, or the precise training, qualifications and professional affiliations of the cook – as it were.

The next proviso regarding 'what works' concerns the 'for what' subsidiary question, to which we should add an 'assessed against what' inventory – with what measure of validity and reliability?

This is now the defining message for assessing the research quality and the convincing nature of clinical recommendations. This in contrast to the earlier style, which could be summed up as 'something called this' was offered to a range of clients with 'something' a bit like this (e.g. depression, anxiety states – which are a *continuum* rather than single conditions) delivered by a range of therapeutic affiliates who said that the following precepts were uppermost in their minds when they were seeing clients, which produced the following 'results' – which typically ranged from verbal reports of recovery, to standardised measures of improvement. These were once then all combined in the meta-analysis 'blender' and whizzed up together, and the resulting concentrate offered up as scientific advice (see Sloane *et al.* 1975; Smith & Glass 1977). We do much better now, and the key principle in health and social care research is that of 'logical fit' between studies of the typical known causal patterns in conditions, a close, diagnostic fidelity (using DSM IV^{TR} and ICD 10 criteria – but also, say, in cases of depression, the Hamilton and Beck scales) to be sure that we are looking at clinically significant manifestations with known prognostic implications (base rates and outcome rates with and without intervention) and then seeing whether we can improve on them.

Then there is another range of factors, not discussed much in clinical manuals, which are sociological in nature. Training courses in the helping professions tend to develop 'most favoured' explanations which are privileged by the various professional tribes. Thus, confronted by an unemployed man with clinical-level depression, most social workers will reflexively consider the lack of work and the threat to identity it brings as causal, not the other way around (why did he lose his job?). Psychiatric nurses are more likely to think in terms of illness and compliance with pharmacological treatments and see the social circumstances as a backdrop. Occupational therapists are more likely to encourage tracking what the depression does to other aspects of health and lifestyle (immobility, lack of social contact, lack of physical exercise, all the items in the cope-ability activities of daily living scales) and take the 'cabin fever' explanation. What is interesting is that at the level of causes, maintaining factors and leverage points for treatment, all three sets of actors exemplified are right to an extent (see Brown & Harris 1979; Thase & Jindal 2004; Creer *et al.* 2004; NIHCE 2007c). The issue before us is how best to integrate services for mental health problems and other conditions – which are usually multiply caused and maintained – and manage and coordinate cooperation so that 'territorial disputes' do not get in the way of evidence-based effective help. In other words, the bulk of the evidence for most conditions should lead us towards a multi-component view of causation, and thus to integrated, multi-professional interventions. This idea of a 'logical fit' between causes, maintenance factors and sympathetic interventions based on outcome research of good quality is the best predictor of positive, clinically useful outcomes in studies of the effectiveness of approaches used in mainstream practice.

Messages from history

The history of psychotherapeutic outcomes/applied psychology/clinical social work research may be divided into three distinct stages:

1   The first basic question was: 'Is it possible positively to influence psychological and behavioural/circumstantial problems by talking to the people who have them?'
2   Next, is the technical content of the discourse important, or do simple attention and expectation effects, combined with a sympathetic understanding of their plight, account for any positive reactions? So-called 'placebo effects' (Latin for *to please*) are an imported metaphor from medical/pharmacological research which still causes us problems, not least because these effects still account for 50 to 60 per cent of effects in RCTs in any field. This leaves the interesting question of what factors account for the other 40 to 50 per cent – because in serious conditions, 20 per cent effect sizes above process factors would be a very cost-effective contribution (see Eysenck 1985; Lambert & Ogles 2004).
3   Now that some of the above basic questions have been answered – yes, talking therapies can be effective; no, although many forms of practice produce some verifiable gains – CBT tends to be more effective than all the other forms (see Craighead *et al.* 1994; Sheldon 1995; Lambert 2004). Thus different approaches are not created equal 'in the right hands'. We know this because would-be helpers from a wide range of professional backgrounds who incorporate these techniques; trained psychotherapists themselves, and even, in some cases, trained and supervised volunteers, tend to do equally well in outcome studies, and it works well in groups, and not only when clients have undivided individual attention (see Barlingame *et al.* 2004).

The methodological standards for both original experiments and systematic reviews are now incomparably better than in earlier effectiveness research. Imagine this kind of criticism being made today:

> It will not pass unnoticed that the findings on patients who had completed psychoanalysis are based on 210 cases out of the original 10,000.
>
> (Rachman & Wilson 1980: 57)

The main problems with early reviews have been well documented. They are: (1) evaluation groups who were almost always evangelists for the approach under study were in charge of the projects; (2) uniform *clinical* significance was hardly ever considered when blending together the results of very disparate studies; (3) attrition rates (particularly high in psycho-analytic studies) were not added into the final statistical tally; (4) self-reports and the examinations of case notes by groups of 'experts' (guess from which backgrounds) were used rather than standardised measures of changes. The literature has changed in character over the past few years, and the 'what works for what and why?' questions are now paramount.

The next stage in outcome research concentrated on *techniques*; that is, do some forms of psychological intervention produce better or worse outcomes for certain conditions or problems? They do, but there was much wrangling over this: (1) because of strong theoretical affiliations; (2) because the 'self-denying ordinance' required for an impartial systematic review was not in place; (3) because some doubts remained that scientific methods were 'appropriate' in this field, and so cosier, more 'sympathetic' (to whom or what, one was entitled to wonder) should be allowed. These reviews are still worthy of some consideration today, so influential were they: Luborsky and colleagues' compilation (1975); the Smith and Glass review (1977), important for pioneering the idea of meta-analysis, and combining individual studies to produce large treated populations so as to increase statistical power – but in this case taking controlled and uncontrolled studies together without due differentiation or 'layering' in results; and the Sloane and colleagues' review (1975). In the excitement at this new idea of combining research results, quality was often sacrificed to (statistically playable with) quantity. This problem is receding, but has not yet quite gone away. The consensus from these early reviews, give or take an emphasis, was the *Dodo Bird verdict* (Carroll 1872): 'All have won, and all must have prizes', or the Snark's view: 'What I tell you three times is true'. Rachman and Wilson's wonderfully forensic review of reviews uncovered many causes for concern, notably the dropping from analyses of results from behaviour therapy with troubled children – a major application of behavioural approaches (but not really 'psychotherapy', the authors decided). They also looked at the methodological quality of individual studies and found many inclusions wanting, even by the standards of the time (see also Kazdin & Wilson 1978). Their re-analyses came up with the following conclusions: (1) not a single comparison showed behavioural approaches to be inferior to psychotherapy; (2) no evidence of symptom substitution was obtained, even in studies specifically designed to uncover it (see Sloane *et al.* 1975); (3) behavioural therapy was found to be more broadly applicable to the full range of psychological disorders than traditional psychotherapy; (4) behavioural therapy is more effective with complex disorders; (5) in four out of five measures of client satisfaction with the *process* of helping, behavioural therapists did better(!) (see Rachman & Wilson 1980: 120–121). Therefore we need to be careful about the current sidelining of this essential ingredient of CBT.

Contemporary evidence on the effectiveness of CBT

Anyone researching the effectiveness of CBT approaches today cannot but be amazed by the number of clinical trials testifying to its usefulness in cases of depression and anxiety disorders, or its promise in obsessive-compulsive conditions, eating disorders and even on psychotherapy's 'Russian Front': the psychoses, such as schizophrenia. Then there are 'externally examined' systematic reviews which bind together these results (see Bergin & Garfield 1994; Lambert 2004; NICHE 2007c), but also remember that, outside the mental health literature featured in these reviews, there are many other secure applications such as in work with troubled and troubling children, where the positive results have never been better before or since these approaches became recognised as the therapy of choice (Kazdin 2004). Therefore, although early enthusiasm for these approaches outstripped their empirical support, there has been a veritable explosion of RCTs dealing with a diverse array of fully clinical populations over the last twenty years.

For the most part CBT outperforms all other psychotherapeutic approaches and pharmacology-only treatments (see Matt and Navarro's (1997) analysis of sixty-three meta-analytic studies of the effectiveness of such approaches, with overwhelmingly positive and robust results, plus Westbrook and Kirk's (2007) large sample study of CBT in routine practice).

Which variant of CBT for what conditions is the next question. In other words, some forms of depression are hard to connect with current environmental circumstances and are more 'endogenous', as we used to say. Therefore a treatment programme combining medications with CBT may be the best approach (see NIHCE 2007a), keeping an eye open for anything psycho-social (e.g. strained family relationships, employment circumstances). Some forms are more easily connectable to current environmental circumstances and previous experiences, and might benefit from a more predominantly psychological approach. Similarly, depressions in adults and depressions in children and adolescents have different features and different clinical and service implications (see Weisz *et al.* 2009). Therefore we have moved gradually through 'works or not' approaches via 'compared to what' questions, to 'for what clinically defined conditions' to a recognition that along the latter multi-dimensional spectra, different approaches may be required according to the client's assessed position on them (see below).

In line with this, the rest of this chapter is, bearing in mind the 'logical fit' point discussed on p. 28 organised around the principle of current best evidence on the causes and typical development of mainstream conditions so far as we know them, followed by recommendations as to which variant of CBT has shown itself to be the most useful, but not neglecting other interventions which might work well alongside it, or instead of it.

Depression

This is the commonest mental disorder. The lifetime prevalence figures for major depressive episode (DSM IV^{TR}) from large community samples (trawling rather than angling) range from 10 to 25 per cent for women and 10 to 12 per cent for men. Two comments: (1) the range for women is unacceptably wide and is probably due to diagnostic uncertainties. Women come forward more readily for help than men, and typically relate their low feelings to domestic/family issues. (2) The higher figures are not accounted for entirely by post-puerperal conditions. 'Men' might be the answer.

Untreated, this condition is episodic with a relapse rate of around 60 per cent and a suicide rate of 15 to 18 per cent. Men are more at risk (the figures are about double); they have a reduced tendency to seek help, tend to disguise and hide symptoms and their consequences – particularly in regard to the effects on their work. Thus stiff upper lips, though occasionally useful in life, also carry dangers. Incidentally, in cases of severe depression the point of greatest danger is not at the bottom of the emotional trough, but when some help has been received and there are early signs of recovery, then motivation (including motivation for self-harm) increases, and the sufferer begins to see that a return to previous functioning is in prospect, with all its additional demands and responsibilities (see the case example on p. 51). I have lost two clients to severe depression; both killed themselves when clearly on the road to recovery. So mental illnesses can kill, and we should take them as seriously as we do the overtly physical illnesses which politicians and service planners can more readily imagine they or their families might get one day. Here is what it feels like to have it. The following words are by Lewis Wolpert (a distinguished embryologist who recorded his struggle with depression in an insightful book *Malignant Sadness*):

> It was the worst experience of my life. More terrible even than watching my wife die of cancer. I am ashamed to admit that of my depression but it is true. I was in a state that bears no resemblance to anything that I had experienced before.

> (Wolpert 1999: viii)

The problem with writing about depression is that there has been 'linguistic creep' regarding the term. The same word is often used for the unhappiness caused by the collapse of a relationship; the sense of panicky helplessness that comes with losing one's job; or the persistent *ennui* that can result from being in the wrong job or the wrong relationship. Thus there is a continuum of effects to consider here. Some people are deeply unhappy but find it hard to point to specific reasons as triggers for their mood. Others have plenty in their lives to justify low mood and morbid preoccupations, but avoid diagnosis and treatment.

In the literature there are some who, though predominantly depressed have occasional bursts of unsustainably elevated mood, though not quite meeting bipolar diagnostic criteria (see p. 38). The physical brain sites being the same (the limbic system) and the biochemistry being similar, the term *varipolar* depression has been coined. I struggle with this idea of 'manic latency' as it were, since many clients/patients *never* show clinical levels of elevated mood and many people who experience hypo-manic or manic episodes never get depressed. In addition, the figures for genetic heritability are different for these different expressions (see McGuffin *et al.* 2005). The terms adopted here will thus be *clinical depression* and *major depressive episode*.

Diagnostic criteria and assessment

Diagnosis remains primarily a medical decision, but assessments from allied personnel (e.g. psychologists, nurses, social workers) increasingly contribute to the process. Therefore, all concerned need to understand both the basis of any categorisation and its implications for treatment and after-care. Professional democracy or something close to it has broken out, and the accuracy and the roundedness of diagnosis has benefited as a result.

Another major improvement that has occurred is the development of taxonomies for mental disorders based on the essentials of given conditions, and based on epidemiology and blind, inter-rater reliability studies. Practice knowledge still has a place, but subjectivity and psychological fancifulness are now more in check. In parts of continental Europe where these frameworks are still seen as professionally style-cramping (perish the thought) Freudian concepts are still in use in diagnoses of depression and schizophrenia, and inter-reliability rates have thus remained poor.

The two catalogues that have been most influential are *The Diagnostic and Statistical Manual* of the American Psychiatric Association (DSM, now in its fourth, text-revised version (DSM IV^{TR})) and *The International Classification of Disease* (ICD 10) produced by the World Health Organisation. There are two provisos to enter regarding the use of these even as *guides*. First, here are degrees of overlap between different conditions – which might be better thought of as a *spectrum* rather then as a set of separate boxes; namely, blue for depression, red for schizophrenia, purple for schizo-affective disorder, but bearing in mind overlapping conditions which are the equivalent of 'mauve' (e.g. depression with paranoid features, panic disorder with obsessive features). Post-partum conditions can start off with depression, and manifest themselves as psychotic later. The timescales here are often short and can catch professionals off guard, particularly where there is no previous history of mental disorder. The point being that with specialist treatment the prognosis is good and this applies to all the diagnoses we shall be discussing; assessments should not be thought of as one-off categorisations. Standardised tests should be the scaffolding against which clinical judgements are made, notably the Beck Depression Inventory (BDI) (Beck *et al.* 1961); The Zung Self-rating Scale (ZPI), and the Hamilton Rating Scale for Depression.

Second, validity and reliability levels are less secure in some of the behavioural disorders of childhood and adolescence and these categories sometimes look uncomfortably tautological as labels (for a sociological critique of classification systems see Boyle 1993; Bolton and Hill 1996).

Diagnostic criteria for major depressive episode

The main criteria are:

1   A period of at least two weeks in which there is either depressed mood or loss of interest or pleasure in nearly all activities (anhedonia).
2   At least *four* symptoms from the following list: changes in appetite; sleep pattern (including early-morning waking); lack of interest in social interactions (which adds up to sitting slumped in a chair for large parts of the day); reporting that there is nothing to look forward to; preferring to be alone; decreased energy; difficulty with/no concentration and/or in making decisions; preoccupation with thoughts of death, illness and/or suicide; irritability and/or an inability to sit still – particularly in cases featuring young people.

Causes

Let us begin with some general, methodological points. Virtually all mental disorders and many psychological conditions are now known to have a familial, i.e. genetic, component. In some cases (e.g. bipolar disorder and schizophrenia), this is substantial (see below); in others they are a background feature affecting susceptibility, course, responsiveness to treatment and relapse rates. Our best estimates for varipolar depression from this comparison are a 37 to 40 per cent predisposition due to these biological factors, but if the mood disorder is even very occasionally bipolar, this risk more than doubles. We should be careful with the popular idea of 'genes for' however, since normally we are considering clusters of interacting genes which themselves interact with environmental precipitators (or are contained by resilience factors) which also have their biochemical and structural effects through the process of physical development which begins, remember, *in utero*.

Our knowledge of such influences comes mainly from four types of study.

1   *MZ/DZ comparisons*: MZ twins are more or less genetically identical; they have 100 per cent of their genes in common, whereas DZ twins have 50 per cent of their genes in common. Even though they are brought up in a common environment, we should see, if the genetic hypotheses holds true, a substantial jump in risk levels for mental illness between the two types as much as we do for many physical conditions (see Tsuang and Vandermey 1980; Winokur *et al.* 1995; McGuffin *et al.* 2005).
2   *Family studies*, which examine increases and decreases in risk among relatives according to their closeness or distance, vs. general population figures. These show that the greater the level of consanguinity the higher the concordance, usually.
3   *Separated twin studies*: in this research identical twins who have been separated at birth and reared apart in different environments are compared. In serious mental illness they indicate a strong biological influence at work.
4   *Cross-fostering studies*: these studies come at the problem from the opposite direction, i.e. they look at collections of twins from families with no known mental health problems, one of whom has been transferred into a family where one or more members has, or

more likely, develops a mental disorder during the placement. Follow-ups show evidence of stress but not of precipitation of mental illness above population norms. Thus bipolar disorder and schizophrenia are not environmentally *catchable* in quite the way that depression is. Children need reflections of personal worth as much as they need vitamins. Yet these outgoing, optimistic, love-affirming responses are exactly what people with depression find hardest to give (see Rutter 2007). The point as in the rest of this discussion of familial factors in mental illness is not that we should see such factors as deterministic but rather as influential, creating an upward gradient of learning from environmental stimuli. For example, most people with depression or bipolar disorder will be able to point to environmental factors which are clearly implicated in their recent relapse, even though these are often normal stressors for most of us, and capable of remediation. Oversensitivity to stressors on the one hand, and due attention to environmental factors and how to manage them, on the other, is the best approach from these literatures on bio-psycho-social *interactions*, since that is what they are.

Psycho-social influences

Studies from medical sociology reveal the following environmental factors to be associated with depression:

1   Class position, and all that goes with it, emerges as a major epidemiological and aetiological factor, not sufficient in itself to produce severe depression, but constituting a powerful mixture of 'provocative' agents in the absence of protective social factors, and associated with a doubling of the rates of continuing depressive illness (see Brown and Harris 1979).
2   Poverty is a major predisposing factor in both mental and physical ill-health (see Black *et al.* 1980; Acheson 1998), since room for counteractive measures and the retention of a sense of self-control is so restricted, which leads to increased tension, and 'nothing works', learned helplessness mindsets (see Seligman 1975; Gilbert 1992).
3   Bereavement, and loss, especially when still a child, and particularly involving the loss of a mother prior to or during adolescence, also produced a noteworthy, statistical association in these data. Just think of the consequences of such events at a developmental stage when most of us are emotionally vulnerable and trying to establish a stable identity for ourselves even without such burdens of grief and loss, and these results are very plausible – more so given findings from the rest of the developmental psychology field on such issues (see Rutter & Hersov 1987; Slater & Muir 1999).

Table 2.1 gives some typical comparison figures for those suffering from depression who had or had not experienced major life events (e.g. bereavement, divorce, abuse, loss

Table 2.1 The relationship between life events and social support in depressed women

	Social support *(% depressed)*	*No support* *(% depressed)*
No life event	1	3
Life event	10	23

Source: Cleary and Kessler (1972) quoted in Brown and Harris (1979).

of employment) in their lives, and who did or did not have compensatory sources of support. There has been much wrangling over these statistics but the differences are so large as to be unlikely to be greatly accounted for by collateral factors. I am quoting this thirty-year-old material since it remains (a) the most comprehensive, and (b) the most scientifically robust that we have.

4   Single parenthood or semi-single parenthood, particularly if there are two or more young children, is the next set of factors to emerge from this research. We normally see children as a gift, except that the view may change when adverse socio-economic and personal factors intrude, and when even their ordinary, developmentally-par-for-the-course demands are misread and turn into last straws. Halsey and Webb (2000) documented the effects of being a poor, single parent in an admirably non-judgemental way via a series of well-conducted studies and reviews. They were pilloried for pointing out the obvious fact that bringing up children alone is, in most cases, doubly demanding and that there are measurable effects on social mobility, education, social exclusion, future employment and later entanglements with the law. Halsey has never said that it *couldn't* be done: many pull it off, some feel better off for it given what they had been through before. Rather, he has argued that *statistically* it was much more difficult, and therefore that social support should be a priority in social policy – as it now is through such initiatives as 'Sure Start' (but see Rutter 2006).

5   Unemployment emerges as a provocative factor in a number of studies and has also been associated with suicide in young males. We rather forgot about it until recently and now it is once again a major social problem – particularly for those with a history of serious mental illness. It is likely to be a major factor in the lives of 80 per cent-plus of these surveyed populations. Apart from its raw economic consequences, it affects any sense of personal control, self-esteem; choice; family relationships, and both mood and behaviour. We currently have 2.5 million people unemployed in Britain, a million of whom are young people. However, if we factor in the 'economically inactive' plus long-term incapacity benefit recipients, the figures are even more challenging – both economically and in respect of aetiological factors known to be involved in depression. It is estimated that 110 million working days are currently lost per year in Britain due to depression. This costs an estimated £9 billion per annum if we combine treatment and care costs and lost economic output. Political puffs celebrating the fact that 'we have never been healthier' concentrate on physical health and tend to exclude mental ill-health – the effects of which cannot be measured by simplistic waiting list times and so on.

6   Happily, alongside provocative factors, there also exist protective ones, most notably in the form of a confiding partner – or even a reliable friend. These counter-effects seem to derive from emotional intimacy, practical support and a willingness to listen and stay involved through troubled times.

7   Practical provision, housing and basic income support have all improved over the past twenty years, but at the expense of emotional support and advice. Time, in-depth knowledge of particular circumstances and problems and a willingness to stay the course with clients are, to the detriment of services, now regarded as a forgo-able 'luxury'.

8   We also know from epidemiological research that women are more likely to seek help with emotional problems and depression than men; and from psychological research that they are more likely to blame themselves for the negative circumstances in which they find themselves. The problem is that if a woman presents repeatedly with symptoms that,

even though their effects may be blunted by medication, are beyond the immediate reach of routine pharmacology, she will tend to be referred to a psychiatrist, and thus labelling factors come into play.

Although vulnerability to depression – particularly in its more severe forms – appears from twin studies to be genetically endowed to the tune of about 30 per cent-plus, environmental circumstances, life events and personal crises therefore play much stronger precipitating and maintenance roles. Furthermore, depression has social and psychological effects of its own on those nearby, particularly upon young children. All forms of mental illness have a severe impact on families, but depression, particularly in mothers and if chronic, has the most insidious effects on child development. Children of pre- and early school age are likely to attribute any supposed blame for it to themselves (see Piaget 1958).

Thus, in the absence of, or in support of, the protective factors reviewed above, professional helpers have two main functions in cases of depression: (1) Advocacy, i.e. to act as negotiators with the various services, including medical and nursing services which can play a crucial role in recovery. This function is highly valued by clients (see Macdonald and Sheldon 1997). It is also worth remembering that not everyone has a GP, and that those who do may sometimes be *persona non grata* with them; not all GPs will undertake reviews of medication unprompted; and not all workplaces live up to their published aims regarding employment conditions. Therefore, having someone on side to mediate regarding these crucial factors is perceived time and again in client opinion studies to be vital. (2) As practitioners we can work directly with children and with families to explain the workings of this illness, and help to dispel common myths. We can also attempt to remove some of the inappropriate self-blame which goes with these conditions. We can also help to harness the available resources and extended family and friends to meet the needs for the support of clients.

Epidemiological and treatment research shows that depression peaks in early to mid-life and then again in old age (an underestimated cohort) but that in a smaller number of cases it can occur in childhood and adolescence, where the simple use of antidepressant medication has come under critical scrutiny as a result of systematic reviews (see Garland 2004). The evidence on the general effectiveness of SSRIs (selective serotonin re-uptake inhibitors) in children and younger adults has undoubtedly been distorted by attempts to hold back a 'grey literature' of negative results. Such medications may thus help some, but may induce suicidal behaviour in a significant minority.

At the other end of the age spectrum, depression in elderly people is under-diagnosed in primary care close on 50 per cent of the time, possibly because of masking effects of other physical conditions and cultural stereotypes.

Effective treatments for depression

The main trends from interventions research suggest the following to be the more effective treatments for depression. Pharmacological treatments are not strictly within the remit of this book, except that social workers, nursing staff and psychotherapists are expected to back up prescribing decisions and encourage compliance with the medication regime prescribed, noting and passing on information about side-effects (the main reason for relapse), and carrying out liaison work to encourage regular medication reviews so that something better than 'prescribe-and-forget' approaches results, so we ought to know something about what we are supporting. The first generation of effective antidepressive medications were the Tricyclics. The dosage safety margins and the side-effect complications were, however, rather challenging for prescribers and there is emerging evidence of longer term dependency effects. These medications have now been largely replaced by a new generation of SSRIs, though both tricyclics and the earlier monoamine oxidase inhibitor drugs still have a role with patients who simply do not respond to the safer, less side-effect burdensome medications. SSRIs act upon mood centres in the brain by reducing the rate of neuro-transmitter 'recycling'. They are an effective treatment and are better tolerated than earlier medications; have fewer side-effects such as lethargy or agitation – but are slower acting, which can be a problem in urgent cases. Phased combinations of psychotherapy, counselling and support, plus appropriate medication appear to be particularly effective in complex cases (see Thase and Jindal 2004; NIHCE 2007a).

Contemporary research on the effectiveness of CBT for depression

The outcome research resources we have are extensive. The ones made use of here include the following:

☐   The NIMH (National Institute for Mental Health) review (see Elkin 1994).
☐   The Hollon and Beck reviews (in Bergin & Garfield (1994) and Lambert (2004)).

The NIHCE (National Institute of Health and Clinical Excellence) review (2007c) plus a Psych Lit. search on effects in controlled trials will also be used (1) to support the other material, but (2) according to the age range and other factors of clients treated, and the variants of CBT featured, and (3) according to their relevance to different points on the spectrum of depressive symptoms. In the background, the work of Craighead *et al.* (1994) with its combination of research on the nature of depression and digests of empirical research on the outcomes of CBT, plus advice on the implications of such findings, has been invaluable. Sources from social care contained in Sheldon and Macdonald (2009) are also summarised here; for health personnel, studies from the work of Creer *et al.* (2004) have been the most influential. Where the results from different professions using CBT are important, then we are down to individual trials (e.g. Vittengh *et al.* 2007).

The first point to note is that there is a convergence of results; a near complete consensus on the utility of CBT – something unprecedented in the literature of the helping professions. This is particularly the case for depression and anxiety-based conditions. The effect sizes are large, and the number needed to treat/intention to treat figures are comfortingly low in cost-effectiveness terms (see Hollon & Beck 2004; NIHCE 2007c).

Here is a summary of the main results from these systematic reviews of controlled trials, beginning with an overview:

> There can be little doubt that cognitive-behavioural methods are effective in the treatment of depression. In particular CBT has been tested extensively in clinical popu-lations and appears to be as effective as medications with regard to reduction of acute distress and quite possibly is longer lasting. In a chronic recurrent disorder like depres-sion, evidence of a preventative effect is most exciting.
>
> (Hollon & Beck 2004: 454)

The British NIHCE (2007c) advice is concordant with the American research. Based also on an extensive systematic review, it goes a step further in giving clear, current best evidence-based guidance on what to do in cases of clinical depression. Here is an interpretation of the recommendations:

☐ There is scope for 'screening' in primary care and general hospital settings regarding high-risk groups (e.g. those with a past history of depression or a strong familial history of the same). In the face of significant physical illness – a major trigger and maintenance factor – particularly among elderly patients, this strongly affects prognosis and well-being. Owing to cultural conditioning, older people are not really *expected* to be happy (the 'good innings' theory of ageing), so depression can be missed. The same applies to depression in children and adolescents, where they are considered to be too young to have enough adverse experiences to trigger it. But then some young lives are filled early on with abuse, misery, parental discord, bullying and physical and emotional neglect enough to last a lifetime (see Macdonald 2001). If such intendedly preventive/'stitch-in-time' approaches are to be extended, then we shall need to monitor the false positives/false negatives ratios. Who exactly is going to undertake this is unclear since evidence-based GP units are not really part-time research centres, and so real, academic research centres depend on the input of reliably categorised data from these sources – which they sometimes get, and sometimes don't.

☐ A nice idea, 'watchful waiting' in cases of mild depression is sensible, but then in my own practice I have often found that one or two clarifying interviews plus a phone call to monitor current state will be enough to divert clients from a more serious decline. The prescription of antidepressants (the reflex action of most GPs) is not recommended for mild depression in the NIHCE review since the benefit/harm ratio does not warrant it. The question is who exactly will be doing the watching, and how awake to troubling signs will they be? The child abuse literature (see Macdonald 2001; Sheldon & Macdonald 2009: ch. 10) could well be summed up in these terms, but then sudden, unexpected crises create havoc within best-laid plans.

☐ Continuing with the theme of early intervention paying dividends, the NIHCE review supports combination treatments of SSRI antidepressants and individual CBT. The problem is that the former are readily obtainable, while the latter will probably require several telephone calls, two or three emails and a funding conversation with the PCT by the referrer (about to change). These, from practical experience, can often be disincentives, and so patients stay on medication with a background hope of something more individual and related to their environmental circumstances – which may or may not materialise. There is now enough acknowledged research evidence to require that CBT for mild to moderate depression should be prescribable as pills. The availability of trained therapists needs to be improved (already in government sights); but also the referral and funding system needs streamlining – this being the major obstacle to ready access. However, GPs often lack knowledge of what they are recommending and conflate counselling, 'eclectic' psychotherapy and CBT (her upstairs) in a way they rarely would with medications. Thus some top-up training for them is the next step (see BMJ 2002).

☐ The results from reviews of CBT effectiveness regarding depression are congruent: whether they are (1) American, British or wider European the results and the implications are very similar; (2) we should not neglect the 'back catalogue' of findings. In short, one can see little in Craighead *et al.* (1994) that differs greatly from the reviews in Bergin and Garfield (1994), from Gilbert's more epidemiological approach (1992), or in Lambert's (2004) take on all of this. Depression and its consequences was much the same then as now, and the international research is *cumulative* in that the protocols for reviews and international trials are now pretty secure (see www.repysch.ac.uk). *Implementation* of findings is the next challenge, not ever-more refined definitions of particular sub-approaches.

☐   The predominant methodological pattern for the many RCTs is to compare CBT with pharmacology alone, or CBT (with or without medication) with other psychotherapeutic approaches (see Bergin & Garfield 1994; Craighead *et al.* 1994; Lambert 2004). If (the point made on p. 29 notwithstanding) we do lack certain kinds of research regarding the treatment of depression, here would be my three main contenders: (1) academic, discipline-consolidating, impartial, expanded studies with *believable* 'placebos', i.e. attention-only controls. We are learning now from methodological research how difficult it is to pull these off, even if normal 'blinding' procedures are used (the careful work of my colleague Edzard Ernst shows this well in the field of 'complementary' treatments in health); (2) there is a case for some well-designed (i.e. fully representative) qualitative research on exactly what ingredients of CBT for depression are primary, or secondary but helpful, or surplus. Hollon and Beck (2004) have produced a useful research digest but this is still very theoretically led. That said, there is *some* information available from studies of effectiveness (mainly but not solely regarding depression and anxiety states) from studies of the *process* of therapy (see p. 69). (3) We have only modest numbers of experiments regarding the use of CBT in clients with severe social problems alongside their psychological/health difficulties.

These *desiderata* aside, any careful reading of this large literature on CBT shows it to be a reliable, cost-effective treatment for mild to moderate, developing depression (the majority of cases); to be a useful adjunct to medical treatment in severe depression, and good results are also to be had in more serious chronic cases via relapse prevention; to work, if suitably adapted, effective for all age groups, and, if the basic protocols are adhered to, to be equally effective whether delivered by trained psychologists, trained social workers or trained psychiatric nurses. The challenge is now, very clearly, that of improving routine, timely access, and incorporating suitable, competency-based training into qualifying courses. There is plenty of space for this when one considers the clutter of non-evidence-based material routinely taught.

CBT and bipolar disorder

Another mood disorder, this is also known as manic-depressive illness. This is a devil's bargain of a condition: the uplifted mood, the energy and the false (or sometimes real) sense of creativity that it brings make it addictive; before that is, the mental collapse into despair that occurs later. So patients often avoid help from dullards, spoilsports and dupes (i.e. friends, family and professionals).

Byron, Van Gogh, Virginia Woolf, Picasso and Sylvia Plath are in a long list of historical figures who suffered from this condition and ascribed many of their achievements to its (unfortunately transient) blessings. The downside was described by Winston Churchill as 'the black dog'. Kay Redfield-Jamison's compelling book, *An Unquiet Mind* (1995), gives frank and deep insights into what it is like to live with extreme mood swings. She is herself a sufferer/beneficiary, but she is also a professor in a department of psychiatry, and co-author of the standard textbook on the illness (see Goodwin and Redfield-Jamieson 2004). Here is a summary of her views:

> The war that I waged against myself is not an uncommon one. The major clinical problem in treating manic-depressive illness is not that there are not effective medications – there are – but that patients so often refuse to take them. Worse yet, because of a lack of information, poor medical advice, stigma or fear of personal and professional reprisals,

they do not seek treatment at all. Manic-depression distorts moods and thoughts and incites dreadful behaviours, destroys the basis of rational thought, and too often destroys the desire and the will to live. It is an illness that is biological in its origins, yet one that feels psychological in the experience of it; an illness that is unique in conferring advantage and pleasure, yet one that brings in its wake almost unendurable suffering and, not infrequently, suicide.

(Redfield-Jamison 1995: 6)

The prevalence rate is around 1 per cent. About 15 per cent of people who suffer from it kill themselves, but this is, statistically, the iceberg tip of the misery it brings; it can also lead to aggression towards loved ones, family, relatives and friends, financial ruin and occupational disasters. Twin studies show a strong familial inheritance pattern, with risk figures of around 70 per cent; higher than for unipolar depression or even schizophrenia.

The symptoms (especially for bipolar disorder – though there are other, less extreme, 'mixed' manifestations) are straightforward, though there are also studies showing diagnostic confusion with florid schizophrenic episodes, particularly where young people and ethnic minority patients are concerned. There is also a risk of confusion with manic episodes triggered by drug misuse. The essentials for accurate diagnosis are:

☐ One or more manic episode – characterised by highly elevated mood, alongside a major depressive episode.
☐ Erratic and untypical behaviour.
☐ Risk-taking well outside the norms of previous behaviour.
☐ Racing thoughts and irritation at the 'slowness' of other people.

During near-manic episodes, sufferers feel highly creative and full of energy until, that is, exhaustion sets in. The major depressive episodes that follow (one or more is necessary for the DSM IV[TR] criteria to be met) are a cruel anticlimax to this and are often anticipated by patients. Therefore, in this illness, there is, on the way down, or on the way up, a window of insight, and it is at these transition points that suicide risks increase. As to causes, anyone who has personally encountered this condition will, if rational, abandon notions that these problems are anything other than brain disorders; the effects are so severe; so independent of social circumstances, and so much more likely to produce family and occupational discord than to be reactions to it – though recall Redfield-Jamieson's words: they *feel* psychological.

Causes

Neuroscientists are making steady inroads into an understanding of mood disorders (see http://www.brainexplorer.org/bipolardisorder-aetiology.shtml). A range of neurotrans-mitter chemicals such as noradrenalin, serotonin and dopamine have been the subject of research studies. The basal ganglion and the limbic system (the mood control 'thermostat' sites at the back of the brain) but also the frontal and temporal lobes and the prefrontal cortex have all been implicated. Cortical areas seem to be the location for the profoundly negative thoughts that compound depressed or elevated mood by adding in cognitive components, and urging behavioural expressions, which in turn impact back on the mood state itself. As we shall see later, it appears that a basic genetic predisposition affects brain chemistry but that this vulnerability is triggered and maintained via environmental factors, both present and past, and by lifestyle factors.

Pharmacological treatments

The reason for the inclusion (above) of a little information on what is known (much isn't) on the effects of brain chemistry on disturbed mood is because pharmacological treatments, in their attempt to control imbalances in this very biologically driven illness, and compliance with such regimes – particularly if they are the subject of regular reviews – is probably the best hope for recovery, providing, that is, there is sufficient psycho-social support to make cooperation tolerable.

Kick and McElroy (1998) in their review of interventions research pick out Lithium salts as 'the pharmacologic cornerstone of treatment for patients with bipolar disorder'. It is an element, not a high-tech chemical formulation, and has been used since the early 1970s to largely good effect. However, this optimistic statement, based on (to date) ten controlled trials and one recent systematic review, requires two riders: (1) Lithium does not suit *all* patients, the effective dose being uncomfortably close to the toxic dose, and there is a new generation of atypical anti-psychotics with fewer side-effects – except for high weight gain, which is regularly present, and not without physical and psychological consequences. (2) The problem with these treatments is that many patients fail to take them as prescribed; in other words, in the manic phase they dislike the idea of being less 'alive' (even though such feelings are usually regarded by friends and relatives as illusory, repetitively self-damaging and unsustainable). Therefore the regular matching of dosage to psychological and social circumstances is time-consuming, but crucial. All staff, from consultants to GPs to psychiatric nurses to social workers, need to involve themselves in such treatment programmes with the aim of securing the best trade-off between family stability, mood stability and toleration of side-effects. The same point holds for the depressive phase of the illness, where patients feel awful, are often suicidal and paranoid, but have neither the energy nor the rationality to continue with the regime unless actively supported.

There follows an account as to what this process of accurate dosage – with an eye to coping with current environmental stresses – feels like from the inside:

> The too rigid structuring of my moods and temperaments, which had resulted from a higher dose of Lithium made me less resilient to stress than a lower dose, which, like the building codes in California that are designed to prevent damage from earthquakes, allowed my mind and emotions to sway a bit. Therefore, and rather oddly, there was a new solidness to both my thinking and emotions. Gradually, as I began to look around me, I realized that this was the kind of evenness and predictability most people had, and probably took for granted throughout their lives.
>
> (Redfield-Jamison 1995: 67)

Psycho-social interventions

From twin studies and follow-up research, between 30 and 40 per cent of precipitation and relapse in bipolar disorder occurs as a result of environmental factors. Therefore, since we can do little at present other than to counter biological factors by medication, what useful alterations can we make to these psycho-social pressures? The research literature currently contains nine type 1 randomised controlled trials (RCTs) testifying to the additional usefulness of psycho-social interventions in mood disorders, enough evidence to be going on with, particularly if considered alongside promising, but less robust type 2 trials and alongside insights from qualitative, client opinion research (see Craighead *et al.* (1998) on influences affecting the depressive state; also Milkowitz *et al.* 1996).

Our best bets regarding such approaches may therefore be summed up as follows:

☐ There is some good evidence regarding the efficacy of psycho-education; that is, simply holding sympathetic dialogues with clients and their families to explore the nature of the disorder and sensitising them to early signs of relapse. Having worked in this field for many years, it is staggering to me that so few clients have been briefed in an evidence-based way on the nature of the conditions from which they suffer – a general point, not limited to mood disorders. The internet may change this, but this is not a controlled medium – its *raison d'être* some would say – but it is therefore occasionally a dangerous source of information to the vulnerable who sometimes select out what they want to believe.

☐ Most studies on relapse prevention in this field feature variants of cognitive-behavioural therapy and family therapy – with a scatter of small-scale qualitative studies on the effects of counselling on medical compliance.

☐ Professionals have a role to play in limiting the damage, both to clients and to their families. In the manic phase sufferers are very likely, for example, to give away money well beyond their means, and to ruin their employment prospects or their businesses. Families, though they usually understand that something is very wrong, nevertheless often attribute such behaviour to malign intent. Therefore, in the early stages, probably the most beneficial interventions that staff can make are via a family conference where early signs of mood disturbance, damage-limitation and family support are at the top of the agenda.

☐ Social workers play a role in preventing and containing the financial ruin referred to above. There is a Court of Protection, purpose-built for such problems – though research suggests that they and families often apply to it too late, when most of the damage has already been done. The evidence here suggests therefore that a more pro-active approach is necessary, which might mirror the 'assertive-outreach' schemes which have proved useful with untreated schizophrenia.

☐ Bipolar disorder can inflict terrible damage on marriages and partnerships. Not only is this condition very hard to live with for non-sufferers but, understandably, high levels of criticism and emotionally charged interchanges are also linked to relapse (see Milkowitz *et al.* 1996). Therefore, counselling and psycho-education approaches for partners may have an immunising effect (see Sexton *et al.* 2004).

☐ Because social services have been somewhat artificially divided between 'adult care' and 'child care' there is a danger that cases which overlap these categories are dealt with by one division or the other, but not by both. In short, people with mental illnesses often have children, and their safety, their development and their life chances are much affected by this fact. To have a parent, particularly a mother, with a mood disorder poses a significant risk, particularly to babies and young children – not that the love isn't there, just that the rationality is not there. This can have severe educational and social consequences for children, a cross-border problem in social services and in health.

Bipolar disorder has been given less attention in the CBT literature than the seriousness of the condition deserves. There are three plausible reasons for this: (1) it is strongly familial (around 70 per cent co-mobility in twin studies) and is therefore viewed as a genetic/biochemical problem best addressed via pharmacology; (2) categorisation disputes regarding whether this is really a separate condition from major (varipolar) depression, given that the brain sites are thought to be the same; (3) Thase and Jindal (2004) in their review suggest that psychiatry may have been resting on its laurels regarding Lithium and later pharmacological treatments. The results from outcome research are also mixed and complicated:

- ☐ Nothing much other than medication has anything close to a dramatic effect in the manic phases and is superior to CBT alone.
- ☐ Some adjunctive positive results have been achieved by blends of CBT, family therapy, social casework and psycho-education in support of family members, partly via supporting cooperation with medical regimes, partly in predicting/anticipating and taking precautions against potential damage to relationships, careers and the welfare of children (see Sheldon and Macdonald 2009: ch. 13).
- ☐ There are some long-standing promising trends (first tried out in cases of schizophrenia: see Vaughn and Leff (1976) and Falloon *et al.* (1984) for the inception of the idea) regarding measuring and then tracking high levels of expressed emotion in families. These are understandably ubiquitous sequelae, but levels of criticism, attempted control, rows and high expectations to behave otherwise, either worsen or trigger a manic episode when clients are on the cusp of developing one. These episodes alienate patients from sources of advice and support. However, there is only limited evidence of CBT *preventing* relapse, either independently or via improved compliance with medication regimes. Our best role is probably to make sure that families are informed and protected; making decisive referrals to medical colleagues, heading off disasters at work by proper liaison, and above all making sure that any 'explosions' are controlled ones. Relapse prevention interventions for the downward spiral towards depression produce better results (see Hollon & Beck 2004).

Anxiety disorders, panic attacks and phobias

Anxiety, though developed through evolution to be an 'intentionally' unpleasant, persistent, precautionary arousal system to put us on watch against adverse experiences, generally, has a benign motivational influence on our thinking, emotions and behaviour. It steers our behaviour via negative reinforcement. It is anticipated punishment below the virtually automatic and extreme effects of more urgent fight/flight reflexes. The cognitive effects are strongly influenced by learning, but also by temperament and personality factors (see pp. 91–99). These are increased watchfulness, hypochondria (see Clark *et al.* 1998), over-representation of threats by 'scanning', worry, rumination and negative misattribution irrespective of regular empirical experience. The emotional experience is of low to mid-level arousal and negative emotions. The behavioural experience is of casting around for things to do that might 'turn down the volume' on the forgoing components: irritability; procrastination over future actions; avoidance behaviour, and inappropriate attribution of problems to others. Unless (heaven forbid) someone with a personality disorder is reading this, so far, so normal. This is everyday human experience. However, when clients find themselves on the shoulders of any number of bell-curves, say, for untoward emotional arousal, conditionability, self-blaming tendencies, or have had a series of life events (learning experiences) that are more adverse than is typical, then these tendencies are more crippling – recognition of which is usually what drives people to seek professional help.

Diagnostic criteria for anxiety-based disorders including phobias

Panic attack/panic disorder is a discrete episode, or series of episodes, where there is a sudden, intense apprehension, fearfulness, horror or sense of impending doom (see DSM IV[TR], ICD 10). Physical manifestations include autonomic nervous system reactions such as heart palpitations, sweating, trembling, shortness of breath, unsteadiness of gait, dizziness, nausea or fear of fainting. Cognitive components are: catastrophic thoughts (e.g. about dying from an induced heart attack or a stroke, expectations that one will go mad, derealisation, fear of embarrassment, hyper-vigilance regarding circumstances thought likely to provoke a reaction (classical conditioning) and of somewhat self-fulfilling monitoring of bodily states (breathing, heart rate, chest tightening, balance)) – a kind of 'microphone feedback' effect where the signals being picked up and amplified intensify these reactions: a cognitive/emotional vicious circle (see Clark & Salkovskis 1991). At the behavioural level, escape and avoidance and/or hypochondriasis (anxiety about small, sometimes random bodily signals) are typical, but create negative refinement effects (for a case example see pp. 104–106). Not surprisingly, panic disorder and agoraphobia often go hand in hand and avoidance of all or most outdoor circumstances via generalisation effects is common (see p. 102), and which, because of fear of loss of control and subsequent embarrassment, may lead to social phobia. Therefore travel (where escape opportunities are curtailed) and contact with friends and relatives (who might be able to offer support) are curtailed – another vicious circle.

Four or more of the above experiences reaching a peak within ten minutes constitute the DSM IV[TR] criteria. Lifetime prevalence for panic disorders with or without agoraphobia (around 50 per cent have both) from community samples hover at around 2 per cent. Clinical samples produce rates of around 10 per cent. Onset is typically in late adolescence to the mid-thirties, though older people are not exempt. Women are three times more likely to suffer from this disabling set of conditions.

Causes

Twin studies (n = 13) show concordance rates of around 40 per cent, with 21 per cent non-additive panic disorder specific genetic variance. There is reported co-morbidity with generalised anxiety disorder and with alcoholism (self-anaesthetisation perhaps). Overall, such data suggest that panic disorder and associated agoraphobia have a noteworthy genetic predisposition. Arguably, this could be transmitted or mediated via personality variables such as conditionability. All of the above figures mirror a major contribution from the environment, i.e. from life events, previous learning or a dramatic, threatening experience. One tends to see many clients who will point to frightening experiences in their life histories, but also, typically, background histories of untoward arousal in general. Fear-arousing experiences thus lead to specific instances which stay in the minds of clients as 'causes'. Outside post-traumatic stress disorder, or combat stress (where the events are enough to psychologically flatten *anyone* – predisposing factors aside) an interaction of familial and learning history and threatening (conditioning) experiences is the model which best matches available data (see Hollon & Beck 2004; McGuffin *et al.* 2005).

Treatment effects

We have many studies across the therapeutic spectrum from behaviour therapy (utilisation of systematic desensitisation, staged exposure) to cognitive therapy (encouraging clients to reinterpret triggering stimuli; whether internal (bodily) or external (environmental)). More often today, a combination of both approaches, from psycho-education to cognitive reinterpretation, to reality-testing behavioural experiments with or without relaxation training, is used. There are a number of overlapping reviews and meta-analyses which look jointly at panic states and agoraphobia. Recovery rates in controlled trials of CBT are excellent at around 80 per cent, suggesting that they outperform pharmacological approaches (e.g. Imipramine, Benzodiazepines) and have longer lasting effects and fewer relapses than in the pills-alone condition (25 per cent vs. 60 per cent is typical). These approaches should therefore be virtually an ethical obligation (see Clark *et al.* 1994; Barlow & Lehman 1996; DeRubeis & Crits-Christoph 1998; NIHCE 2007a).

Generalised anxiety disorder

Years before the merger between cognitive and behavioural methods for anxiety-based disorders, behavioural approaches alone had an enviable track record of effectiveness, as revealed by numerous controlled trials – except in one area, that is, Generalised Anxiety Disorder (GAD). With 'simple phobias' – as they were inappropriately called – making them sound easy, recovery rates over controls were in the 65 to 70 per cent range with very good rates of non-relapse (see Emmelkamp (2004) for a review).

However, GAD proved much harder to treat via graded exposure and relaxation-based reciprocal inhibition, although some worthwhile gains were reported. The problem was that the targets (circumstantial triggers) for disabling anxiety were shrouded in a fog of routine, unconsidered misinterpretations, worry and routine generalised avoidance, so widespread and interconnected that to attack one aspect left many others in place, and had a limited impact on overall psychological welfare. The issue was taken up by critics as evidence of symptom substitution – which it was not, since most of these other sources of anxiety were already known and on the case record. The hope was that in selecting worst-fear scenarios and ameliorating them there would be a positive generalisation of effects. It helped a little (see Sheldon 1982, 1995; Emmelkamp 2004), but was too small an overall effect to be viewed as a reliable clinical benefit.

There has been a reconceptualisation of this disorder over the past few years from pervasive arousal, to the role of worry and apprehension:

> With the recent emphasis on chronic and pervasive apprehension and worry, the core features of the disorder are now seen as being even more cognitive.
>
> (Hollon & Beck 2004: 457)

Thus it now appears that it is not multiple exposures to anxiety-provoking stimuli that create an inter-linking series of mini phobias, but a learned, partially inherited mindset with adverse emotional consequences (e.g. affective/cognitive feedback loops) which sensitises clients to many stimuli; and never encourages him or her to see any but the most secluded and controlled circumstances as 'safe'.

A summary of the DSM IV[TR] diagnostic criteria for GAD (and its close cousin Overanxious Disorder of Childhood) follows:

☐   Excessive anxiety and worry (apprehensive expectation) occurs more days than not, over a period of six months about a number of events and activities. This untypically high arousal, multiple referents for this, and mid-term chronicity, are the primary criteria.

☐   Whatever their thoughts about its origins or reality, clients/patients find the problem difficult to control.

☐   Anxiety and worry are accompanied by at least three symptoms from the following list: restlessness, fatigue, lack of concentration, irritability, muscle tension, disturbed sleep.

☐   Impairment of social and or occupational functioning.

Alternative diagnoses (e.g. substance misuse, the fall-out from panic attacks, overreacting or pervasive generalised features of post-traumatic stress disorder (PTSD)) are discussed in DSM IV[TR], p. 473.

This disorder is characterised by a set of fears and apprehensions that are well out of proportion to the actual likely consequences, even if these worries were to be realised. The precautions, cognitive and behavioural, and the emotional costs, are rationally not worth it, given that what is feared will occur is quite unlikely to do so (see p. 172 for a case example). Another background feature to watch out for in assessment interviews is that often there is great (almost systematic) importance given to very small, anticipated failures. The pressures of modern life, with ever-increasing expectations from schools; daily health scares in the media – 'One cup of coffee a day can damage your heart', 'Have you been tested for Chlamydia? It could prevent you from having children . . .', 'If you drink more than one glass of wine a day, it could increase your risk of mouth cancer by three times' (no base rates are ever given, so from 1 in 100,000 to 3, or 169 in 100,000 to 347 is never reported, but note that few French and Italian towns contain people over the age of 45).

A young client of mine who could not sleep in his own bed, use a telephone, dry his hands on a towel, or eat a meal in company (the diagnosis was Aspergers syndrome and GAD) used to download hundreds of pages of heath and safety advice from government websites on dire threats from infected kitchens in schools, his university, or in cafes and restaurants, and send them to me. He was a physical science student, so it was possible to discuss the numbers, but of course all this was really resistance to a desensitisation/exposure scheme. A more cognitive-behavioural approach which began with the question: 'Do you not have an immune system then?' made some headway, but simple controlled exposure had the most impact. CBT results are mixed to say the least for this condition (see Lopata *et al.* 2007).

The aim of the health and safety industry is to motivate the population to ever greater watchfulness without regard to the side-effects of all this, and has gone well beyond the prudent and sensible. The three quotes given above are used relentlessly on British television. Thus we live in increasingly anxious times, even if (in Western countries at least) the threat of hunger has disappeared, we have an extensive health service based on reasonable evidence; we are no longer going to be bombed to oblivion by the Russians and so on. Thus there is a cultural context to anxiety as there is to eating disorders (see p. 52), a 'going rate' for it in our society. We have never been safer, but we have never felt less safe. Paedophile attacks on our children have not risen since 1946 per head of population, but childhoods have been changed forever (my proposal for compulsory critical appraisal skills training for all journalists has so far been ignored).Without reverting to the idea that societal circumstances *cause* mental illness they certainly influence their inception and course and the way they are interpreted.

The point is that what the individuals portayed in Figure 2.1 overleaf probably fear most (catastrophic cognitions) is that they may one day inhabit Edvard Munch's more iconic painting *The Scream* (you will already have the image in your head).

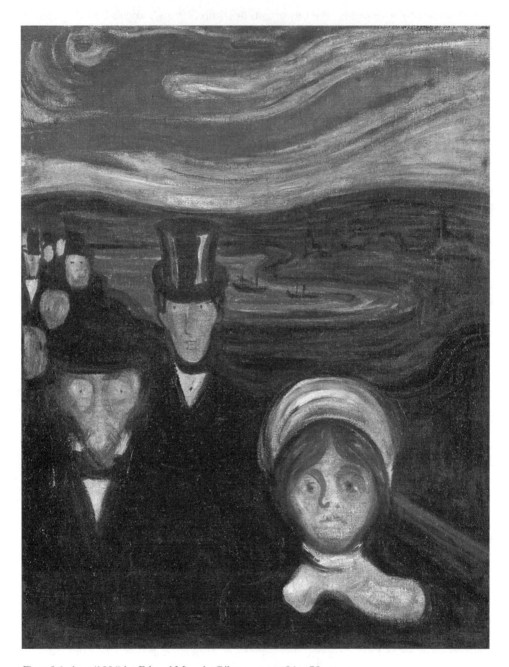

Figure 2.1 *Angst* (1894) by Edvard Munch. Oil on canvas, 94 × 73 cm.

Source: Munch Museum, Oslo. © Munch Museum/Munch Ellingsen Group/DACS, London 2010.

Prevalence and course

The lifetime prevalence rate is 5 per cent. The general pattern in clinical practice is for clients/patients to report that the condition for which they are seeking help has earlier precursors; 50 per cent report an onset in childhood or adolescence – not all can nail this down to *specific* events, though it is tempting for them to do so in consultations since this is what therapists like to hear. Onset can also be in the twenties. Thus, this is often a long-standing, background condition, perhaps a personality-based condition (see Eysenck 1960; Claridge 1985) made worse not by *actual* life events, rather than by the fear of them (see the case example on p. 172).

Causes

The evidence for genetic predisposition is mixed, though the DSM IV^{TR} concludes that there is a familial pattern (p. 474). The problem is that early twin studies, few of which have large samples, concluded that there was none. Later, larger, more methodologically robust studies concluded that there was moderate evidence of heritability. There are two further problems in interpreting this material: (1) diagnostic criteria were tightened up between DSM III and IV; (2) more widespread attempts to separate out GAD and GADC (Generalised Anxiety Disorder of Childhood) from other conditions which include generalised anxiety were made (e.g. phobias – where generalisation often occurs; hypochondriasis, and in post-traumatic stress disorder). Further genomic investigations suggest that gene positions and activities for bipolar disorder (highly heritable) and GAD are similar. The most sensible (non-ideological) path out of this methodological tangle is to look at recent, large sample reviews and analyses (see McGuffin *et al.* 2005). The ongoing Virginia Twin Registry results show heritability of around 30 per cent. Such meta-analysis typically comes up with co-morbidity rates of between 20 and 30 per cent, which suggests a substantial environmental influence.

The main contenders here are (1) an interplay with broader personality factors; for example, 'punishment sensitivity', problems with sociability; and developmental learning factors; i.e. it is possible to learn, via classical operant conditioning, and over an adverse childhood, that the world is a dangerous place, and that watchfulness and avoidance 'pays' (see the example discussed on p. 45). These influences can be either continuous, unrelenting features of childhood (see Macdonald 2001) or, as in post-traumatic stress disorder (PTSD), single or short sequences of dramatic events.

Effective treatments

There are at the time of writing three systematic reviews of RCTs testifying to the effectiveness of cognitive-behavioural therapy for this condition (see BMJ 2002). Given the multiple, potential targets (often too many for exposure/desensitisation approaches to work) *cognitive restructuring* approaches (see p. 234) which encourage a rational reinterpretation of all threatening stimuli and cues, plus motivation enhancing *experiments* to empirically test out beliefs, have been found to be beneficial. Relaxation training may be a helpful *adjunct*, but used alone produces inferior outcomes (comparisons from other treated RCTs with, for example, non-directive, experiential, group anxiety-management therapy, found substantially better results for CBT with even larger effect sizes as against waiting list controls. The research on children and adolescent manifestations is even more robust, which may just be due to more being done with this group or because not yet fully established forms of the condition are more treatable.

The case for early intervention looks convincing (see Kazdin & Weisz 1998; Kazdin 2004; and for encouraging results for CBT with social phobia see Herbert *et al.* 2005).

Pharmaceutical treatments

Most work has been done on the Benzodiazepines, which undoubtedly have some useful effects; they are quick-acting, but carry side-effects (typically sedation/drowsiness, and concentration problems which have social, mobility and occupational consequences) and there are also studies showing dependence effects. As with minor tranquilisers and with Busprirone (which has fewer side-effects) there is little or no evidence of continued gains past the initial relief phase (see BMJ 2002; Lambert 2004: 457–458) and may not be well tolerated. Nor do they confer lasting benefits, as does CBT (see Hollon & Beck 1994). The case for the routine use of CBT in this disabling disorder is clear, as is the case that the main point of attack is the systematic, diffuse, non-evidence-based cognitive tendency to overestimate/ misinterpret signals of possible risk and danger and to underestimate coping abilities in the face of distracting worries. Ready access to CBT is again the largest challenge in both primary and secondary care, and with both adults and children – the latter in particular are prone to have their anxieties located in family life and so reflexively get family therapy. Where you live is of course where problems will largely manifest themselves, but this is not to say that they are *caused* by that environment.

Obsessive-compulsive disorder (OCD)

We all have small obsessions in our lives (think back to your childhood), but some individuals are completely taken over by them. This is the fourth commonest mental disorder, with a lifetime prevalence rate of 2.5 per cent, and it can have ruinous effects on the quality of life of both sufferers and their families. This imprisoning condition occurs in both males and females with, typically, an earlier onset in males (6 to 13 years) and a later onset in females (20 to 29 years).

Diagnostic criteria

To meet DSM IV^{TR} criteria, clients must have experienced the following:

- Repetitive behaviours (e.g. hand washing, extreme checking, or a rigid observance of strange rules and rituals). Minimally, these must occur for at least an hour a day.
- These behaviours and their obsessive cognitive components – which can be equally distressing – are aimed at preventing some feared event (such as contamination, infecting loved ones, not preventing disasters). Thus there is a strong negative reinforcement element, in that behaviour is precautionary well beyond cultural norms or half-way rational approaches to everyday risks.
- At some stage, most sufferers recognise that these compulsions in both their cognitive, behavioural and emotional forms are unreasonable and excessive – but nevertheless feel trapped by them.

Causes

These are not fully known, though there are candidate areas in parts of the brain that are thought to control impulsivity and alertness. There is also a strong familial pattern, with large increases in vulnerability according to kinship. Monozygotic twins have a much higher incidence than do dizygotic twins and so it is reasonable to conclude that this is partly an inherited disorder but also one in which stress factors and obsessive cognitions play a part in precipitation and maintenance (see McGuffin *et al.* 2005). High and pervasive levels of anxiety in parents can help to create this condition in children, so it is a 'catchable' disorder

Genetics and environmental factors

The literature on the genetics of OCD is surprisingly sparse given the damage that it routinely does. The best interpretation of the evidence that we do have is of a 30 per cent-plus rate of heritability, which of course leaves a lot of room for developmental/environmental factors.

Obsessions are part of the human condition. Indeed, it is an evolutionary success story that human beings are alert to, and take precautionary action against, harbingers of danger, which through learning become established in our behavioural repertoires. I have taught research methods and pushed the idea of more rational approaches to psychological and social problems for more than thirty-five years but I still wave at single magpies to forestall widowerhood (the worst of things) by means of a small gesture (the easiest of things). We all have childhood memories of not walking on the cracks in the pavement so that the bears don't get us (there *are* no bears in Britain outside of zoos, and few squared-off pavements in Yellowstone Park where there are).

One comes across cases, such as those below, where simple learning theory is enough to account for the condition, as with (1) that of a late middle-aged woman who as a child was evacuated from a city to a farm during the Second World War, treated with routine cruelty and pushed into a hen coup for a day as punishment for wetting the bed. She emerged covered in fleas, and said: 'Over all these years I've never felt clean since.' The problem was that her children, who would walk into the room like surgeons, hands aloft, were not allowed contact with her after school until they had wiped themselves down with neat disinfectant, and that they had acquired her habits – her reason for her referral *of them*; (2) a young woman with regularly changing diagnoses, normally qualified with the term 'schizo' – or 'borderline' or 'personality' (she did have preoccupying ideas of reference). The worst set of these were that the indicators on cars in the street were flashing in rhythm which reminded her of sexual intercourse (she had never experienced it, but did masturbate and felt very ashamed of the fact). The therapist (me) persuaded her among other things to think about the family life of the car factory worker, and what he would say to his wife if asked what he was doing that day. 'We are all busy putting indicators on cars so as to intimidate Laura, I don't know who she is, but . . .' was the candidate answer. No mental implosion; the first laugh ever, and the idea of thinking about intrusive thoughts and their origins and functions was established.

Such 'heretical' practices (challenging delusional thinking) largely from people who had given up on psychoanalysis and were practising as behavioural therapists, eventually resulted in new models of the origins and potential tractability of both delusional and obsessive thinking (see Birchwood & Tarrier 1992; Wykes *et al.* 1998). No, I haven't mixed up my mental disorders, for the very same orthodoxy, namely, challenging obsessions, is now being used in the treatment of obsessive-compulsive disorder, with very good results.

Returning to the role of the environment (i.e. of learning), look back at the picture on p. 46 by Edvard Munch (a wonderful artist but a troubled man). Here is an account of his upbringing from a recent biography:

> The children's smallest misdemeanour called forth the reminder that Mama saw them from heaven – and grieved. After the beatings Christian (father) would be overwhelmed

by remorse but his sense of proportion was unbalanced by his isolation and his severity towards his children was spurred on by his desperately sincere religious conviction.

(Prideaux 2005: 15)

I have seen many cases of obsessive-compulsive disorder where childhood experience (i.e. *learning* experiences) are more than enough to account for their hyper-vigilance in adulthood. Human beings typically underestimate the power of environmental contingencies over character and blood.

Pharmacological interventions

There are effective medical treatments, and there are many randomised-controlled trials testifying to this fact. The prime indications are the SSRIs and tricyclic medications. Up to 60 per cent of patients respond well to these, but numerous studies also show that cognitive-behavioural approaches and social support schemes enhance their effectiveness considerably and surpass pharmacology-alone results (see Chapter 7).

Psycho-social interventions

The more methodologically robust studies, including systematic reviews of RCTs, are clear that variants of CBT are the methods of choice (as recently concluded by NIHCE 2005a).

The key therapeutic ingredients for effective practice with CBT for this condition are: (1) explaining the irrationality of obsessive-compulsive thought patterns and excessive precautionary behaviour; (2) empirical testing with therapeutic support – testing out the hypothesis that anxiety and fixation will eventually fade and that nothing that was feared has actually happened.

Here is a good characterisation of this disorder:

> According to Cognitive theory, obsessions typically involve the recurrent perception that one has placed oneself or others at risk through some action (or failure to act), and compulsions consist of attempts to undo this risk through some type of subsequent action. From a cognitive perspective, the issue of personal responsibility looms large; it is this theme that is believed to distinguish (OCD) from the other anxiety disorders.
>
> (Hollon & Beck 2004: 460)

Effective treatments

Pharmacological approaches (usually SSRIs; e.g. Sertraline), which are what GPs typically go for on first contact, produce some relief quite quickly, but there is a high and quick relapse rate once the course finishes. Behaviour therapy (desensitisation and relapse prevention, with relaxation training in the background) has been found to be effective (see BMJ 2002), as has CBT (see NIHCE 2005a). Cognitive therapy too has been found to be effective, but then the cognitive approach, if it is used, should contain a substantial element of exposure, and behavioural therapy should also try to address the catastrophic thought patterns of clients/ patients. There is no point in ducking this issue any longer: there are few users of cognitive therapy who do not urge and oversee behavioural experiments, and there are few behaviour therapists who do not take stock of how clients *interpret* provocative stimuli. We should call all versions of this approach *cognitive-behavioural therapy*, and drop tribal symbols and sectarian affiliations.

CBT is an effective treatment for this condition (see Rosa-Alcazar *et al.* 2008); CBT plus medication (e.g. Fluoxamine) improves results. CBT typically maintains it gains over a two-year follow-up period (four systematic reviews, and double-blind trials compared to medication alone) (see Franklin *et al.* 1998). No harms are ever reported, as is the case throughout CBT literature – not bad. Case example 2.1 shows (1) the complexities of this condition and the ruin it can bring in its wake; and (2) how cognitive, behavioural, emotional and social factors must be taken together.

CASE EXAMPLE 2.1

This case involves a young man with two children. To say that he was estranged from his wife is to distort the facts, yet he did live away from home and was something of a recluse. Nevertheless, he loved her and, by all accounts, she loved him. He had decided to separate 'for the good of the children' – but this was not the usual sort of 'good'. He suffered from a severe form of obsessive-compulsive disorder which involved excessive attention to hygiene, and various rituals which dominated his life, but above all, from ruminations about 'bad thoughts' and a strong feeling that one day he might act upon them. The worst among these involved the sexual abuse of his own children. The case records contained no example of anything of the sort happening, but there was an ever-present fear that it *might occur* if he lost control.

The history revealed persistent attempts to secure help. The *dramatis personae* were two GPs: the first one could not hide her revulsion and found a way to remove him from her list; the second confessed himself 'baffled' but nevertheless prescribed cocktails of medication which either sent his client to sleep or made him even more agitated. Enter a consultant psychiatrist, who did not think he could improve upon the existing regime, but regretted the fact that he could no longer procure aversion therapy. (Even if it were valid on ethical grounds, it is ineffective.) The consultant saw the patient at three-monthly interviews for 'reviews' but was useful only in referring him on to other specialists. These included a psychologist who gave up after one session and referred the client back to the psychiatrist, who recommended a course of ECT (he was not depressed but deeply unhappy). The patient undertook this almost as a form of deserved punishment or 'exorcism'. Apart from memory loss, there was no effect. Meanwhile, someone in the surgery, which was located in a small village, leaked the story of the reasons behind the separation, and a campaign of 'outing' this client as a potential paedophile began. He was ostracised by many, and became even more reclusive. Eventually the possibility of cognitive-behavioural therapy was hit upon (more by chance than from a reading of the research) and he was referred to the present author, who saw him on seven occasions. What emerged was a childhood history of buggery at the hands of his stepfather, with, he suspected, the partial collusion of his mother, and the fact that his obsessions began in his early teenage years and grew worse later.

The patient reported finding the CBT approach useful, particularly discussions of his childhood experiences, and of the non-rational aspects of his patterns of thought. The contents of his history that concern us here are: (1) a feeling of *despoliation* arising from his sexual abuse and a feeling of betrayal by his mother; (2) a feeling that he had been 'chosen' for a bad life and had come from 'bad blood', and (3) the steady onset of his obsessional preoccupations with the *worst thing that could happen* and the fear that these impulses could attach themselves to just about anything. Therefore there was a consequent preoccupation with suicide; (4) fantasies about a 'cure' that would not involve him too much in trying to understand his illness, but would take the form of something *done to* him, ideally involving surgery; and (5) a strong feeling that however much support he was given, 'something' would soon 'snap' and would lead him to 'his destiny'.

The patient had more understanding and self-forgiveness by the end of the CBT sessions and thought he had made some progress with deflecting obsessive thoughts. He also went out more, and sought and received the support of two old friends. Then, one evening, after a sleepless night full of 'the worst thoughts', he drove into a nearby wood and gassed himself with exhaust fumes. The message he left explained that it was 'best' for his children and for his wife, and that although 'people' had been very helpful, he now realised there was no real cure and that he would have to fight his demons for the rest of his life and was too tired to do this.

The priest at the crematorium chapel gave a brisk, coded sermon about the perils of mental illness, and how much more (unspecified) help should be made available to sufferers. Then he hastily left. From his behaviour one found it hard not to think that he saw himself as committing a potential sinner to judgement thankfully sooner rather than later.

Not all cases are as dire as this, or so filled with loss, but it does need to be recognised that OCD tends to infiltrate lives, and only rarely presents as a small, inconvenient, hang-up about a simple set of circumstances. A case study with a happier outcome can be found on p. 242.

See Bagley and Ramsay (1997) for a good account of suicide risk and prevention.

Eating disorders

These conditions are included in this chapter because anxiety and chronic cognitive misrepresentation play a major role in their inception and course. They involve deliberately restricting the consumption of food, or binge eating and then vomiting (bulimia). The commonest condition is 'anorexia nervosa of unspecified type' (50 per cent in community samples – much higher rates of anorexia nervosa in clinical studies). This contrast represents a classification failure. That half of a population of sufferers should end up in a head-scratchingly residual category cannot be right (see Treasure *et al.* 2010).

Diagnostic criteria for anorexia nervosa

☐   Refusal to maintain body weight at or above a minimally normal weight for age and height (e.g. weight loss leading to maintenance of body weight less than 85 per cent of normal; or failure to make expected weight gain during periods of growth, leading to body weight less than 85 per cent of normal).

☐   Pervasive fear of gaining weight or becoming fat, even though patently underweight.

☐   Disturbances of the way in which one's body weight or shape is experienced; undue influence of body weight or shape on self-evaluation, or denial of the seriousness of current low body weight.

☐   In post-menarcheal females, amenorrhea (i.e. the absence of at least three consecutive menstrual cycles).

Types

☐   *Restricting type*: During the current episode of anorexia nervosa, the person has not regularly engaged in binge eating or purging behaviour (i.e. self-induced vomiting or the misuse of laxatives, diuretics or enemas) but continues to restrict the intake of food.

☐   *Binge-eating/purging type:* During the current episode of anorexia nervosa, the person has regularly engaged in binge-eating or purging behaviour (i.e. self-induced vomiting or the misuse of laxatives, diuretics or enemas).

These eating disorders, which predominantly affect young women (at a figure ten times greater than in males) and have a death rate approaching 20 per cent, have been heavily politicised in the past, with feminist psychologists seeing them as a form of 'hunger strike' against patriarchy. Questions have also been raised regarding the influence of advertisements featuring sylph-like models who are obsessive about their body shape. It is interesting to note that in countries where the food supply is precarious, anorexia is much less common, even though it does have a strong familial pattern worldwide. Twin studies show predisposition levels up to 70 per cent (see Tierney 2004). In much of the literature, there exists a false dichotomy between biological/developmental and socio-cultural influences. Genes produce a wide range of phenotypical expressions, which at the level of 30 to 40 per cent constitute strong inhibiting or enhancement effects. Therefore, the 'ideal shapes' in the old 'Bollywood' films favoured chubbiness, since this was a sign of socio-economic standing. Then as economic prosperity improved, Western-style thinness has become more fashionable. Biology, culture, societal factors and psychology thus all *interact* here, as they do throughout the spectrum of mental health conditions.

It is hard to escape the conclusion that what we are dealing with here is a variant of obsessive-compulsive disorder which, via socio-cultural factors, happens to latch on to food and body image (research tells us that 70 per cent of women polled are unhappy with their size, weight, shape and appearance).

Psychological studies of starvation effects (interestingly, conducted on conscientious objector volunteers in the USA during the Second World War) revealed that the first few days of food deprivation are characterised by intense feelings of hunger, indeed by ever more minute preoccupations with food; by dreams about food; by conversations about little else, and even by visual hallucinations about food. Then, steadily, appetite recedes and a state described by some as 'ascetism' or as 'transcendental' takes over – as recorded by practices of fasting for religious reasons throughout the ages. Alexander Solzhenitsyn (1967) in his semi-autobiographical novel *One Day in the Life of Ivan Denisovich*, recalls the experience in the Gulag of being put into solitary confinement on 'punishment rations' (a small bowl of gruel once a day) and hearing whispered advice from the next cell *not* to eat it, lest the pangs of hunger become intolerable. Complete abstinence for a few days would make the desire for food less preoccupying. Something similar to this extinction of appetite effect seems to occur in anorexia.

Effective interventions

We now have good systematic reviews of interventions for anorexia nervosa and its sister condition, bulimia nervosa – which is typified not by not eating food in the first place, but by binge eating followed by self-induced vomiting and purging (see NICE 2004).

Pharmacological interventions for bulimia are much better documented and are more methodologically secure than for anorexia nervosa. This is probably because the latter condition was long seen as a primarily psychological problem. Tierney's review offers a corrective to some of the confusions of symptoms and causes – which once held up in similar fashion, our understanding of schizophrenia.

Antidepressant/anti-anxiety medications are widely used for the treatment of anorexia nervosa, often in combination with family therapy and cognitive-behavioural therapy, but whether single interventions in either direction are superior to combinations is as yet unclear from controlled trials. Pre-post tests and client opinion studies however point (tentatively) to such combinations (see below). Qualitative studies of the experiences of clients undergoing treatment reveal the following common features:

☐ Diagnosis is often faltering, as clients regularly attribute their weight loss to external factors (e.g. problems at school, failed relationships, disagreements with parents). These influences are as likely to be symptomatic as causal, but interactive sets of complex difficulties blur the picture and many GPs have little clinical experience with eating disorders.

☐ Family therapy and cognitive-behavioural approaches are most effective when the diagnosis is firm and the focus is on harm reduction. The harnessing of family support and giving the client a voice should be the main foci of interventions.

☐ Family therapy approaches which carefully expose the various 'games' and avoidance strategies usually at work in this disorder are often (though sometimes retrospectively) valued. That is, if a loved one is apparently starving herself to death in front of her parents, then the temptations to become increasingly coercive, or to feed by stealth, are understandable but are likely to be viewed by the young person as the *cause* of her aversions rather than as a well-meant attempt to help.

☐ Therapeutic regimes must, of course, allow the experiences of all parties a certain priority, but weight gain and improved body mass index measures *must* be the final measure of improvement, not self-reported well-being, lest this too becomes part of a manipulative trade-off.

☐ Time-limited focused, quite intensive interventions do better than less structured interventions (see Crisp *et al.* 1991; Tierney 2004). People with anorexia are often socially isolated, having exhausted much of the patience of their families, friends, schools or employers. Therefore, sympathetic advocacy is valued by clients.

In these cases, anxieties are over getting fat, even though all the objective evidence points to self-starvation or binge eating and self-induced vomiting as being the main causes for concern. Different routes to the same distorted ascetic 'ideal'. Genetics research (see McGuffin *et al.* 2005) suggests that interactive gene clusters very similar to those found in obsessive-compulsive disorders predispose individuals towards these conditions.

Next, let us remove from serious consideration the treatment most likely to be used in the early stages: dietary advice from a primary care nurse ('eat more') which in one study produced 100 per cent withdrawal from the programme. Indeed, early contact with non-specialist staff often leads to disengagement from treatment.

Bulimia nervosa, though a more dramatic illness, seems, oddly, to be more susceptible to treatment. Cognitive-behavioural approaches are effective (see Lambert 2004; NICE 2004). In anorexia, which quickly becomes embedded in family 'games' to coax food into the sufferer on the one hand, and to be ever more vigilant against these incentives on the client's part, no form of psychotherapy emerges as clearly more effective (except that we can rule out psychoanalytical approaches as being clearly unhelpful). However, some gains have been made by harnessing family support via family therapy, particularly if cognitive-behavioural in emphasis. There is no evidence that antidepressant medication, either alone or in combination, makes for clinically significant improvements. One factor worthy of mention, however, is that whatever the approach used, a weighing scale in the background to monitor progress, though usually resisted, is essential. CBT in these cases is unlikely to break through highly rigid belief systems about the ideal of being painfully thin/not remotely fat. Cognitive therapy alone does as well as behavioural therapy alone. The CBT-based family therapy approach does not only address false beliefs of the client, but is a means of reining in high expressed-emotion reactions. The danger here is that such therapists are ideologically programmed to look for *causes* in families – who often exhibit frustration, and patterns of miscommunication with their daughters. There are often rows; draconian restrictions on freedom; attempts to feed surreptitiously, and code messages about weight loss and appearance. But then, as in the case of schizophrenia under R.D. Laing's influence (1960), these are not the *causes* of the condition, but the fall-out from it. 'Tread lightly, for you tread on distorted but deeply-held beliefs' is the best advice. The retention of love and support in a form that the young person can accept, cooperation-building with the family, and some gentle, straight talking with the client, is about the best that we can do. If CBT is factored in, there is a chance that this might improve things further in younger sufferers.

CASE EXAMPLE 2.2

As a keen amateur ballet dancer, Sarah, aged 15, decided further to restrict her diet for art's sake. Over a few months people started to comment on her dramatic weight loss. It eventually came to the point where she was made to see her GP by her parents. He diagnosed her as anorectic, an opinion that was hard for Sarah to accept:

'I didn't think there was anything wrong. I couldn't understand what all the fuss was about.'

Despite Sarah's unwillingness to acknowledge that she had a problem, her GP suggested she saw the practice nurse. However, Sarah did not find this particularly helpful:

'She wasn't really experienced in treating people with anorexia. She just talked to me about what I should be eating but I ignored what she was saying because I thought she just wanted to make me fat.'

When Sarah's weight loss continued, her GP realised that she needed more expert assistance. Therefore, she referred Sarah to a specialist eating disorders service, where she received cognitive-behavioural therapy. Sarah found this helpful because it challenged her negative thoughts and encouraged her to think about things differently. It also made her feel that she was regaining some control of her life. Sarah also noted that it helped to talk to someone who understood her condition:

'She [the therapist] didn't just think I was attention-seeking or dieting. She knew that this was a real problem for me and that made me realise I had to do something about it.'

The specialist service also arranged for family therapy sessions which she found helpful, though there were times when she felt the experience artificial, with everyone being 'on their best behaviour'. But then:

'In family therapy I was able to say things to my parents that I hadn't said before. They listened to me instead of shouting and they started to understand what I was going through.'

Six months on, Sarah is still receiving individual therapy, but she is gaining weight. She also still attends regular group sessions at which she meets other young people with anorexia to talk about her problems.

Psychotic conditions

Most schools of psychotherapy/applied psychology, despite initial aspirations based on their own preferred theoretical interpretations of causes, learned quickly to steer clear of these very biologically embedded, chronic and occasionally dangerous conditions. Let us first look at the diagnostic criteria, and then at the outcome research done for various approaches, including CBT.

Schizophrenia

An awkward term, which we have been stuck with since Bleuler coined it in 1908, meaning, literally, 'split mind', and referring to a disconnection between thinking, emotion and environmental experience. Epidemiological studies show a worldwide prevalence of just below 1 per cent of populations. However, such diagnoses amount typically to 40 per cent of the case loads of mental health staff. Social anthropological research shows that all cultures have a special name for it, whether with benefit of psychiatry or not, and these cultural definitions place emphasis on delusions, social disconnection and on unwanted feelings of external control, which are seen not to be the fault of the sufferer. An eighteenth-century physician referred to it as 'the most solitary of afflictions' (see Scull 1993). The condition has been known throughout history, and a number of famous and talented people have been afflicted. The nature poet John Clare (1793–1864) – though there is more to him than that – was probably a sufferer, though schizo-affective disorder (a mixture of manic-depression and schizophrenia) has also been put forward. He spent much of his life in the Northampton asylum, and now psychiatric wards across the country are named after him. It is worth noting here that it was the medical superintendent who was responsible for bringing his poems to light.

John Clare's life bears testimony to the fact that even if there is something innate at work in the condition (before we had a name for it), environmental/experiential influences are also at work. He had a lost first love, 'Mary' (Mary Joyce), who was, in his imagination, half mythical, half real, and whom to his dying day he was sure he had married. That he felt himself too sensitive to live in the rough world is evident in his work. This feeling of social disconnection and different-ness is at the centre of this condition, and the first generation of psychiatrists were aptly called *alienists*. Here is a verse from John Clare's poem 'I am':

Into the nothingness of scorn and noise,
Into the living sea of waking dreams,
Where there is neither sense of life nor joys,
But the vast shipwreck of my life's esteems;
And e'en the dearest that I loved the best –
Are strange, nay, rather stranger than the rest.
(John Clare 1821)

So much for the inside-out experience, but if we want to help we have to turn next to outside-in factors.

Diagnostic criteria

The first thing to note is that we are not dealing here with a single illness, but with over-lapping syndromes. However, there are core characteristics and it is sensible to begin with these.

Schizophrenia is a major, debilitating mental illness owing to its severe effects on the lives of sufferers and of those around them. It is a psychotic condition, in that the client's insight into it, the false perceptions which accompany it and the irrational attribution of symptoms and their original causes, are sometimes or often impermeable to rational discussion. I say 'sometimes' because one regularly meets patients who, if one accepted the first premise – 'my body is being interfered with by outside forces'; 'people whom I have never met mean to destroy me' – then their odd-seeming, precautionary measures can look like rational defen-siveness, except that the premise for them is patently false.

This condition usually comes with *positive* and *negative* symptoms. The former reflect overt distortion of normal functions (e.g. bizarre and grossly inappropriate behaviour; disturbed speech which is tangential and illogical; false beliefs, and in the most serious cases, a tendency to act upon these beliefs). The term *negative symptoms* refers to an absence of, or a severe diminution of, normal behaviour (e.g. profound social withdrawal, a flattening of affect, and a lack of volition), so that there is little in the way of speech or behaviour to sustain ordinary social interaction.

The more specific DSM IV^{TR} criteria for this diagnosis should guide our understanding and may be interpreted as follows:

☐ Hallucinations: seeing things that are not objectively there; smelling odours (usually noxious ones) that no one else can smell; feeling bodily intrusions that no one else can find any cause for; or more commonly, hearing voices which seem to the patient external to him or her.

☐ Delusions: thoughts which often carry imperatives for behaviour. These are often bizarre, erroneous beliefs, which are strongly held and resistant to reason. They may be persecutory ('people follow me wherever I go'), or they may take the form of 'ideas of reference' wherein commonplace objects and events acquire special significance. In a case known to me, the sight of a salt cellar on the breakfast table meant 'I have been sexually assaulted in the night', 'a salt . . .', etc. The difference between schizophrenic cognitions and our own everyday tendencies to misinterpret stimuli is (1) the degree of bizarreness; (2) its imperviousness to later reflection or rational discussion; (3) its persistence in the face of contrary evidence, and (4) a sense of loss of control over the processes of mind and body due to external, manipulative forces.

- ☐ Thought insertion: ideas that are felt to be put inside the head from outside; or thought withdrawal, the idea that private thoughts are being 'removed', and possibly broadcast to others.
- ☐ Incoherent speech is often a manifestation of thought disorders and false perceptions. Typically, patients lose control of the structure of any particular narrative, going off track, failing to complete points, exhibiting loose associations which have considerable meaning for them but not for listeners. In serious cases there is frank incoherence or what has been called 'word salad' where no normal syntactical, grammatical or logical sentence construction rules are evident.
- ☐ Schizophrenia can also manifest itself in grossly disturbed behaviour, from childlike silliness to extreme agitation without apparent external provocation, to bizarre dress (mind you, in the old psychiatric hospitals, ill-fitting trousers, boiled sports jackets and bizarre colour schemes were more to do with institutional indifference than illness-driven choice).
- ☐ Catatonic behaviours: immobility and staying in strange postures until moved are rarer these days, since effective pharmacological treatments exist, but in the early stages of serious, untreated cases these can still be seen.

As to negative symptoms (i.e. absence of usual and appropriate behaviours), the following patterns are regularly seen:

- ☐ Affective (emotional) flattening: the blunting of the usual forms of emotional expression. There is often a lack of facial expression (but note that this can also occur in cases of clinical depression); reduced body language and general social disconnection.
- ☐ Apathy, and an avoidance of stimulating circumstances, particularly an avoidance of emotionally demanding social circumstances.
- ☐ Disconnection from family and friends, however helpful and supportive they have been.

Within this general picture several aetiologically and epidemiologically distinct subtypes of the condition may be detected (see Table 2.2).

Table 2.2 Subtypes of schizophrenia

Subtypes classification	Main symptoms
Paranoid type	Persecutory ideas and feelings and/or profound jealousy without cause; religiosity or grandiose behaviour (but note that these may be a feature of bipolar conditions).
Disorganised type	Disorganised speech and/or behaviour; inability to engage in everyday tasks; strange speech patterns, inappropriate laughter.
Catatonic type	Marked psycho-motor disturbance; immobility; echolalia – repeating whatever is said by another person.
Undetected type	All of the above symptoms may play a part but are mild or episodic in their presentation.
Residual type	This diagnosis requires at least one episode of schizophrenic behaviour, but is without prevalent psychotic symptoms, though with some negative symptoms such as poverty of speech, flattened affect or avolition.

Source: Adapted from DSM IV[TR] criteria.

☐   A further problem with diagnoses based partially upon negative symptoms relates to the effects of pharmacological treatment itself. First-generation, neuroleptic medications were notorious for producing side-effects which many patients regarded as worse than the disease: weight gain, heart problems, salivary dribbling; tardive dyskenesia (strange, high-stepping gait), neck rigidity, constant drowsiness. Second-generation medications have fewer side-effects. Relapse rates with such treatments are 20 per cent per year; but 80 per cent per year off them. Dosages and tolerance levels need to be regularly reviewed. Health and social care staff have a role in alerting medical colleagues to such problems, since the commonest cause for relapse, alongside excessive stress, is the side-effects from prescribed medications.

Causes

The first thing to acknowledge is that there is much that we do not know. Of all the mental illnesses, this one has been the most controversial. There are (not very convincing to me) social-anthropological and sociological studies which have sought to depict schizophrenia as a form of socio-cultural rebellion and a better manifestation of true sanity than most of the bourgeoisie can rise to. The Marxist philosophers (Foucault, Sartre) depicted the condition as a psychological *cri de coeur* against the alienating pressures of what they called 'late capitalism'. The psychoanalysts vaguely saw the condition as rooted in childhood psycho-sexual conflicts (what isn't for them) but now steer well clear of these patients since the symptoms are, clinically, too extreme to justify even their less fanciful notions as to aetiology. Nevertheless, they did have an even vaguer, broader influence. Bateson *et al.* (1956) put forward the idea of the *schizophrenogenic* mother (think Bates motel); R.D. Laing mistook family tensions accompanying the illness for the causes of it, recanting these views later (see Laing 1960); Thomas Szasz (1961) doubted the very existence of mental illness. Such treatises still have minor cult status on some social work training courses.

The problem facing attempts to disentangle the strands of biological inheritance and environmental experience is that usually the parents who confer the genes also provide the upbringing. Thus, even though studies have concluded for decades that mental illness runs in families, and that the greater the consanguinity (blood-relatedness) the greater the risk, we could never be sure what the transmission routes were. More secure data come from the three different research methodologies discussed on p. 32. However, it appears from these later data as if you cannot 'catch it' – though one could well have one's life chances influenced by the social, psychological and economic consequences of it – as is the case with any serious disability. However, symptoms of schizophrenia in parents seem to be recognised by older children as something completely different, as troubling but non-rational, and so not a cause for self-blame.

A set of identical twins, separated at birth, met by accident at a volunteer fire officers' convention (see Figure 2.2 below) when someone who knew one of them asked the other how he had managed to get into the bar since he had just passed him walking in the opposite direction. Both are firemen, both are married to schoolteachers, coincidentally I hope, both wives are called Doris; their hobbies are close-on identical; the books they own are amazingly similar, and they are both halfway through building the same kit canoe for the hunting trips that they both enjoy. Scary.

The question is, supposing that one of these twins (and many others in a sample) had a secure diagnosis of schizophrenia: what would be the chances of the other acquiring it? Table 2.3 displays a pooled-data table typical of many others, showing levels of actuarial risk for schizophrenia (p. 61).

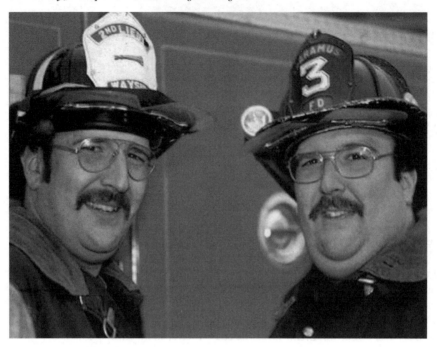

Figure 2.2 Twin brothers

Source: Reprinted courtesy of The Image Works/Encarta

Table 2.3 shows three things: (1) that the greater the level of consanguinity, the greater the likelihood of a diagnosis of the same disorder in a relative; (2) that there is a substantial leap in risk for MZ twins versus DZ twins which is well beyond chance for decisive environmental influences (see line 7 of Table 2.3), but that (3) this still leaves about 40 per cent-worth of environmental factors to be accounted for. We in the helping professions tend to be educated to look preferentially at these influences (things we can do something about), though it is worth noting that society has made no more progress with completely environmental problems such as racism, ageism and gender-discrimination than with some partially inherited ones.

Let us look next at how biological, psychological and social factors *interact* – for this is the key word – to produce precipitation and relapse. The best model of such influences that we have was thought up by mathematicians familiar with psychiatric data – a good example of the benefits of disciplinary conciliance.

Figure 2.3 is best thought of as a 3D graph in the shape of a piece of paper with a fold in it. The three axes are: (1) genetic burden, from low to high; (2) environmental stress levels, from low to high, and (3) the actuarial likelihood of being counted among those diagnosed as schizophrenic. Better still; think of the surface plane in terms of the coordinates that could be drawn across it. Thus if a line is extended from the genetic axis, and intersects a line drawn from a point on the environmental stress axis, where they cross, and how close to the 'snowbank' precipice they are, determines the likelihood of precipitation or relapse.

The stress axis in Figure 2.3 is made up of secure results from medical sociology (see Brown & Birley 1968; Leff *et al.* 1982) from psychology and from social psychiatry (see Falloon *et al.* 1984; Birchwood & Tarrier 1992; Sheldon 1994). Although it would be very easy to

Table 2.3 Level of risk to relatives of schizophrenics

Relation	Risk (%)
First-degree relatives	
Parents	4.4
Brothers and sisters	8.5
Brothers and sisters, neither parent schizophrenic	8.2
Brothers and sisters, one parent schizophrenic	13.8
Fraternal twin, opposite sex	5.6
Fraternal twin, same sex	12.0
Identical twin	57.7
Children	12.3
Children – both parents schizophrenic	36.6
Second-degree relatives	
Uncles and aunts	2.0
Nephews and nieces	2.0
Grandchildren	2.8
Half-brothers/sisters	3.2
Third-degree relatives	
First cousins	2.9
General population	0.86

Sources: Based on figures from Slater and Cowie (1971); Zerbin-Rüdin (1967); Shields and Slater (1967); Tsuang and Vandermey (1980).

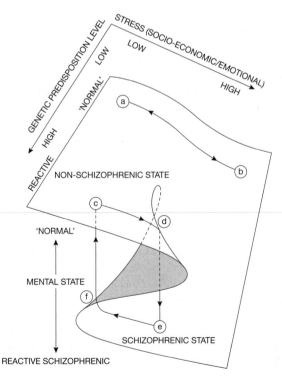

Figure 2.3 Relative impact of genetic and environmental variables in schizophrenia

Note

This model encompasses the suggestion that a high level of genetic predisposition requires only a middling level of environmental precipitation to produce a strong risk of disorder (c-d-e). Similarly, a middling level of genetic burden requires a high level of precipitating stress to manifest the disease (a-b). When the stress is relieved the patient returns to a period of relative normality (e-f-c).

Source: Woodcock and Davis (1978).

gather the impression from station bookstalls that 'stress' is a condition which afflicts mainly the employed middle class, in fact, stress – that is, being required to come up with demanding behavioural responses against a short timescale, against which circumstances conspire, and therefore feeling disablingly emotionally aroused, worried, and fearful about failure – falls disproportionately upon the poor, the psychologically troubled, and the mentally or physically disabled. Social-economic findings also show that if one was not poor before becoming mentally ill, one is almost certain to become so afterwards. Indeed, the social conditions in which most seriously mentally troubled people live add up to: being on one's own; probably without a partner; with few if any friends; with no employment or even occupation; with few if any relatives or carers to lend support; subsisting in a voluntary housing scheme; being precariously welfare benefit-dependant, and on the receiving end of a meagre 'care in the community' service (see Leff 1997; Macdonald & Sheldon 1997). The experience is that one has few if any options, and a feeling that little that one does will have an impact becomes internalised. It also becomes self-fulfilling.

However, there is another type of stress, more psychological than socio-economic, co-represented along the top axis of Figure 2.3. This is called *expressed emotion* (EE). This finding emerged in early psychiatric rehabilitation studies (see Olsen 1984) when relapse rates were found to be higher among those patients returning home to their families as opposed to sheltered accommodation or even boarding-houses. Families care on the whole for as long as they can, and they naturally want to encourage away a dehabilitating condition which strikes at the heart of family life. The resultant emotionally laden urging is exactly what people with schizophrenia find most difficult. For example, there are two ways to get someone up and out to the day centre: 'John you are doing it *again;* you *promised* me, why do you *always* let me down?', or 'John we need to get going, breakfast's downstairs'. Families, themselves under great pressure, tend to increase the emotional 'heat' on their loved ones whose 'emotional thermostats', as it were, are damaged by this illness and so readily 'click out'. Research has long shown that people with schizophrenia benefit most from 'cool', supportive, uncritical environments.

Expressed emotion can even be measured. Where up-against-it families and carers score highly on EE scales, the stress, as measured by galvanic skin response (GSR) reactions (a measure of electrical conductivity changes in the skin due to arousal, and part of the leftover, primeval fright/flight mechanism, which the brain has decided still applies in Surbiton in the twenty-first century) in patients goes up and stays up even when encounters are over (see Birchwood & Tarrier 1992). Relapse rates in high EE environments were found to run at 50 per cent, but at only 9 per cent for low EE in one study (see Falloon *et al.* 1990). Therefore this is no vague sociological concept-like *anomie;* it affects physiology, psychology and social well-being.

Let us turn now to experiments which have tried to lower stress in living conditions resulting from too much emotional demand. We have a dozen or so of these, all with positive results (see Falloon *et al.* 1990; Pharoah *et al.* 2006). Figure 2.3 is one such example; it contains a comparison between a family-based carer education and EE-lowering programme, and routine, individual after-care. The difference in relapse rates is obvious. Such interventions, though known about for some years, are not routinely available outside specialist centres (see Centre for Reviews and Dissemination, University of York).

Lifetime, age-adjusted averaged risks for the development of schizophrenia-related psychoses in classes for relatives differ in their degree of genetic relatedness (see Gottesman 1991). Sharper DSM-derived diagnostic criteria for schizophrenia produce even greater concordance (see McGuffin *et al.* 2005; and Figure 2.4).

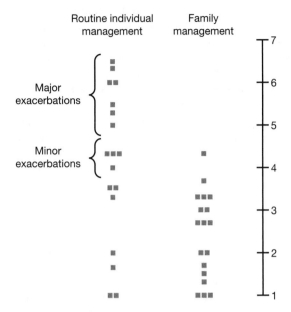

Maximum target rating (blind) during the 9 months of treatment

Figure 2.4 An experiment with expressed emotion
Source: Adapted from Tsuang and Vandermens (1980).

A role for CBT?

Not so long ago, health and social work staff and psychologists were sternly cautioned by psychiatrists that in the 'functional psychoses' it was pointless or even dangerous to try to get clients to analyse their thought patterns and delusions, since these were, under the influence of psychoanalytical theories, deemed to serve as self-protective, ego-protective functions. To encourage patients to examine their irrationality or empirically to experiment with them was to invite worsened derangement:

> To many readers the idea of trying to modify a delusion will seem at least futile and at worst harmful. Medical and nursing professions in the UK have long advised students and staff that delusions cannot be modified and that the best practice is to avoid discussing them with clients. In this section we apply a cognitive therapy style challenge to these beliefs, and suggest that the intransigent thinking may lie more with some professionals then clients.
>
> (Chadwick *et al.* 1996: ch. 4)

Only 15 per cent of sufferers experience chronic deterioration and 25 per cent experience only one episode and then recover; most illnesses take an episodic course with readily observed links to social and psychological crises. A few case examples of my own spring to mind, for exampe, a sound engineer who, after an episode of paranoid schizophrenia, managed to return to work, but the company was 'downsizing' and he 'knew' he would be one of the first to go. He constantly sought reassurance from this wife that he was loved and valued but never accepted the freely given reassurance. He wired their house with sensitive microphones to listen for the sounds of dalliances with 'someone'. Doors opening, sounds and creaks on the stairs were almost convincing, but wildly over-interpreted (they had a dog and a cat). The idea of an empirical comparison was suggested (i.e. reviewing the tapes for three days when his wife was away at her mother's). They sounded identical and on this basis he was willing to consider that these thoughts came from his insecurities and were not the *reason* for his insecurities.

Current evidence suggests a gentle, non-EE-raising CBT approach which indicates to clients that however much their delusional thinking or auditory hallucinations *seem* real, they may not be *valid* experiences. This hypothesis-testing approach works quite well in all but the most serious, chronic cases, where we have to rely almost solely upon medication and social support (see Emmelkamp 2004).

'Second-generation' antipsychotic medications (e.g. Loxapine, Nolindare, Respriridane) are as effective or more effective than earlier medications (e.g. Chorpromazine) and have the blessing of fewer side-effects. This is an important finding, since the commonest reason for relapse and re-hospitalisation, or harm to self or others, is abandoning medication.

There is only limited evidence that CBT improves compliance, but better evidence, particularly in early-course cases, that CBT can have a relapse-prevention role. Thus, CBT-related approaches have a reasonably good track record in relieving negative symptoms and may have a role in persuading clients to reattribute positive symptoms in the early stages (seventy-five RCTs and two systematic reviews suggest that this is so). However, reliable social support is also vital.

There is nothing wrong with targeted symptom relief; crisis prevention, carer support, advocacy, social skills recovery, medication compliance, etc. It would be nice to see more direct effects on the illness, but the more secure the methodology of studies, the less likely are promising claims of this sort. The Cochrane systematic review by Jones *et al.* (2004) compares screened trials with CBT vs. no treatment; CBT vs. other psychological interventions; and CBT vs. medications (n = 19). The results were: CBT is useful as an adjunct to management in the short term; does not reduce relapse rates; did improve mental state in the medium term against standard measures; did reduce the risk of lengthy stays in psychiatric units. In other words, this is a useful adjunct treatment but is far from being a panacea – but then nothing is in this disabling, difficult to remedy condition. More trials of CBT-incorporated care vs. standard supportive care are recommended, since 'no treatment' (see above) does not mean none, just no CBT component.

Personality disorders

These are not common, except on the case loads of social workers and community psychiatric nurses. Such clients usually end up 'doing the rounds'. I didn't really believe in this 'condition', even less in the associated diagnosis of Munchausen's Syndrome by Proxy, until debating this question with a social work student on placement in a hospital paediatric unit, and being shown a video from covert CCTV observation of a grandmother stifling her (apparently adored) newly born granddaughter with the bedclothes and then calling for medical help with 'unexplained' breathing difficulties. Now, with caution, I do.

These conditions have long been recognised as syndromes but the debate as to whether they are genuine mental illnesses or not has never gone away. The Royal College of Psychiatrists played the 'treatability' card a few years ago (i.e. since no effective treatments exist, and since these conditions are largely quantitative exacerbations of average personality characteristics, these patients should thus be (guess what) passed on to Social Services). In recent mental health legislation this position has rightly been reversed since there are many medical conditions for which no effective treatments exist, but for which we still have responsibilities (nice try, no thanks. We have to be in this *together* – it is the only thing that comes close to working: see Dowson & Grounds (1995)).

Personality disorders may be defined as:

> A severe disturbance in the characterological constitution and behavioural tendencies of the individual, usually involving several areas of the personality, and nearly always associated with considerable personal and social disruption. Personality disorder tends to appear in late childhood or adolescence and continues to be manifest into adulthood. These types of conditions comprise deeply ingrained and enduring behaviour patterns, manifesting themselves as inflexible responses to a broad range of personal and social situations.
>
> (ICD 10: 1992)

'Personality' is a construct, a recognisable pattern in behaviour, inferred cognition and inferred emotional patterns which are semi-independent of circumstances: inside-out factors.

H.J. Eysenck (1965) has produced the most enduring, empirically tested set of dimensions. You have to imagine, not a 2D bell-shaped curve, but actually a 3D bell shape; from side to side lies the introversion (stimulus-shy), extraversion (stimulus-hungry) continuum – the nearer the middle, the more statistically typical; from back to front, the neuroticism/psychoticism continuum. It is on the statistical shoulders of the bell curves that the serious cases of personality disorder exist, so that on one side there is a pervasive withdrawal from routine social responsibilities and opportunities, on the other, an aggressive, manipulative urge towards self-gratification at almost any cost to others (i.e. lack of an adequately functioning conscience). In the middle section is something called 'normality'.

The underlying features of these maladies are manifest in the usual stage-progression of moral development (see Kohlberg 1981) and of moral conditionability. These statistics also show a strong environmental component. Soldiers can, after all, be trained into psychopathic behaviour in the circumstances of conflict. Young people, whose status in gangs boosts their fragile identities, can behave in uncharacteristically depersonalised and aggressive ways. The point at issue is that not even in the most extreme environments, not *everyone* does behave in such a way, and so genetic predispositions come into play (see Kendler & Evans 1986).

Types of personality disorder

Table 2.4 is adapted from DSM IV^{TR}/ICD 10 reflecting regularly found pattern ranges and their different names at the extremes of personality, from the profoundly attention seeking, hypochondrical, manipulatory and dependent, to the self-gratifyingly, manipulatively exploitive, or aggressive.

Personality disorders have been shown from large community samples to have a lifetime prevalence range of 0.5 per cent to 3.5 per cent with more men than women affected – a wide variation made worse by low inter-reliability rates whether using clinical judgement alone or DSM protocols. They produce only around 58 per cent diagnostic agreement (which is pretty hopeless). This situation persuaded the authors of earlier versions of DSM to conclude that this was 'almost a diagnosis not worth making' but that we are still stuck with the problem and have to live with the 'almost'.

Table 2.4 Personality disorder types

DSM III^R and DSM IV category	Corresponding ICD 10 category
Paranoid	Paranoid
Schizoid	Schizoid
Antisocial	Dissocial
Borderline	Emotionally unstable
Impulsive type	Borderline type
Histrionic	Histrionic
Obsessive-compulsive	Anankastic
Avoidant	Dependent
Dependent	Dependent
Personality disorder not otherwise specified	Mixed and other

Source: From DSM IV^{TR}/ICD 10.

Effective interventions

There are few, if any. Behaviour-modification regimes (see Sheldon 1982, 1995) such as token economies worked well enough in closed institutions in the 1960s and 1970s, but then, surprise, surprise: since lack of generalised conditionability is at the heart of these problems, on discharge, most patients/clients reverted to doing what came naturally. Cognitive-behavioural approaches and their offshoots are now making clinically noteworthy inroads today and are cautiously challenging the 'untreatability' orthodoxy (see Dowson & Grounds 1995). Nevertheless, the most effective outcomes come from treating symptoms, either pharmaceutically in cases where high anxiety is the motivator, or psycho-socially, where social avoidant responses predominate, or with anti-psychotic medications plus social support where acting upon paranoid/aggressive cognitions poses the worst risks to self and to others.

However, from my own professional experience (nothing more) there is a further set of considerations that I believe are worthy of discussion. Namely, that since these clients, whether fully knowing it or not, tend to depend upon, but often exploit and misuse, health and Social Services support we need to work together. Typical cases show a phenomenal ability to manipulate, indeed to *parasitise* services and exploit their good intentions, complaints systems, etc. So here we have a classic case of intermittent punishment, negative reinforcement, plus small rewards, applied to whole organisations. The only thing I have seen to work is a cast-iron multi-disciplinary approach with a decisive case conference to plan and deploy services when they are not being demanded under threat, a reinforcement of cooperation, with no question of organisations failing to make a contribution because they are currently on 'respite'.

Complications

All of the mental health conditions reviewed above, but the psychoses in particular, are made substantially worse by co-morbid addictions, which influence precipitation and relapse. This problem is now so widespread that many inner-city psychiatric units have dropped previous 'dual diagnoses', since most or nearly all of their patients have these dual afflictions. Class A drugs have the worst effects, particularly the use of crack cocaine in patients with schizophrenia, but Class B drugs (e.g. cannabis) also affect course, relapse rates and recovery, as does overuse of alcohol, particularly in bipolar conditions. The problem in this field is that nothing much on offer, neither pharmacology, nor counselling, nor CBT, approaches the instant, but of course very temporary, relief from symptoms and daily life pressures that these addictive substances have. Cognitive-behavioural approaches can play a role when clients/ patients have recognised the problem *as a* problem, through (1) identifying the triggers and frustrations which lead to use; (2) substituting alternative activities to deflect cravings; (3) controlled, decreasing use – i.e. harm-reduction strategies rather than total abstinence advice; (4) taking note of the influence of peer group pressure; and (5) dealing with the cognitive and psycho-social circumstances which lead to the need for self anaesthetisation – the most promising approach (see Dowson & Grounds 1995; Beck 1999). However, once physical dependency is established, there is no substitute for treatment in a specialist unit rather than in routine mental health care.

I cannot confine our tour of research on the effectiveness of CBT only to mental disorders or clinical psychological difficulties, since there are other fields where this approach has had considerable impact, nowhere more so than in the treatment of behavioural disorders in children.

Behavioural problems in childhood

This is where behaviour therapy cut its teeth. Its results were later improved by the inclusion of cognitive approaches.

I have some reservations about the current fashion for dividing up the problems of childhood with quasi-medical syndromes (see DSM IV[TR]) and prefer (I think on good evidence) to see them as mainly due to maladaptive learning experiences; failures of adequate parenting; poor education, and adverse peer group influence. Although taxonomies are an essential first step in understanding, giving something a name on the basis of its surface features and then implying that this is the *cause* does little to advance our clinical under-standing. Not that there aren't real syndromes (e.g. autism; Asperger's syndrome) (see Sheldon & Macdonald 2009: 314), nor that there are not background biological predis-positions, but rather that *most* children with behavioural problems are where they are as a result of *environmental* influences.

The good news is that in the face of these childhood-blighting, family-disrupting problems, we now have around 1,500 controlled trials of the efficiency of therapeutic interventions (see Macdonald 2001; Kazdin 2004). W.H. Auden's poetic comment that *those to whom evil is done do evil in return* about sums up the challenge of most cases; other less serious ones are more likely to be due to adverse experiences, family conflict, incapacity and a lack of parenting skills – some of which are remediable by therapeutic interventions, some less so (see Kazdin 2004).

The first point to make is that if we define a child as a person under 18 years old, then some of the serious mental disorders reviewed above have their first onset in childhood (e.g. schizophrenia, autism, Asperger's syndrome, plus a significant level of childhood depression) (see Weisz *et al.* 2009). Treatments, both pharmacological and psychological, which do quite well with adults, often do less well with children. There is a general, positive effect from early intervention, before problems solidify, but this depends on suitable *adaptations* to the differ-ent social and psychological stresses and different power relationships of childhood and adolescence. These are not always routinely made.

The main messages from meta-analyses of psychological interventions with children and teenagers are as follows:

☐   Medium to high effect sizes regularly appear in treatment vs. no treatment comparisons. Thus the effectiveness of these interventions is equal to that in the literature on adults (see Kazdin & Weisz 1998; Kazdin 2004).

☐ Cognitive-behavioural approaches are regularly recommended in reviews for a range of childhood problems. The emphasis on mainly cognitive factors through to mainly behavioural emphasis varies with the condition/problem; for example, in anxiety and fears there is an emphasis on desensitisation; in childhood depression, upon cognitive maintenance factors; in obsessional conditions, on parent-based, management training; in conduct and oppositional disorders, on problem-solving skills training via CBT and on self-esteem (see Taylor & Montgomery 2007).

☐ CBT (1) produces efficiency gains over other interventions, and (2) appears to have longer lasting effects.

☐ There is enough evidence from reviews and from the overlapping professional literatures of health and social care (see Herbert 1978; Gambrill 1997; Cigno & Bourn 1998; Macdonald 2001) to back the recommendation that CBT techniques should be routinely integrated into the mainstream professional practice of psychologists, social workers, specialist nurses and health visitors. This last point, with the aim of improving access to evidence-based help in mind, is probably the greatest challenge for the next few years, at least equal to that of training more specialist CBT therapists. However, there is one further, overriding problem that will require concentrated action by all professionals who would like, on the evidence, to provide something more than vague 'support':

☐ Remember what happened to the British dental service in the last thirty years? It was forced and enticed to go largely private, and its connections as a branch of medicine and as a part of NHS provision were deliberately loosened; thus it has become something closer to a branch of the cosmetics industry. As a practitioner of CBT, I would hate for something similar to happen to us as a result of the welcome expansion of CBT qualifying courses, many of whose graduates will head for private practice (almost universally so in the USA). Most things that happen are not intended, but my hope is that this very effective approach will retain its roots in mainstream health and social care practice, aiming to help the most troubled and vulnerable, not as a lifestyle adjunct for the well-off, as psychoanalysis has become (just as well perhaps). NHS/social services/private *collaborations* are a different matter.

Other applications of CBT

There is considerable research literature on the use of CBT in physical health conditions – which often have psychological components not just as a reaction to illness or disabilities, but as a problem-maintaining role too. Examples are obesity – where many self-damagingly overweight clients have semi-magical ideas regarding how the weight goes on in the first place ('glands', genetics), which fly in the face of the laws of thermodynamics. Weight-loss maintenance research suggests good effects for CBT.

In cases of chronic pain, where everything pharmaceutical, mechanical and surgical has been done, some benefits can be obtained by (1) looking at how pain is *perceived* (e.g. as an alarm function, as evidence of damage, as the harbinger of even more serious deterioration); (2) examining with patients how they respond to it; a panicky response as opposed to as relaxed an approach as possible being more likely to intensify it; (3) looking at the circumstances in which pain worsens and what the early antecedents are via 'pain diaries' and ABC charts and to take the diversionary actions which might have worked before (see Ecclestone *et al.* (2009) for a systematic review).

Another field of application is couples therapy. The methods are much the same, but these are in the face of problems where unlocking greater mutual happiness, or a better life for children, lies in the dynamics of the two main players (see Sexton *et al.* (2004) for a review).

Process factors

The 'Bible' of psychotherapy outcome research (Lambert 2004) devotes three chapters to this issue, and it is present throughout most of the rest of the guide. The 'Waller hypothesis' – 'it ain't what you do it's the way that you do it, that's what gets results' – taps into our own experience of professional effects. I achieved a dismal 33 per cent in my final school maths exam. Later I found the subject, particularly statistics, interesting (relax: I have put in the remedial work), but no thanks to Mr Davis, who had a particular line in sarcasm – sarcasm is somehow better in a Welsh accent, but *I* also found it funny, even at age 12. I could appreciate the light humour, even if not the dark numbers: 'Let me explain this idea just once more, so that *even Sheldon* might be able to understand it' [laughter from the girls on the other side of the classroom, two or three of whom I thought I might marry one day when they came to their senses]. 'You have an *Eng. Lit.* brain, boy, that's your trouble, see.' Possibly, except that I got 94 per cent for geometry, taught by the kindly Miss Fuller who didn't have this approach. Technical effectiveness is one thing, the 'carrier wave' on which it is delivered quite another. Thus when we move house and need to find a new GP, we ask the neighbours (admittedly not a secure sample frame) who tend to say 'go for Dr Henry, he's pleasant, kind and he never fusses'; not, note, 'go for Dr Smith, he's the best qualified doctor for miles, and he *lives* on the Cochrane website'. There are noteworthy historical influences on this debate – which many in clinical psychology and psychiatry saw as mere 'placebo effects': (1) the analysis of process factors by Truax and Carkhuff (1967), and (2) the influence from 'humanistic psychotherapy' (e.g. Rogers 1951), and from social casework (see Sheldon and Macdonald 2009: ch. 6).

There are however problems with this enduringly preoccupying research endeavour: first, it is presented within the face of modest (translated by proponents as 'encouraging') rates of inter-rater reliability (e.g. whether helpers are under- or over-challenging of given cognitive interpretations; whether they see empathy, etc.). These rates vary from coin-tossing levels to 80 per cent – which of course leaves behind 20 per cent of doubt as to *what* is going on and how tied into outcomes it is.

The second problem is that the categorising of therapist behaviour and demeanour are *qualitative* factors, requiring the judgement of experts, who of course bring with them theoretical predispositions. When qualitative judgements acquire numbers (72 per cent, 80 per cent) they acquire an air of certainty which directs our attention away from the fact that they are judgements, not facts, and may not be *causally* related to outcomes. The weasel word 'association' is often used, meaning simply that something co-varies somewhat with something else, nothing more.

The third problem is the proliferation of factors which *might* be influential. Hundreds of different factors and interrelationships between them are urged on us and I defy anyone to tell me that *all* these balls can be juggled above an encounter with a troubled client; two or three, possibly.

My conclusion therefore is that a look back at therapist variables research tells us the following:

☐   We like these ideas because we like to feel that we are 'naturals' at this work; that the rich resources of our caring personalities and mere experience transcend 'recipes'. To continue the analogy, can you imagine a chef who, upon gaining his second Michelin star, said, 'It was quite straightforward really, I just followed the recipes.'

☐   The main influential factors, first operationalised by Truax and Carkhuff from the work of Carl Rogers, have stood the test of time (i.e. non-possessive warmth, genuineness, accurate empathy, to which might be added reliable advocacy). Let us look at what these attributes entail. Non-possessive warmth consists of (1) getting across to clients feelings of respect, understanding, caring, acceptance and concern, but (2) managing to do this in a non-threatening way, so that there is no sense of them being 'managed' or taken over and no question that willingness to continue trying to understand depends upon coming up with approved-of responses.

☐ *Genuineness.* The best description of this attribute follows from saying what it is not. To be genuine is not to be 'phoney', not to hide behind a professional façade or image; not to be defensive in the face of challenge; not to resort to 'special voices' intended to signal empathy but widely and rightly lampooned in the media; not to play Rogerian word games, meant to clarify but irritating to most: 'talk normal'.

☐ *Accurate empathy.* Positive feelings and a desire to understand are of little practical use if they dwell inside the therapist; they are a category of verbal and non-verbal *behaviour* and need to be communicated. The elements are: an accuracy of understanding; having a 'ghost' of the feeling inside oneself that the client has inside them; an ability to put oneself in the shoes of another – despite courses of action that they have taken which look to us self-defeating, illogical or even stupid – and then demonstrating that this is the case. All this depends on *active listening*, often a novel experience for clients. I am fond of Bernard Levin's advice on listening to music: 'Do with your ears what you do with your eyes when you stare.'

There follows a section of an interview transcript (this relates to the case discussed on p. 236) which gives the client's reaction to CBT in a case of serious depression:

> Well at the start, it was all new to me because I've spent so long hiding the truth from other people – I was ashamed I expect. But I learnt in our talks that I could say *anything* – what I mean is that you wouldn't fall backwards off the chair if I told you something awful or something I was ashamed of. But then I also liked it when you didn't let me get away with anything (laugh). I had lots of complications in my life and you got me to think again about them. You never *made* me do these things, but I soon got an idea of where you thought I should be heading. Somehow I got it into my head that all the knocking about was something to do with me; that I must have 'asked for it'; *made* it happen somehow. Now I know that I must have been mad to put up with it and that *nobody* should be treated like that. But it's only when you stand back and start to say to yourself, 'hey, I'm a person too, what about bloody *me?*'
>
> (Sheldon & Macdonald 2009: 114)

Most clinicians will tell you that the *way* in which issues have been handled in cases has influenced their outcome. Most researchers will give an 'up to a point' verdict based on the difficulties of separating out methods from interactional processes and assessing the relative weight of each. The sensible conclusion seems to be that process factors are a necessary but not a sufficient condition of recovery.

3   Philosophical implications

Do not all charms fly at the mere touch of cold philosophy?

(John Keats 1820)

I hope to show not; for although the greater part of this book is devoted to technical matters, it is not my intention to persuade psychotherapists or health and social care staff who make use of CBT to become mere technicians. Given the complex and controversial nature of the problems confronting them, it is vital that they should be able to think for themselves and make clear judgements about what their actions – even their allegedly commonsensical and non-theoretical actions – assume about the person needing their help, and about the most effective way of providing it. Therefore, they cannot afford to be philosophically naive. However, there is another purpose behind this brief excursion other than to persuade would-be helpers to keep in view a broader picture of the human condition than the latest set of guidelines on 'maintaining excellence', etc. require. Euphemisms are always lies. Just say no, otherwise you will find yourself needing more and more of them:

> Alice laughed. 'There's no use trying' she said: 'one can't believe impossible things'. 'I daresay you haven't had much practice,' said the Queen. 'When I was your age, I always did it for half an hour a day. Why, sometimes I've believed as many as six impossible things before breakfast.'
>
> (Carroll 1865: 184)

The main reason why cognitive-behavioural psychology and its derivatives are not taught as an essential ingredient of the knowledge and skills which students in the helping professions need to understand and to be able to carry out is vague, ideological opposition, usually from academic staff. We teach our students in a strange way. Despite yards of guidelines from governing bodies, what you get as a student is still much more likely to be defined by the interests of the academics in charge and their previous training, as is what is available in the university library apart from set books which purport to cover everything you will ever need to know.

Applied psychology, particularly in its behavioural and cognitive-behavioural forms, has thus always had a tough time getting into the curriculum and on reading lists as compared to more heart-warming ideas – 'person-centred' this, 'humanistic' this or 'holistic' that. Thus, in this chapter I seek to challenge the still widespread view of this research, and these techniques, as being in any way 'narrow', 'mechanistic' or limited in application.

The setting up in many universities of dedicated, undergraduate and postgraduate courses on CBT is to be welcomed and will, since they have more control over their curriculum, in time spread their influence to mainstream professional education. The mirror-image concern is will this include anything sociological, or social science-derived where it is pertinent? Will courses take account of culture, race, gender or include anything social-psychological?

The first set of questions concerns the processes by which behaviour is instigated, influenced and controlled. For new behaviour is the ultimate test of useful change. If people worry less, have greater self-esteem, have fewer suicidal thoughts or see their children differently, it will almost always be reflected in what they *do*, *don't do* or do *differently*.

Mind and behaviour

The common view held of behaviour in our culture and most others is that it is a surface manifestation of a much more complex and interesting process going on somewhere inside our heads. Further, that (except in the case of a few bodily reflexes) a non-material, non-detectable 'something', obeying none of the known physical laws, manages nevertheless, to control, via its host organ, the brain, the sum total of our behaviour. I refer, of course, to the concept of mind. So much is obvious, you might think. But however natural-seeming and taken-for-granted such notions are, they raise a number of awkward logical problems. How, for example, *can* a non-physical, quasi-spiritual entity (product, perhaps) give rise to something as tangible as behaviour? Speaking metaphorically: what kind of cerebral 'clutch mechanism' connects and disconnects mental activity and physical activity? How can an event of any kind, even a thought, arise spontaneously out of nothing as an *uncaused* happening? Certainly such things are not within our everyday experience of the rest of the material world. So why do we suppose that we are not bound by the same laws that appear to forbid such things elsewhere? Part of the answer is that given the anticipated complexity of having to account scientifically, that is materially, for something so enormously divergent as human behaviour, there is an almost irresistible temptation to assign the whole question of causality to the action of some magical 'black-box' phenomenon within, thereby short-circuiting the whole vexing issue, or moving the discussion to a metaphysical plane. This done, we are left to contemplate only whether 'the mind' is a unity, or how it is different from 'the soul'; whether it has 'faculties' or an unconscious area; how it can get 'diseased' or 'unbalanced', and so forth. In the same way, it is easier to explain the origins and development of life by inventing another supreme being, a marvellous version of ourselves, who fortunately views us as His favourite creation. Then we can assign to Him responsibility for everything (see Dennett 2006). Similarly, some prefer to account for their daily fortunes by the movements of the stars and planets. We do it because, despite appearances, it is *easier*. The baffling alternative is to try to work out the myriad complex interrelationships between our actions and the forces of the environment and previous learning, to which we respond – and which respond to us.

The notion of man as a physical shell, piloted from within by little *homunculi*, has been caricatured for years in the *Beezer* comic's Numskulls. 'Brainy' is the controller of other little creatures who have ear trumpets if in charge of hearing; wind open eyelids with a handle and refer all the time to 'our man'. The trick is to try to imagine what these *homunculi* have inside *their* heads, controlling *their* actions. This is not so far away from the idea of 'a self' inhabiting the brain; although we all have the strong feeling that there is one.

An early advocate of this idea of man as some kind of complicated machine, driven from within, was the seventeenth-century philosopher René Descartes. In trying to square his interest in scientific materialism and his Christian belief, he invented the doctrine of dualism. Here is the first half of it:

> I desire, I say, that you consider that these functions (respiration, sight, hearing, ideas) occur naturally in this machine solely by the disposition of its organs, not less than the movements of a clock.
>
> (Descartes 1664)

As to the other half of this duality which so mysteriously influences the 'clockwork' at every click and turn, no knowledge was claimed of it beyond the certainty of its existence. Descartes saw thinking as the main evidence for it, and a surer guide to his own existence than the inferred sensations of his physical body. Hence his famous dictum: *cogito ergo sum* – 'I think, therefore I am'.

Descartes made his analogy with the most complex machine available to him: the clock. Today, behaviour is more likely to be seen as resulting from the operation of some cerebral super-computer – the most complex machine available to us. But even in this contemporary version, 'the computer' is usually thought to be controlled from within by the magic of mind, by a 'ghost in the machine' (Ryle 1949). Ryle argued that this problem of the mind–body relationship is less a scientific conundrum than a philosophical one. In our terms it is an error of attribution, or in his terms a 'category mistake' and a 'philosopher's myth'. He offers the following illustration:

> A foreigner visiting Oxford for the first time is shown a number of colleges, libraries, playing fields, museums, scientific departments and administrative offices. He then asks 'But where is the University? I have seen where the members of the colleges live, where the Registrar works, where the scientists experiment and the rest. But I have not yet seen the University in which reside and work the members of your University.' It has then to be explained to him that the University is just another collateral institution, some ulterior counterpart to the colleges, laboratories, and offices which he has seen. The University is just the way in which all that he has already seen is organised. He was mistakenly allocating the University to the same category as that to which the other institutions belong.
>
> (Ryle 1949: 17–18)

Accepting that attempts to define mind as an independent entity with self-generating causative properties have fallen into this 'category mistake', it is possible to see how much more logical it is to infer mind from observable behaviour. This is the view of behaviourism which, proponents suggest, may best be thought of as the philosophy of the science of human behaviour (see Skinner 1974), and which is seen by detractors as a philosophical and methodological dead-end. But then, the emerging branch of psychology twinned with biology, *neuroscience*, has produced some disturbing findings: (1) that the idea of personal control over actions might be an illusion – human beings are very bad at sorting out causality when different stimuli and responses cluster together; (2) it may actually have become beneficial to us over evolutionary time to take personal responsibility for what are essentially routine, automatic operations of the brain, since this leads to increased alertness, and to greater learning from consequences, plus the possibility of suppressing reflexes in the cause of more cortically-generated, pause-and-think reinterpretations (see Dennett 2003).

Here are some awkward findings for those who continue straightforwardly to accept that there is a 'self' in charge of brain operations which directs thoughts and then initiates patterns of behaviour based on them. Brooks provides a useful survey of a series of experiments involving the electrical stimulation of brain sites which took advantage of clinical (surgical) procedures to further academic understanding. The patients were conscious throughout:

> Most of these responses were simple movements of the body. I say *simply* as if that weren't extraordinary enough. Fried and his team were applying currents to specific regions of the brain and evoking movements – sometimes just one joint would flex or one muscle group in the face would contract. Sometimes they could evoke a larger response: the patient would assume a posture, extending her neck then retracting her head. . . . But it wasn't the most extraordinary thing. What really shocked the researchers was the patients' reports that they were feeling 'an urge to move my right arm'. 'An urge to move my right leg inwards', 'an urge to move my right thumb and index finger' and when the researchers ramped up the current a little on each case, that's exactly what happened: the urges turned into actions, the very action that the patients had reported wanting to perform.
>
> (Brooks 2009: 156–157)

The point being that most of us would report the cause for reaction as the 'urge', not the urge as a delayed part of it. Daniel Dennett's (1991) concept of stimuli triggering 'multiple drafts' regarding potential reactions, some of which remain unconscious, and some of which get passed upstairs to the cortex under the influence of prior learning, as priorities, is our current best explanation of this strange inversion of what it feels like to decide to do something.

Traditional behaviourism further suggested that since behaviour occurs as a phenomenon within the physical universe it must therefore obey the same laws of cause and effect. Behaviour is seen in this philosophy as an organic adaptation to an ambivalent physical and social environment. In turn, human behaviour acts upon this environment, changes it, and so provides a source of stimulation for others and of feedback for the individual.

Behaviourism further proposed that, contrary to the established view, the cognitive processes which we call consciousness are an interesting by-product of this relationship between body and environment, if you like: *ago ergo sum* – 'I act, therefore I am' – and think about it before, during *or* afterwards.

The experience that we have learned to categorise as 'mind' is the experience of our brains at work, processing sensory stimuli, and, through the use of language, encoding, classifying, manipulating and storing in symbolic form, information about the contingencies in our environment and the likely effects of our future behaviour upon these. Given that this organ, a wondrous super-computer made of meat, has around a hundred thousand million nerve cells, and complex interconnections between them which strain mathematical imagination, we really have no need to resort to 'ghosts in machines'. A 'machine' of this incredible complexity is likely to have some pretty ghostly properties of its own:

> Each cubic inch of the cerebral cortex probably contains more than ten thousand miles of nerve fibres, connecting the cells together. If the cells and fibres in one human brain were all stretched out end to end they would certainly reach to the moon and back. Yet the fact that they are not arranged end to end enabled man to go there himself. The astonishing tangle within our head makes us what we are. Every cell in the cortex receives on its surface an average of several thousand terminals from the fibres of other cells. The richness of interconnection makes each neuron a Cartesian soul.
>
> (Blakemore 1977: 85)

Consider Colin Blakemore's 'astonishing tangle' point further; question: Why are five-inch-high tubs of pot noodles still too hot to eat after fifteen minutes? Perhaps we should fill our radiators with this stuff. The answer is that they have an astonishing curled up surface area. Similarly, the brain, which weighs about 3lb, accounts for around 3 per cent of the body's weight, yet consumes about 20 per cent of its energy.

Popper and Eccles (1977) – a philosopher collaborating with a neurologist – described the effects of the almost unimaginably complex development hinted at here as 'materialism transcending itself'. Their view is that a quantitative extension of function to this near-infinite degree results 'without any violating of the laws of physics' in qualitatively different feedback effects.

Behavioural psychology, neither in its original nor in its newer forms, does not seek to deny the subjective importance of consciousness, but rather to challenge views of this phenomenon which represent it as some sort of disconnected causal entity, impervious, when it chooses, to environmental influence:

> The objection to inner states is not that they do not exist, but that they are not relevant in a functional analysis. We cannot account for the behaviour of any system while staying wholly inside it; eventually we must turn to forces operating upon the organism from without.
>
> (Skinner 1953: 55)

The point being that while I can have direct(ish) access to my own conscious processes, I cannot have ready access to yours. What you may tell me about the goings-on inside your head is subject to all sorts of internal and external pressures and distortions before it reaches me. The poet Peter Porter's lines (1983: 771) spring to mind: 'Which words will come through air unbent / Saying, so to say, only what they mean?' A genuinely scientific account of the relationship between thinking and doing must therefore, it was/is argued, concentrate as fully as possible on the doing part of the equation:

> Whenever we ask about a sentence, 'What does it mean?' what we expect is instructions as to the circumstances in which the sentence is to be used; we want a description of the conditions under which the sentence will form a true proposition, and of those that will make it false.
>
> (Schlick 1936: 340)

I am not speaking here of absolute truth or of absolute falsehood – such definitive states are difficult enough to come by in the hardest of sciences – but rather of the ruling out, as far as possible, by logic and by methods of empirical observation, of obvious errors. We can never be certain of our propositions: 'despite what she says, this child has been sexually abused'; 'this young man knows exactly what he is doing, really'; we can only be temporarily encouraged or discouraged according to the results of tests which rein in the tendency of the human mind to fill in the spaces between observations. For example:

> I found that those of my friends who were admirers of Marx, Freud and Adler were impressed by a number of points common to those theories, and especially by their apparent explanatory power. These theories appeared to be able to explain practically everything that happened within the fields to which they referred. To study any of them seemed to have the effect of an intellectual conversion or revelation, opening your eyes to a new truth hidden from those not yet initiated. Once your eyes were thus opened, you saw confirming instances everywhere: the world was full of verifications of the theory.
>
> (Popper 1963: 5)

When references to possible interior goings-on seem to help the investigation along – as perhaps with the concept of 'attitude' or 'personality' – the inference should always be kept at the lowest possible level. This position on what counts as evidence in the assessment of human behaviour gives findings in this field their relatively greater robustness and replic-ability. But, however heuristically useful, are they a true account of human experience, or even of the necessary limits of scientific enquiry?

The problem with radical behaviourism is that it fails to distinguish between the person who sits, head in hands, on a railway platform for ten minutes because his train is late (again); and the person who sits in exactly the same position for exactly the same amount of time, who has recently lost a loved one, and may or may not jump under the next incoming service. The behaviour is the same, though the latent distinction may become clearer twenty minutes later. The task of prediction for the Samaritans, railway police and psychologists is the same, for if asked what they were doing, both subjects are likely to reply: 'waiting for a train'. Nevertheless, we *know* that the interior experience of these two people is different, and may be implicated in what happens next.

In the past we were forced to choose between the rampant subjectivity of mentalistic psychology – the idea that thoughts arise spontaneously from the conscious or unconscious mind and direct our behaviour (which is rather like saying that appetite causes eating); or the 'self-denying ordinance' of behaviourism, confining ourselves to exterior observations of eating time and speed, salivary flow, etc., ruling out all interior states from peckishness to ravenousness, including disguising one's hunger for reasons of social propriety, developed long ago as a hierarchy-preserving device in times of shortage.

Recent developments in psychology suggest that a science of cognition may not be the contradiction in terms it once seemed. Dennett (1991), a philosopher with a prodigious knowledge of biology and psychology, has laid out the ground rules for such a project in a wonderfully provocative book:

> (1) No Wonder Tissue allowed. I will try to explain every puzzling feature of human consciousness within the framework of contemporary physical science; at no point will I make an appeal to inexplicable or unknown forces, substances, or organic powers.

> (2) No feigning anesthesia. It has been said of behaviorists that they feign anesthesia – they pretend they don't have the experiences we know darn well they share with us. If I wish to deny the existence of some controversial feature of consciousness, the burden falls on me to show that it is somehow illusory.

> (Dennett 1991: 40)

The old joke about what two behaviourists say to each other after making love runs: 'That was good for you, how was it for me?'

Studies of human perception (see Gregory 1970; Dixon 1976; Sheldon 1987), and of the effects of localised brain damage (see Sacks 1985); research on artificial intelligence, and work on consciousness by neuroscientists are giving rise to imaginative theories regarding the nature of consciousness – but, and this is what is new, these theories are grounded in a developing body of *empirical* research. The model of consciousness that is emerging has the following features.

The importance of evolutionary pressures is underlined, not only in respect of our basic physical reflexes, but for cognition too. Edelman's (1987) concept of 'neural Darwinism' (not so very far off from Homme's (1965) attempts to apply operant conditioning principles to thought via the concept of 'coverants') suggests that set patterns of information-processing are governed by early experience while our brains are still developing. Particularly productive neural 'firing' patterns and combinations are laid down by the influence of the environment on brain microstructures and 'preferred' neural firing combinations (these 'pathways' work to produce adaptive behaviour and thus a developmental feedback loop). They are the reason why you shouldn't sit your toddlers in front of the TV all morning under the influence of negative reinforcement. It just makes the urgent developmental task of learning to infer what other (real) people might be thinking or feeling much more difficult later.

All this moves us even further away from the concept of the free-thinking 'I', in charge of all decisions – 'the Central Meaner', as Dennett describes this hypothetical entity. Rather, consciousness is a multi-layered activity, much of it automatic. There is no 'screen in the head' on which all options can be flashed, because if there were, there would be 'no one' to watch it:

> There is no single, definitive 'stream of consciousness', because there is no central Headquarters, no Cartesian Theater where 'it all comes together' for the perusal of a Central Meaner. Instead of such a single stream (however wide) there are multiple channels in which specialist circuits try, in parallel pandemoniums to do their various things, creating Multiple Drafts as they go. Most of these fragmentary drafts of 'narrative' play short-lived roles in the modulation of current activity but some get promoted to other, functional roles in swift succession, by the activity of a virtual machine in the brain.
> (Dennett 1991: 63)

Dennett introduces a small experiment at this point: try it. Imagine a crossword grid; the words down are Gas, Oil and Dry: what are the words across? No conferring, no doodles on paper, just look at them on the screen in your head and calculate the answer. Most students in the psychology class have considerable difficulty with this – to their surprise. Most will confess to, say, looking at window panes to fill in the squares; virtually all report the desire for a piece of paper and a pencil to work out what they *know* is obvious but can't quite hold still in consciousness long enough to 'read it'. We long for an external set of referents to put the problem back into our brains from the outside.

We all have these experiences; though we think our memories are clear, and are reinforced by emotional attachments. The question: 'What did Auntie May look like?' is likely to produce discord at family gatherings. I sometimes have this experience when I am invited/ dragged out on clothes shopping expeditions. After half an hour I wander off and then come back. No wife in sight, so I ask after her (probably in the trying-on cubicles); 'What does she look like?' ask the shop assistants. 'Well, sort of tall [she's 5ft 3in, but carries herself well].' 'What was she wearing?' 'Well, sort of dark clothes. . . .' Not a good witness statement, yet I saw her dress and I've been married to her for nearly forty years. So where, regarding this most familiar and precious of objects in my life, is the definitive 'photographic' image in my head – or in yours in like case?

Consciousness then is 'future-producing', designed to answer the question, vital in evolution: 'What do I do next?' Consciousness is no 'free-floating entity'; it is highly dependent on 'hard-wired', endowed circuits and on more adaptable 'preferred channel' ways of problem-solving, based on experience of the effects of our cognitive/behavioural/arousal experiments.

Consciousness is thus less free of contemporary sensory input than many psychological models would suggest, and thinking is less free of 'yesterday's environments' with their attendant successes and failures than we may imagine. Much of our behaviour is unconsciously formed in line with the above points. Range and complexity disguise the automaticity of set thinking patterns and set responses, the analysis of which is a central feature of cognitive-behavioural therapy.

Does all this mean that we are 'machines' after all? Let us examine the question, and consider the next obstacle to acceptance of cognitive-behavioural models, the charge that these procedures assume that people are, when you get down to it in the MRI scanner, really just programmable entities, which, it is alleged, denies the essential humanity of both ourselves and of those who come to us for help. Here is a summary of a powerful experiment which examines the fundamental attributional error (see Jane Elliot (videotape); Peters 1987).

Shortly after the murder of Martin Luther King a teacher in a predominantly white school in Iowa (Jane Elliot) decided to experiment with the controlling features of her young pupils' attitudes to difference, testing the hypothesis: Do we *learn* to hate? She divided her class by eye colour, saying that blue-eyed children were smarter and better behaved. These children were deliberately praised more, given privileged access to the lunch counter, and first pick of the apparatus in the play area. Brown-eyed children were held up to minor ridicule: 'Isn't that *typical* brown-eyed behaviour, class?' Brown-eyed children became visibly unhappy, underperformed, sat in little sad groups, and deferred to blue-eyed pupils without being asked – they had *learned* their spurious status. Next, the categories were reversed; brown-eyed children were told that *they* were more intelligent and deserved privileged treatment, and *exactly* the same reactions occurred (the film is still available and remains the most powerful way to absorb this testimony to the often-unrecognised power of environmental contingencies – plainly arbitrary ones in this case) over thinking, emotion and behaviour. Follow-up groups show the subjects, now adults, speaking of the benefits of the moral lessons they learned: gripping, but unlikely to get past an ethics review today.

Free will versus environmental control

All new heresies which suggest that human beings (or in this case, the experience of an inner conscious 'I') may not necessarily be at the centre of the universe, give rise to uncomfortable feelings. Furthermore, they appear to defy common sense. I know that the world revolves around me, and that I spontaneously cause things to happen in it, just as I know that the sun revolves around the earth and that the earth is flat; I can tell instantly that the table on the left in Figure 3.1 (opposite) is longer and narrower than the one on the right. But get out a ruler and check.

Similarly, I know that my will is free and that if I wanted to, really wanted to, I mean, I could leave this writing table now for a nice walk outside. The fact that I forgo this opportunity and continue to write is because 'I want to'. Clear enough? It shouldn't be. As an explanation of my present actions it is pure tautology. It says nothing about causes, and does little to advance the reader's knowledge of the factors leading to my present behaviour. A more complicated explanation is that in the past I have had pleasant, or anxiety-reducing experiences (which I have learned to connect with comfort or excitement, feelings of satisfaction, control over my circumstances and so on) as a result of doing things like this at the expense of other, more immediately pleasurable things.

So again, because of my learning history, as I sit here I have emotions that arouse images of similar future events: hearing again the lovely sound of a manuscript hitting the bottom of a post-box; holding a bound copy one day; a favourable review perhaps; the approval of colleagues; the image of an interested reader and so on. These are the reasons why my present behaviour continues (but note that I need never have learned to

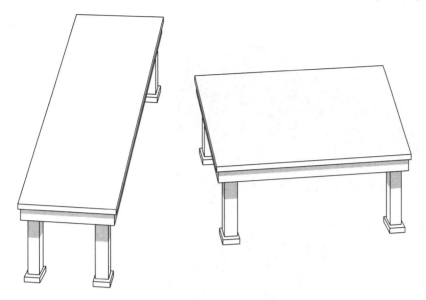

Figure 3.1 Turning the tables

value any of them). In addition, there is the anticipation of aversive consequences lying in wait for me, should I do anything else: walking my dog across a field *but as a wastrel* ('mental camera' pans back to reveal lonely figures in a bleak landscape – after David Lean). My behaviour is following a pattern, as does all behaviour, though it is not always an easy task to identify the controlling factors, especially not from the outside, where, in the present case, it might look as if I were just sitting at a table wearing a fixed expression on my face.

Were one of these controlling factors to change, or a new one emerge – the noise from outside my window of a low-flying aircraft, or the news that the deadline for this book has been extended – then my behaviour might change and fall under the control of a new set of variables. Does this mean that I am a robot? I certainly don't feel like a robot, nor do I experience the behaviour of other people as robotic, and it may be that this is the important thing about free will and determinism. We have the experience of free choice, though we do not choose our choices, nor do we choose the thought patterns which accompany their prospect and execution.

Skinner (1974) argues that the absolute prediction of human behaviour from its causes would be a task similar in complexity to that facing a physicist trying to predict the individual trajectories of all the droplets in a rainstorm (probably a gross underestimation of the problem). But the fact that it cannot be done does not mean that such trajectories do not exist or that they are not the result of known forces. Nor does it mean that we should not go in for the psychological equivalent of 'weather forecasting'. Nor does it mean that we should not look at local conditions so long as we remember that our little maps of hypothetical cause and effect are part of larger ones. First there are small problems of helping a person with a learning disability to acquire skills in self-care (local weather); then there is the wider problem of discrimination in society (climate). All this talk about causality tends to ignore central problems – the one that Einstein criticised classical physics for, i.e. where is the imaginary observer to stand to make such measurements, and over what timescale? Even with the aid

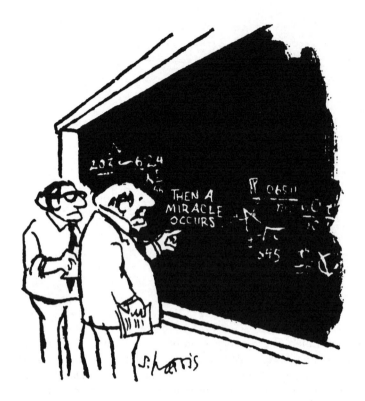

Figure 3.2 Sydney Harris, 'I think you should be more explicit here in step two'

Source: By permission of *American Scientist*.

of the most advanced super-computer, or even some even more advanced, future versions of it, we could never calculate the myriad combining influences that make an outcome the only one that could possibly happen given *all* the circumstances. Such 'perfect knowledge' is completely unachievable – even in economics which relies on the idea – as we have recently seen to our cost. The best we can do is to regard ourselves (and our clients) as having an *experience* of free will, which assumption is presumably good for us and for society. Imagine a legal system which assumed genetic and environmental determinism. There would be no punishing consequences, which themselves are part of the causal blizzard. I am reminded of a case in London a few years ago, of a psychology student charged with serial shoplifting. He argued that his genetics, his upbringing and regular reinforcement determined his behaviour (he was caught only late in his career). The judge said that he found this (self-)defence intellectually convincing, but that sadly, given his *own* genetic inheritance, life experiences and indoctrination in law, *he* too had no alternative than to sentence the defendant to three months without the option!

Rather than fretting over the issue of free will or questions of self-determination, the concern of those of us who wish to use psychological knowledge for good should be to widen the range of possible responses which the individual can make to his or her environment – including responses which seek to change it.

In response to such a discussion Dr Johnson once said, striking a rock, 'we know our will is free and *there's* an end on't!' (Boswell 1740). With due deference, given what we have learned from behavioural psychology and cognitive neuroscience in the last century, it would be more reasonable to argue that our 'will' is an inference from our behaviour – which is not free. However, given the enormous complexity of this interaction of stimulus and response, we *feel* that it is (and there's an end on't?). As before, a quantitative change from one single, simple reflex to a multiplicity of stimulus–response connections produces a qualitative change in appearance, and behaviour turns into a process in the same way that a series of film stills is turned into movement and drama by the rapid motion of the movie projector. The stills are there all the time and are the invisible components that give rise to the perception of a *flow* of behaviour on the screen. Action and interaction become a stream of events. Thus, if we say that the Second World War was caused by the Treaty of Versailles, though influential, this is only part of the picture, as is saying that Mr X's depression was caused by redundancy when in most cases many other predispositioned biological and social factors are likely to be included. However, we need to remember that even streams have their component parts, right down to the individual molecules of hydrogen and oxygen that are their building blocks. At this micro-particle level we are increasingly led to believe that 'building blocks' is quite the wrong sort of term, and that chaos rages (see Gleick 1988). But this may have less to do with indeterminism than with *indeterminability*, though as an empiricist I have to accept that the two are effectively the same, for now. The view of interaction taken here is that discrete elements in this process of influence by the environment, and reinfluence by the individual in society, are blurred by the speed and complexity of events. Such a view acknowledges multiple causation and recognises that what is often regarded as the cause of something is merely the last, or the most conspicuous part of a great many preconditions necessary to its occurrence (Verworn 1916). In this way it may be said that operating the switch *caused* a light bulb to illuminate, but in fact many other complex factors were at work to bring this about, given the immense interactivity of causal influences.

Consider the cosmologist Car Sargan's question: 'How to make an apple pie from scratch?' Answer: 'First, create your universe.'

Thus, for prediction purposes, we live in a highly interrelated, probabilistic environment. Thus, I can state with a conviction as close to certainty as we will ever get, that *you* are not going to win the Euro Millions Lottery, not that *no one* is, that someone will is a certainty, but that *you* won't. To get a feel for this, next time you buy a ticket, use the numbers 1, 2, 3, 4, 5, 6. Psychologically, this decision to lengthen the odds would seem foolish, but then statistically (probabilistically) this sequence has as good a chance of winning as your child's birth date. You are *much* more likely to be run over by a bus.

Karl Popper (1982) suggests that a proper challenge for determinists is to predict the exact moment at which his cat might jump on to his writing table, and to draw the exact outline of paw marks where it will land. It can't be done; yet how equally silly to see this as a completely *indeterminate* sequence. Cats are genetically equipped for jumping; their instincts make them feel safer when high up, they learn readily to associate places where their human food- and comfort-providers sit, mainly in the mornings perhaps, and so forth. In any case, I fancy that had B.F. Skinner been given a day or two with this cat we might have seen something worth watching.

It is often said that social care and health staff should be *practical* people, which is often simply politician-speak for 'shut up and do as we tell you'. It is true that we are mostly concerned with the nearby causes of unhappiness ('local weather'). These influences are usually the most predictable and the most tractable, but they are not the only ones with which we should be concerned. We also have a duty to persuade our clients to think more rationally, less self-punishingly, about larger scale sociological and political factors ('climate'). A case in point is unemployment. This causes depression, family and relationship difficulties, increases crime, adversely affects health, damages the welfare of children, and produces widespread social dislocation (watch this space). It is usually discussed by politicians (where they feel that they can do nothing much about it) as a macro-economically determined phenomenon (a curious convergence of view, this, between conservatives and old-style Marxists). Yet most public measures taken against it are individual, psychological and motivational in character; for example, relabelling the unemployed (in true Orwellian fashion) as 'job-seekers' – are the homeless soon to become 'flat-seekers' one wonders? What little help is provided often reinforces a view among victims that it is *their* fault, not that of gambling bankers, that they should try harder, present themselves better, update their CVs and so forth. A little positive cognitive-realignment and reattribution in such cases, based on the facts, is the opposite of shaping individuals into social conformity and denial of choice, provided that this is not *instead* of personal help but in addition to it. I can think of two or three cases where, to the clients' initial surprise, but then to their relief, I have advised that 'You are not mentally ill; you are psychologically up against it because of the behaviour of your employers; thus, you don't really need a psychotherapist, you need a good employment lawyer; let's see if we can find one' (see p. 214).

Being a bit utopian at heart, members of the helping professions tend to have a fickle relationship with theories. Any sniff of a constraining implication and they are set aside for something more supportive of the best in human ambition. Thus behaviourism, even when served up in a cognitive suspension, is a 'closed-system', is 'determinist', is 'controlling', is 'dangerous' in the wrong hands – where other therapeutic approaches, however ineffective, are somehow not. This chapter (and see Chapter 9 on ethics) is offered as a corrective to such views in the hope of persuading readers that these are matters to be wrestled with, not selected for comfort's sake.

There are several further points to make here:

1   The more a therapist can persuade clients to reinterpret stimuli; the more reliable, evidential information is made available, the more problems can be seen from more than one fixed point of view, and the less black/white thinking predominates; the more clients can be encouraged and supported to make small experiments based on their beliefs and their typical reactions, the broader the range of responses available for future reinforcement and the less narrowly reflexive and detrimental is the behaviour. The research literature also regularly tells us that if this can be pulled off there is an 'immunisation' effect, so that *new* stimuli and *new* problems can be more successfully dealt with (positive generalisation: see Chapters 4 and 7).

We must next consider the recent findings from cognitive theory and cognitive neuroscience and try to predict how they will influence cognitive-behavioural practice. This burgeoning literature is so large that a considered survey with pointers is all that is possible.

2   Earlier work on 'definitive, all-powerful brain sites for . . .' has been replaced (in the same way that 'genes for . . .' interpretations are now regarded as somewhat naive). The latest research takes stock of *interconnections* (though there *are* initiating sites) between, say, an emotional kick-off which is automatically referred upstairs for cortical interpretation, and,

if it is not, through genetic influences and learning experience, we start dealing with threats automatically, thinking about them later. When this goes wrong, as in combat stress and post-traumatic stress disorder, then the role of the CB therapist is to try to encourage a pause, and then to analyse and interpret this automatic sequence with the client.

3   Cognitive appraisal, itself constructive in nature through learning and selective perceptions, is not separate from emotional arousal. Few thought patterns are without an emotional 'soundtrack' and thoughts too are, as a result, subject to classical and operant conditioning influences (see Chapter 4). For although psychology teachers still put up stimulus-response diagrams, outside animal laboratories (and hardly within them, as Pavlov discovered) stimulation virtually never occurs as an individual quantum of information; we swim in a sea of stimuli, and through learning, selectively respond to them – sometimes usefully, sometimes self-defeatedly (which is where we come in). Behaviour gives rise to thoughts *and* emotions. Emotion gives rise to thoughts *and* behaviour, or to inaction, in an *integrated* way. We separate out these parts of the evolved human brain only for teaching purposes and compartmentalise them to the detriment of our discipline (see Damaisso 1994). Thus, there is nothing 'mechanical' about our learning relationship with the environment; the patterns are immeasurably rich and reciprocal. It has taken us quite a while to come to know what (from anthropological studies) Australian aboriginal people have always assumed.

4   The function of consciousness, the 'virtual machine' in the brain, is warily to review environmental contingencies, but also (until recently a neglected feature) to maintain the internal world of the body. Over-monitoring and over-interpreting internal events is where panic attacks, hypochondria and anxiety states come from. We have an environment inside us too.

5   There have been some recent attempts to correct fashionable excesses in psychology (one is here reminded of the differences between *haute couture*, and what it is reasonable to wear in public). In this vein, Steven Pinker (2004) has reminded us that however undemocratic-sounding the idea, biological and genetic interactions in particular have more influence on behaviour than we feel comfortable with – hence the discussion of familial patterns in this book. But I myself have no notion of genetic *determinants*, rather of genetic-environmental *interplay*.

6   We must not neglect the role of language (see Pinker 1999), which is the main tool of social cooperation – which, unthinking ants aside – *homo sapiens* excels at, and which has changed our fortunes remarkably in the evolutionary stakes. We also 'talk' to ourselves inside our heads (see Vygotsky 1962); we comment to ourselves about what potentially negative, or potentially pleasant and useful, stimulus clusters might *actually* mean, and these informal 'conversations', if we have a little time to spare before we *must* act, are an example of the phenomenon of consciousness. They turn calculations about rewarding and punishing experiences inwards. In other words, consciousness does not just scan the external environment; it monitors our position in it and reactions to it.

7   Regarding the role of emotion in human behaviour and cognition, two insightful treatises on the much neglected (by cognitive psychologists) theme of emotion and its influence on consciousness, Damassio's *Descartes' Error* (1994) and Le Doux's *The Emotional Brain* (2003), suggest that there is an internal positive and negative reinforcement and punishment system within ourselves, influencing memory but above all operating through conditioning. The rush of emotion felt by Marcel Proust in response to the madeleine cake (the famous example in *À la recherche du temps perdu*) was sudden and overwhelming. Actually thinking about what had triggered the powerful reaction took him a number of

hours. Here is an interesting experiment: Le Doux discusses a patient suffering from a form of dementia following a brain injury, who would greet the therapist pleasantly with a handshake, but had no recognition of him at the next meeting and no memory of what had passed between them at their previous meeting. He taped a tin tack to his hand and, pricking his hand, the patient recoiled; at the next meeting, there was still no memory of who the therapist was, or what he might want, but the patient refused to shake hands without knowing why (see Le Doux 2003: 180–181).

We can all have this experience after receiving an electro-static shock from our cars; no matter how much we think about the next encounter, how rare this is, how it depends upon dry weather, how harmless it is, etc., we approach next time with trepidation.

However arcanely solipsistic it may seem now, philosophers in the eighteenth century were very concerned with the question of whether the external world was real or a figment of our imagination – a question of logic. Dr Johnson sums up my views, i.e. (in paraphrase): if you meet a solipsist, punch him on the nose, and see if he remains one!

Remember that Descartes was a product of the 'Age of Reason', and that there might be such a thing as 'cultural conditioning'. Here is Descartes' justification of his *Philosophy* – of which he was very proud: 'A proposition so enduringly true that no amount of skepticism will shake it':

> From that I knew that I was a substance, the whole essence or nature of what it is to think, and that for its existence there is no need of any place, nor does it depend on any material things: so that this 'we', that is to say, the soul by which I am what I am, is entirely distinct from the body, and is even more easy to know than is the latter; and even if body were not, the soul would not cease to be what it is.
>
> (Descartes 1637)

Visit any funeral service or graveyard and you will see that this is our fondest hope. Talk to anyone untutored in psychology and you will soon find out that this view of a 'ghost within the machine' is still the predominant view of mind and its influences. However, as Damassio observes:

> This is Descartes' error: the abyssal separation between body and mind, between the sizeable, dimensioned, mechanically operated, infinitely divisible body stuff, on the one hand, and the unsizeably, undimensioned, un-pushpullable, nondivisible mind stuff; the suggestion that reasoning, and moral judgement, and the suffering that comes from physical pain or emotional upheaval might exist separately from the body. Specifically: the separation of the most refined operation of the mind from the structure and operation of a biological organism.
>
> (Damassio 1994: 249–250)

Conclusions

'We can never escape from philosophy', observed Dr Johnson. However unused we are to thinking in that way; however suspicious of airy-fairy theorising we *practical* men and women are, it will always come back to bite us. For our everyday 'practical' actions are suffused with assumptions about the nature of the human condition, and how those who share it with us and are in trouble, might best be helped.

The argument here, and throughout this book, is that we need to recognise the inter-relations of biology, cognition, emotion and behaviour, and the back catalogue of experiences which will probably be defining current problems and the acceptability of proposed solutions. All these elements, and a close understanding of them above the level of therapy training manuals, should be incorporated into our practice, since each offers a potential leverage point for useful change. Let us therefore, for both ethical and technical reasons, eschew affiliations to one or other parts of this matrix of influences, and in every case consider this as an *integrated* system a long time in the making.

Part Two

Psychological theory and research

4 Learning theory and research

As more and more of the behavior of the organism has come to be explained in terms of stimuli, the territory held by inner explanations has been reduced. The 'will' has retreated up the spinal cord, through the lower and then the higher parts of the brain, and finally, with the conditioned reflex, has escaped through the front of the head.

(Skinner 1953: 48–49)

This chapter will review the different theories and research studies on learning, from which the techniques known collectively as cognitive-behavioural therapy are derived. Such an account is necessary for two reasons. First, so that the person applying the approach will understand the reasons for what he or she is doing, rather than just dipping into a bag of therapeutic tricks and hoping to come up with the right one. Second, so that a proper assessment of the client's problems can be made. In this field, there are no general purpose procedures, and decisions about which approaches to use are based upon certain well-established findings as to how behaviour (including problematic behaviour) and its cognitive and affective accompaniments or even *causes*, come to have their influence in the first place.

Most of what makes us truly human, most of what makes us individuals rather than 'clones', most of what gives us a discernible personality – made up of semi-predictable patterns of behaviour, emotional reactions and thinking styles – is the product of learning. We get a little help or hindrance from genetic endowment, but are far from being *tabulae rasae* – blank slates (see Pinker 2004).

Natural selection has, to a unique degree, favoured *homo sapiens* with immense behavioural flexibility, with memory and with foresight. The advantages of these gifts for an otherwise physically unpromising primate are that we are less caught out by environmental change – either over time or through forced change of location – and that we can multiply our influence many times over through advanced forms of social cooperation. Archilocus observed in his parable of 650 BC that 'The fox knows many little things – the hedgehog one big one'. Fine for *Erinaceous Europeanus* over several millennia, until, in the late nineteenth century, Herr Benz decided to pursue the production of horseless carriages.

Thus there is an interplay of biological, developmental and environmental factors which influence what we learn and how easy or difficult it is. However, outside these predispositions, and our possession of a few 'hard-wired' drives towards what Dennett (1991) has called 'The four Fs' (flight, fight, food and procreation) our actions and their internal concomitants are largely the products of experience.

Here is a list of the basic research-derived assumptions:

☐   By far the greater portion of the behavioural repertoire with which individuals are equipped is the product of learning. This vast range of possible responses is acquired through lengthy interaction with, and adaptation to, an ambivalent physical and social environment. We alter the environment and in turn the environment alters us in endless, reciprocal fashion.

☐   Genetic and other physiological factors also influence behaviour in a more general sense, and there is an interaction between these and the environment through inborn influences on intelligence, temperament and personality, and through predispositions to mental disorder (see Eysenck 1965; Thomas *et al.* 1968; Caspi *et al.* 2003; Sheldon and Macdonald 2009: see ch. 13).

☐   Two broad processes of associative learning account for the acquisition and maintenance of motor, verbal, cognitive and emotional responses. These are: *classical or respondent* conditioning, based on the work of the great Russian physiologist I.P. Pavlov, and *operant or instrumental* conditioning, based on the work of the American psychologists E.L. Thorndike (1898), and B.F. Skinner (1953). To these influences must be added vicarious learning, or modelling, which process contains elements of both classical and operant associations (see Bandura 1969).

☐   Consciousness, and the ways in which we process information about past, present and predicted future environments – which bundles of stimuli, contingencies and imaginings include self-observation and appraisal of our own behaviour – are a deeply mysterious but not a mystical set of phenomena. Thinking too follows patterns and is rarely far removed from the effects of external influences. In other words, above the level of simple reflexes, we do not simply *respond* to stimuli, we *interpret* them first, but not haphazardly (see Bandura 1977; Dennett 1991): 'There is nothing good or bad but thinking makes it so' (*Hamlet*, Act 2, Scene ii). This is generally true, particularly in the social world, but I am not convinced that it covers a strong smell of aviation fuel in the cabin at 30,000 feet; my money is on Pavlov there.

☐   Behaviours that we judge to be 'maladaptive', 'abnormal' or 'self-defeating' are learned in exactly the same way as those that we are disposed to call 'adaptive' or 'normal'. Any apparent differences between the two are mainly a property of the attributive and evaluative judgements we make about behaviour, rather than of the properties of the behaviour itself or its origins.

☐   The behavioural and cognitive-behavioural therapies owe their existence to learning theory – a vast body of experimental evidence on how humans (and other animals) adapt themselves to their environments by a process akin to 'psychological natural selection' – by which strains of action, patterns of thoughts and feelings thrive, perish or lie dormant according to the *effects* that they have. Each dimension of learning has given rise to therapeutic approaches logically consistent with the basic research.

☐   Properly applied, these therapeutic derivatives have a direct and beneficial effect on a wide range of problems and are not threatened by a re-emergence of 'symptoms' in some different form.

The next concept of which the reader needs to be made aware is that there is not one master learning theory from which all these principles are derived, but different, overlapping theories, some of which have led to broad theoretical consensus, and others to continuing disputes. However, before we can proceed to examine these differences, we need a general definition of learning. There are many available but the common ground between them is that the concept of learning applies to the *associative processes* whereby new and relatively durable responses are added to the individual's repertoire. The following simple outline will meet our immediate requirements (those with an appetite for extended technical definitions should consult Hillner (1979) and/or Grey (1975)).

> Learning may be defined as a relatively permanent change in behaviour that occurs as the result of prior experience.
>
> (Hilgard *et al.* 1979: 18)

Three qualifications are immediately necessary to this short definition. First, and contrary to the everyday meaning of the term, there need be no intention on anyone's part to *impart* learning for it to take place. Nor need there be any *intention* on the part of the learner to acquire new information or behaviour. Second, we must exclude all effects due to fatigue, illness or the influence of drugs. Third, the effects of learning may not be immediately apparent. A newly acquired potential for behaviour can be stored in memory until circumstances are propitious for its performance.

The next question is: *How* do organisms learn? Five related influences are usually cited:

1   Classical conditioning: whereby the temporal-spatial association of one stimulus with another – already capable of producing a certain response – leads eventually to responding to either stimulus alone.
2   Operant conditioning: where the acquisition of new responses occurs as a result of our experience of the rewarding, punishing or relief-giving consequences of behaviour.
3   Vicarious learning: where new responses are acquired by observing the behaviour of others and the outcomes that their actions produce.
4   Cognitive influences governing the *interpretation* of stimuli.
5   Genetic–environmental interactions, whereby learning some things is easier or harder than others.

Let us now examine the implications of what has been proposed so far in more detail, beginning with factors rooted in our biology.

Genetic influences

Mention the possibility of innate influences on behaviour at some interdisciplinary conferences and you are likely to hear the background hissing once reserved for the characters with black hats and moustaches in the old western films. There are good Pavlovian reasons for such irrational reactions. (1) The mistaken identification of all genetics research with right-wing political ideology (eugenics), and the manipulations of Sir Cyril Burt in particular – he made up most of the data on which the 11+ selection exam was based (see Eysenck & Kamin (1981) I failed mine, largely because I couldn't readily work out what the shape on the left if rotated would most be like the one on the right. I didn't know and I still don't care, apart from the fact that I had to go to night school after work to gain university entrance qualifications. Am I bitter? Irritated, rather, that in all the debates over selection, so little emphasis is given to the validity and reliability of the means). (2) A perceived conflict with allegedly more 'democratic' notions of social engineering to secure the needs of individuals. (3) Unflattering professional implications for would-be helpers who, if such influences were overriding, would be condemned to struggle vainly against fixed human potentialities. These views are plain wrong. Modern genetics research stresses biological and environmental *interaction* (see Gottesman 1982, 1991; Berger 1985; Pinker 2004; McGuffin *et al.* 2005). However, if there *are* predispositions within us that make some things easier to learn and adjust to, and some things harder, then arguably we had better know about them – for ethical as well as technical reasons, as Case example 4.1 reveals.

CASE EXAMPLE 4.1

I once interviewed a single mother with an 11-year-old autistic son who (with limited professional assistance) had worked out a rough-and-ready behavioural management scheme for herself. It worked reasonably well when applied consistently, but left her feeling guilty. She felt guilty about 'regimentation', guilty about having occasionally to resort to medication and guilty that she and her ex-husband might have failed to cooperate fully with a recent course of psychoanalytically flavoured family therapy which they had found bizarre. Focusing on the irrationality of such feelings and their deleterious effects; congratulating her on her skills as an amateur behaviour therapist, and putting her in touch with a regional support group, produced considerable relief. There was little else apart from greater consistency that could have improved upon her existing approach, nothing to do except to reinforce it, and to try to remove from her any irrational feelings over the limits of her influence on a substantially biological, developmental condition: 'not your fault' was a key message.

A knowledge of genetic influences is important, therefore, in telling us what *not* to do, or to imply, through our professional behaviour, but to substitute *compensatory* learning-based approaches in the face of something we can do little about; the same is often true in cases of dementia.

Innate influences on childhood development

The word 'sterile' often appears before the phrase 'nature/nurture debate' in textbooks, indicating, to me at least, that the authors have given up on one of the most important topics in psychology. Understandable but regrettable, and largely due to the immense methodological problems involved in unravelling the cable-knitted strands of these influences. Yet significant work has been done that avoids the simplistic approaches of early research, and the balance of probability has steadily shifted away both from the sporting environmentalism of the 1960s and 1970s and the a priori genetic explanations of an earlier era, towards the centre, the point at which two strong sets of influences interact to produce typicalities in behaviour, cognitive styles and emotions. The careful and persistent longitudinal work of Thomas and colleagues which began in 1968 represents this shift rather well.

Here is the issue – a brave one to take up at the time:

> As physicians we began many years ago to encounter reasons to question the prevailing one-sided emphasis on environment. We found that some children with severe psychological problems had a family upbringing which did not differ essentially from the

environment of other children who developed no severe problems. On the other hand, some children were found to be free of personality disturbances although they had experienced severe family disorganisation from parental care.

(Thomas et al. 1968: 2)

Thomas *et al.* observed (with acceptable levels of reliability) substantial qualitative and quantitative differences in the behaviour of a sample of young babies (n = 181) and blind-rated them along the following dimensions:

- [ ] The level and extent of motor activity.
- [ ] The 'rhythmicity', or degree of regularity of functions such as eating, elimination and the cycle of sleeping and wakefulness.
- [ ] The response to a new object or person, in terms of whether the child accepts the new experience or withdraws from it.
- [ ] The adaptability of behaviour to changes in the environment.
- [ ] The threshold of sensitivity to stimuli (a major theme in Soviet psychology at the time).
- [ ] The intensity, or energy level of responses.
- [ ] The child's general mood or 'disposition', whether cheerful or given to crying, pleasant or 'cranky', sociable or otherwise.
- [ ] The degree of the child's distractibility from what he or she is doing.
- [ ] The child's attention span and degree of persistence in a given activity.

They then classified the children (according to the profile created by their positions on these continua) as 'easy', 'slow-to-warm-up' and 'difficult', and followed them up over the next twenty-one years. They were concerned to see whether children who exhibited, for example, low levels of conditionability and high levels of fractiousness early in childhood posed greater problems for parents as they grew up, and whether patterns of over-representation in referral for psychological help would emerge. Here is a summary of their findings now augmented by later research:

- [ ] Temperamental characteristics tended to remain stable over the years, 'slow-to-warm-up' babies growing into quiet schoolchildren, active, outgoing babies into active, outgoing teenagers. We now have further research on this hypothesis (see Caspi *et al.* 2003) wherein 10,037 children pre-assessed on temperament classifications such as undercontrolled, inhibited, confident, reserved, and well-adjusted, were assessed twenty-three years later. This highly quantitative comparison research depends of course on the validity and reliability scores at T1, T2 attrition rates (but the authors retained 96 per cent of their original sample), and reliability checks on the largely qualitative/observational judgements originally made. These show high concordance accuracy regarding subsequent correlations. Here is a summary of the authors' conclusions:

> When observed at age 3, some children were classified as undercontrolled (10%) were rated as irritable, impulsive, emotionally labile and impersistent in tasks. At age 26 they were intolerant and scored high on traits indexing negative emotionality: they were easily upset, likely to overreact to minor events, and reported feeling mistreated, deceived and betrayed by others . . . When observed at age 3, children classified as inhibited (8%) more shy, fearful, and socially ill at ease. At age 26, they were characterized by an overcontrolled and non-assertive personality style, they

expressed little desire to exert influence over others and reported taking little pleasure in life.

(Caspi et al. 2003: 510)

- ☐ The categories employed by Thomas *et al.* had considerable predictive value. For example, 70 per cent of the children from the 'difficult' group (parents did not know of this classification) developed behavioural/emotional problems requiring professional intervention, whereas only 18 per cent of the 'easy' children did.
- ☐ Temperamental–environmental clashes were readily understandable in terms of the child's early behavioural profile and were often tractible once a consistent, 'with the grain' environment or set of contingencies was engineered. For example, active, outgoing, hard-to-condition babies, who moved on to controlled classroom conditions, tended to kick over the traces. Children from the 'difficult' group generally exhibited many problems of frustration control and needed extra help to acquire a tolerable measure of this.
- ☐ Attempts by parents to counter adverse temperamental tendencies were often effective. However, the further down the shoulders of the distribution curve the child was in early life, the greater the effort and persistence required to modify this as the children grew up.

This important research, part of a series, with findings well-replicated elsewhere (see Hetherington & Parke 1986; McCrae *et al.* 1997), does not carry the authority of a separated twin study. It does not, for example, control for experiences in the womb (where foetal exposure to drugs and alcohol can have severe consequences in later life – as shown in studies of adoption outcomes (Sheldon & Macdonald 2009: 240–246)). What it does is reinforce something that parents have been saying for years, namely that children are *different* right from the start, that they are not just pieces of organic blotting paper, soaking up environmental influences; rather they are active contributors to the process of interaction with their parents. A growing body of evidence counsels us to take more seriously the child's individual contribution to the learning equation:

> At a very early age, human babies show signs of a strong urge to master the environment. They are limited in what they can do by the slow development of their skill in controlling their own movements. Thus it is fair to call them 'helpless' in the sense that they cannot manage the environment well enough to survive unaided. This makes it all the more interesting to discover that the urge to manage the environment is already there at the time of this helplessness and that it does not appear to derive from anything else or to depend on any reward apart from the achieving of competence and control.
>
> (Donaldson 1978: 110)

The upshot of all this is that we must realise that some expectations and some plans will be easier for some children to go along with than others. Here is what most parents think they are going to get when they have a baby:

> John was my touchy feely baby. From the first day in the hospital he cuddled and seemed so contented to be held that I could hardly bear to put him down . . . We took him everywhere because he seemed to enjoy new things. You could always sit him in a corner and he'd entertain himself. Sometimes I'd forget he was there until he'd start laughing or prattling.
>
> (Hetherington & Parke 1986: 85)

And here is the kind of testimony about the realities of child-rearing that we should perhaps be listening to more open-mindedly; let us call this child Damien:

> Nothing was easy with him. Mealtimes, bedtimes, toilet training were all hell. It would take me an hour and a half to get part of a bottle into him and he'd be hungry two hours later. I can't remember once in the first two years when he didn't go to bed crying. I'd try to rock him to sleep but as soon as I'd tiptoe over to put him in his crib his head would lurch up and he'd start bellowing again. He didn't like any kind of changes in his routine. New people and new places upset him so it was hard to take him anywhere.
>
> (Hetherington & Parke 1986: 85)

The disappointment and guilt created by such experiences can lead to the pathologisation of temperamental differences, the blaming of the victims, and to a vicious circle creating or adding to a risk of maltreatment – as Case example 4.2 shows.

CASE EXAMPLE 4.2

A breathless member of the public telephoned Social Services to say that her neighbour, a young woman, was pacing the garden in the rain rocking her baby with exaggerated movements and yelling at it to be quiet, and that she feared for its safety. The subsequent interview revealed the following:

☐ Since bringing the baby home three months ago he had slept irregularly and unpredictably, crying most nights and throughout the day.

☐ The parents had tried both attempting to regulate feeding by 'demand' approaches, and ignoring fractiousness – but were always defeated by the child's persistence.

☐ The child had been examined by a paediatrician, and the Health Visitor had called regularly to advise on the removal of obvious provocations for the behaviour.

☐ The parents were tired, angry, disappointed and beginning to row. The mother especially felt that the problem was due to some failure of hers. Medical staff unwittingly reinforced this view by telling her the obvious – none of which advice worked.

☐ More worryingly, the mother admitted to growing hostility towards the child and to a difficult-to-dispel feeling that he was crying on purpose and choosing his moments for maximum disruptive effect. She confessed to shaking the child and coming close to hitting him.

The main point of intervention in this case was the vicious circle that had been set up by the child's behaviour, producing anxiety, guilt and strife between the parents, making them in turn less reliable and consistent. A joint approach was organised involving the paediatrician, health visitor, GP and social worker, and formal records began to be kept – which identified (1) a very challenging level of fractiousness, but (2) that the mere keeping of records reduced these problems a little and made the parents feel more able to cope. Probably the most telling impact came from the paediatrician who again examined the child, found nothing medically wrong and voiced the opinion

---

that the problem was 'constitutional' and had little to do with the standard of care available. This authoritative 'reframing' of the problem greatly increased the willingness of the mother to help draw up and stick to a hyper-reliable set of routines rather than casting around for different solutions. She also felt able to ask her mother for help, which previously she had been too ashamed to do. The baby continued to be difficult to pacify, but the parents coped with increasing confidence, sharing the care more equitably within a preplanned framework. Most importantly, they had the knowledge that some babies are just like this, a challenge that has to be survived.

Biological influences on personality

The most powerful influences affecting the kind of people we become are experiential. Yet, in a strange way we each become more or less than the main drift of our experience would predict. We develop a discernible 'personality' quite early on in childhood. Although we speak (often in a circular way) of someone's personality as if it were another kind of organ inside them – 'David's gregarious behaviour is a product of his outgoing personality' (which we know is the case because of his outgoing behaviour) – all that can be said for the term is that there *do* appear to be roughly reliable, seemingly unique patterns and consistencies to our behaviour which are somewhat independent of local environments (contingencies) which others use as a basis for attributions and predictions about how we might behave in particular circumstances and what we are likely to do next. We also make concordant judgements about the thinking patterns and emotions of others which we infer from their behaviour – sometimes accurately, sometimes not.

The main clue to personality factors at work – whether predominantly due to biological difference, a particular pattern of learning, or both, is when behaviour and emotional expression appear to *transcend* contingencies – the pressures and temptations of the here and now. This in turn depends upon the strength of these contingencies (see Plomin *et al.* 1977, 1999). Thus, although *extroverts* ('stimulus-hungry' individuals) may be less noticeable than usual in the examination hall, they will probably suck in louder breaths, ask for more windows to be opened/closed than others. Similarly, although *introverts* ('stimulus-shy' individuals) are usually less visible all round, the right combination of deinhibiting social conditions (alcohol, music) can produce untypically outgoing behaviour. (I once had a favourite picture of my normally quiet co-author Professor Geraldine Macdonald dancing a Highland reel over crossed salad servers while under such influences, but, mysteriously it has gone missing.)

This concept of extroversion–introversion (Eysenck 1965; Gray 1975) has proved remarkably robust in experimental tests. Its mixed reputation is based upon a misunderstanding that it is a theory of *types*; that is, that the human race contains two different kinds of people, the inward-looking and the outward-going. Rather, we should think of a bell-shaped distribution of traits, with most of us in the middle demonstrating a well-adapted and flexible mixture of behaviour, and smaller and smaller numbers on the steepening shoulders of the curves showing less and less current-contingency-inspired flexibility in our actions.

On the one side of the curve we have what might be thought of as 'stimulus-hungry' individuals, prone to sensation-seeking behaviour on the basis of nervous system differences which automatically reduce external stimulation. The signals from the environment are 'filtered' and therefore they seek to pre-amplify them by outgoing behaviour. On the other hand, some people are 'stimulus amplifiers'; that is, prone to sensation shyness given the prospect of 'overload'.

An analogy might help here: some people appear (as it were) to possess 'Ferrari nervous systems', wherein a little right-hand pedal stimulation threatens to drive up arousal to uncontrollable levels. Some of us, on the other shoulder of the curve, appear to possess 'Citroen 2CV nervous systems', where considerable stimulus input is required to produce slow acceleration and buildup with a limited top-end range. Counter-intuitively, the Ferrari NS model applies to the *introverts* who are stimulus-response reducers so as to prevent themselves from firing up to uncomfortable emotional levels. The Citroen 2CV NS reaction belongs to the *extroverts*, who in order to obtain enough stimulation have to stamp on the environmental gas pedal and seek to pre-amplify stimulus inputs. Most of us, in the middle of the curve are Ford Foci, capable of occasional bursts of speed when the conditions are right, and tootling along when not. Galvanic skin response (GSR) measures in extroverts (as assessed on the Eysenck Personality Scale) show that there is a distribution of hard-to-achieve condition-ability to stimuli, and on the introversion side, to punishment-sensitive reactions. All the rest depends on interaction with the environment and how we typically approach it. (Eagerly? Trepidatiously? There are, in old Hollywood terms, some people who tend to ask *'Why don't we put the show on right here in the barn?'* And others who want to check the fire insurance policy.)

We thus appear to inherit and, through experience, develop these optimal arousal ranges (see Scarr and McCartney 1983) and much of our behaviour and our planning is dedicated to keeping ourselves comfortably within them. Therefore some learning tasks are more difficult for some people to address – anything requiring persistent self-control and delayed gratification on the extroversion dimension; anything requiring overcoming inhibitions and acting on first impulse on the introversion dimension. There are, therefore, *gradients* of learning for all of us. Sometimes acquiring new behaviour is a downhill 'feet off the pedals' affair, sometimes a long, hard climb.

Note that no particular combination of personality and environmental configurations is more favourable. Introverts find reflection, planning and considered action easier, and the demands of sociability harder. Extroverts find impulse control more difficult but spontaneity easier. Either predisposition can get one into trouble or frustrate the process of getting out of it. Both wings of the continuum require that we adjust the demands of our therapeutic programmes, consider the difference of approach required for the impulsive, somewhat paranoid young man described on p. 174 and the shy, almost phobic young woman whose case is outlined on p. 220 and the point should be clear.

Condensing the essential ingredients of personality has been methodologically challenging. Allport (1937) started with dictionary definitions of common trait descriptors; Cattell and Eysenck condensed the brew further over the next few decades. The consensus that we have arrived at today is that there are five sets of factors ('The big five') that repeatedly turn up in empirical measurements of cross-situational tendencies to think feel and act in patterned, semi-independent ways:

1   *Extroversion*: Talkative, energetic and assertive, versus quiet reserved and shy. Yes, I know that you flit between these options according to free-spirit choices, and you may even be in the majority, but there are still daily environment-transcending *likelihoods*. Thus the phrase 'I met Jeremy Clarkson for the first time the other day, we had a quiet chat about environmental issues, and he served up the most wonderful Tofu salad for lunch'; or 'I remember well when we, just a group of Eng. Lit. students, turned up unannounced at J.D. Salinger's house in New Hampshire. He invited us all in and we partied and talked

about his new work into the early hours. Then he insisted on a group photograph', now you know immediately that this is all made-up. But why do you (since neither you nor I have ever met these people)? Cognitive, behavioural, emotional consistency is the long-known answer. Be aware of it in your work is my not-so-simple advice.

2   *Agreeableness*: Sympathetic, kind and affectionate versus cold, quarrelsome and vindictive. We all know people whose first impulse is to say 'Yes, anything I can do, just name it' and others who want to know the full details of your predicament before giving highly qualified offers subject to 'terms and conditions'. (If you've never met the latter, then I suggest you stay working where you are.)

3   *Conscientiousness*: Organised, responsible and cautious versus careless, frivolous and irresponsible. There are some people who, statistically speaking, will always pre-plan against a task they see as demanding, and others who will 'just go for it'. I confess that I bend towards the 'Let's just head north then ask the way' group, rather than the 'AA printout plus Sat Nav group', but make no claim to superior efficiency. The problem with conscientiousness is that it can easily overspill into procrastination. To repeat the point, either tendency can be self-defeating, depending on the circumstances.

4   *Emotional stability*: Stable, calm and contented versus anxious, unstable and temperamental. The word 'temperamental' here means that such a person is more likely to be driven by emotional arousal than by a rational appraisal of circumstances. I would say that this untoward tendency accounts for about 50 per cent of all the clinical work of cognitive-behavioural therapists. The point on a continuum of observed threat seems to vary consistently from cognitive appraisal and planning in the ascendancy, to 'flight/fight' emotional reactions being semi-automatically in the ascendancy. I have treated clients whose emotionally driven reactions are just about plausible in conditioning terms (e.g. after a car crash or being trapped in a lift for twenty minutes) and others who have endured far worse experiences (e.g. in combat situations), and who, though traumatised, somehow know that they will recover their equilibrium with a little support: different self-concepts.

5   *Openness to experience*: Creative, intellectual and open-minded versus simple, shallow and unintelligent. Many cases come our way where the main focus of help is to encourage clients to see their difficulties from a different angle or as interactive, not mono-causal; to experiment with new experiences, etc. Without doubt, some people find this easier or harder than others, but we tend to see those in the latter category: 'If you always do what you've always done then you may well get what you always got' is a good starting point for such discussions.

The high probability that there are innate factors at work in influencing the dimensions of personality is shown in Figure 4.1.

We are in an awkward position with such data however, since trait expressions are strongly influenced by environmental contingencies. As with all predispositional/environmental interaction, the interplay is often complex and it is hard to disinter the elements and proportions in research statistics. One thing is certain: we humans have a strong tendency to underestimate the behaviour and even the thought-shaping power of the environment and its reinforcement contingencies – remember the vows of continued contact at 'leaving dos' which aren't quite realised in the face of other preoccupying factors, or the railway timetable. As therapists, therefore, we should never underestimate the power of contingencies and the possibilities for modifying these.

Next, in line with the list on p. 90, we turn to the processes by which, against this biological backdrop, learning occurs.

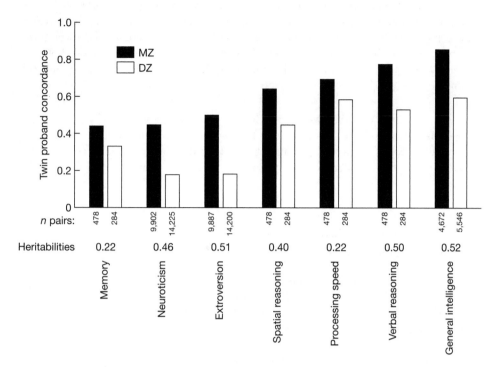

Figure 4.1 Twin concordance rates for common attributes

Note
Identical (MZ) and fraternal (DZ) twin intra class correlations for personality neuroticism, extroversion, visual reasoning, processing speed, IQ, etc.

Source: Adapted from the work of Plomin *et al.* (1999: 83).

Classical conditioning

Classical conditioning is a term first applied to the work of Pavlov by Hilgard (1948) to distinguish his principles from those of the developing *operant* model. An alternative term for this process of stimulus association is *respondent conditioning*. Few readers on encountering the name 'Pavlov' will not have conjured up an image of a bearded man in a lab coat accompanied by a bored-looking dog – which is quite a good example of classical conditioning and might, as we can now say, 'ring a bell'. Pavlov's work dates from the turn of the nineteenth and twentieth centuries, and his real achievement stems from his painstaking methodology and his careful analysis of results; from the detail and the accuracy of his findings rather than from their novelty. People throughout history have felt their mouths water at the thought of food, though none is present. Animal owners throughout the centuries have banged food pails and watched their animals come running. But then, apples fell from trees for thousands of years before Newton.

This chapter will review the results of a series of seminal animal experiments. This is necessary to get the 'psychological grammar' of conditioning theories right before we move on to the much more complex interactions that human beings have with their environments. Everything discussed in this chapter has been repeated in analogue form with humans, with the same results.

Pavlov's experiments were designed to settle an argument over the nature of certain 'psychical' secretions from the salivary glands of animals. 'Psychical' here refers to secretions of saliva present *before* the presentation of any food – a reaction presumed to originate spontaneously from the mind of the animal (Pavlov 1897). Crossing into the psychological domain, Pavlov soon found himself lacking a satisfactory means of investigating this phenomenon:

> In our 'psychical' experiments on the salivary glands, at first we honestly endeavoured to explain our results by fancying the subjective condition of the animal. But nothing came of it except unsuccessful controversies and individual, personal, uncoordinated opinion. We had no alternative but to place the investigation on a purely objective basis.
>
> (Pavlov 1897: 183)

Pavlov's procedure was as follows. A dog underwent a small procedure to facilitate the collection of saliva directly from the cheek gland. The dog was then trained to stand quietly in a harness. The laboratory was soundproofed and the experimenters observed the proceedings through a one-way screen. Thus there was no possibility of extraneous sounds or movements distracting the animal. The sequence of the experiment was: a bell is rung – the animal reacts only slightly to the new noise. No salivary flow is recorded. Next, a quantity of meat powder is delivered to a food tray in front of the dog. He salivates and eats it. After a few pairings of the bell (or light, or range of other originally neutral stimuli) with the food, the dog begins to salivate to the sound of the bell alone. He continues to do this over many trials, even though no food is guaranteed. The dog has learned a new response. My dog listens intently for *The Archers* on the radio. When the playout music is heard, he sits in front of me, salivating: 2:15 p.m. is when he is fed. The Sunday morning Omnibus edition causes problems.

Let us look at this process of associative learning schematically, to see what is involved (Figure 4.2). The association between the unconditional stimulus and the unconditional response exists at the start of the Pavlov experiment and does not have to be learned. The association between the conditioned stimulus and the conditioned response is a learned one. It arises through the pairing of the conditioned and unconditioned stimuli followed by an unconditional response (salivation to the proximity of food). The conditioned

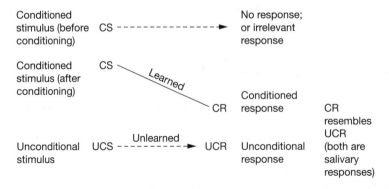

Figure 4.2 A diagram of classical conditioning

response (salivation to the bell) resembles the unconditional response (though they need not be identical).

An example of the progression from animal to human experiments is to be found in the celebrated study of fear acquisition through classical conditioning, carried out by Watson and Raynor (1920). The subject of this study was a toddler known to history as 'Little Albert' (in parody of Freud's celebrated analysis – via his father and by post! – of a boy with a phobia of horses, called 'little Hans'). Freud's theories of phobia acquisition held sway at the time. These identified repressed castration anxieties as the likely cause, the horse acting as a symbol of powerful masculinity. A less florid explanation emerges from the fact that Little Hans had once stood next to a dray horse which had dramatically collapsed and died in its shafts. Watson and Raynor wished to challenge the received 'wisdom' by seeing whether a phobia could be created in the laboratory. The procedure was as follows. A tame white rat (CS) was introduced into a playpen containing little Albert, and the latter began to play with it without apparent fear. (Fear of small animals is not innate in man, though see (1) below.) However, during subsequent trials, whenever the rat was introduced, a fire gong suspended over the pen was struck vigorously to produce a loud noise (UCS). A fear reaction to sudden loud noises *is* innate in humans, and so this produced an unconditional fear response (UCR). Soon little Albert became distressed just at the sight of the small animal, even when its presentation was not accompanied by a loud noise (CR). A new, conditioned response (fear and avoidance of small furry animals) had been acquired. Classical conditioning is particularly important in the acquisition of new emotional responses.

While in the field of conditioning there is plenty of evidence that new fear responses can be generated by simple contiguous association, it is erroneous to assume that all fearful responses develop in this way. Later work (see Seligman 1975; Bandura 1977) suggests that conditioning is a less 'mechanical' phenomenon than envisaged by Pavlov. In this research there are three important trends to note:

1   If Pavlovian concepts were universally applicable, it should be possible to condition a fear reaction to anything. The fact that certain kinds of objects (CSs) can set up conditioned reactions much more easily than others, and that some pose formidable difficulties, raises questions about the simple paired-association model. It appears that perhaps, as a result of natural selection, there are certain stimuli (e.g. heights, enclosed spaces, animals and insects or other mobile, intelligent, scurrying organisms with an adaptive, potentially-predatory capacity) of which we are especially prone to learn to be afraid. Further, that there are other objects and events where associations will not easily stick. The idea of a continuum of 'preparedness' and counter-preparedness is increasingly important in research on this topic.

2   Some investigators have raised doubts as to the distinctness of classical learning procedures and have put forward single process theories (favouring an exclusively operant analysis of learning). Later in this chapter the reader will see that the two models do overlap at certain points (see p. 111). In this book the view that there are two overlapping but still fairly distinct learning processes is retained, because, as yet, the research that once threatened this position has been insufficiently replicated to justify a radical reappraisal.

3   Since it is possible for human subjects to have powerful fears of circumstances and animals which they have never encountered and are unlikely to come across (e.g., snakes in Britain), it is clear that cognitive variables are involved in fear conditioning. Thus, in the absence of any real snakes (they kill more people than any other kind of animal abroad, but are scarce

in the UK, though there are plenty of reptile phobics), we acquire a fear of an *image*, presented to the accompaniment of distaste or anxiety. Here perceived parental distress or distaste may be the original UCS: the child's anxiety in the face of this the UCR, the snake image, the CS, and the eventual fear reaction to the *idea of* snakes, the CR.

The strangest phobic reactions I have ever encountered were a pair of identical twin students both with a fear of (wait for it) buttons, and a curiosity about the fact. Both were revolted by the idea of wearing any garment with buttons on it. Both wore only clothes with zips or velcro. The GSR ratios of both went through the roof when asked to touch a button. Neither had any idea where this phobic reaction came from but said it had started in early childhood. You won't see many of these clients in your clinics or departments; the remit here is that they are technically interesting. One could advance a theory that buttons act as CSs, for being dressed when one doesn't want to be in early childhood, of being, as it were, 'swaddled' through the agency of buttons (but then the Hopi Indians in anthropological studies were thus confined until they were six months old, and quickly regained any developmental losses). The problem cannot simply be a genetic/evolutionary one because buttons haven't been around for long enough. A puzzle: a simple attention-seeking device against getting dressed, which means abandoning close contact and suckling, a conditioned negative reinforcer (see below). Leaving the centre of your universe as a small child (mother) and going somewhere else where slightly frightening things can happen begins with being buttoned into your outdoor uniform. I can just about entertain this. However, at least the treatment (controlled exposure) was easier than the explanation. Case example 4.3 describes something more usual.

CASE EXAMPLE 4.3

I had little fear of thunder and lightning as a child until I went to stay with my grandmother and observed her storm preparations. At the first sniff of ozone (S^d – discriminative stimulus) she would open the front and back doors to facilitate the easy entry and exit of thunderbolts; turn off the electricity ('because it attracts lightning'), turn all the mirrors to the wall for similar reasons, and retire to a cubby hole under the stairs, just as she had done during air raids in the Second World War. My thoughts were: if this strong, competent, seventeen-stone lady on whom my well-being usually depends is running for cover, then I had better join her fast. Diagrams in the *Boys Book of Science* and a little natural exposure put paid to this nonsense later.

Stimulus generalisation

Let us return to Watson and Raynor's work since the next stage in the experiment illustrates a clinically important phenomenon called *stimulus generalisation*. Once the conditioned response was established, similar responses could be obtained to a variety of like stimuli; for example, other small animals, parcels of furry material, or allegedly (though this is disputed) Raynor's fur coat. This effect was noted also by Pavlov who found that having conditioned dogs to salivate to the sound of a bell, the same kind of response could then be induced by other signals.

This phenomenon of generalisation gives us a clue to the biological purpose of stimulus association. It has great survival value for the organism, and anything that confers a biological advantage is likely to have been selected in the evolutionary process. Clearly, the conditioned reflex is a winner in this respect, since nature cannot 'foresee' all eventualities and therefore it can work only to a limited extent through specific genetic endowment. Faced with the problem of changing, highly variable, danger- and satisfaction-infused environments, nature instead conferred *conditionability*, or, if you like, *programmability* – the ability to learn about the functional relations between objects and events. Thus, well before the food enters the dog's mouth, its upper digestive tract is prepared for it and is ready to break down large glucose molecules via the enzyme Ptyalin for their energy value. The earlier this process begins, the shorter what would once have been a highly vulnerable feeding episode (the best time to invade Britain is still 1.30 p.m. on a Sunday), and so the better from the point of view of survival. If an animal can learn to respond to stimuli which reliably precede the opportunity to feed and have the digestive process underway, so much the better. Try it yourself:

> It is a crisp autumn morning, and standing in the garden, you smell Sunday lunch cooking – roast lamb and mint sauce (vegetarians can substitute mushroom flan, or, if all else fails you can imagine licking half a lemon).

If the conditions are right, the response that will have taken place (saliva filling the mouth) is another example of classical conditioning. This particular response is established through the past pairing of actual food with images of food, and words that eventually come to represent and signal the likely presence of food or the need to find some.

Because stimuli naturally impinge in groups, it is biologically advantageous for those reliably associated with each other to have the same general effect. Imagine a member of a primitive species of *homo erectus* not endowed with this facility thinking to him or herself: *'Now I've seen those large stripy beasts before and I know they can be quite nasty, but I wonder what the smaller spotted ones do?'* and the long-term value of stimulus generalisation should become clear. Once an association has been formed, it can itself form the basis of new learning. Thus the process of classical conditioning 'strings together' stimulus connections, and an absence of birdsong in a clump of trees can eventually come to evoke a fear reaction consistent with the above example. If all this seems arcane in terms of today's sophisticated living conditions, imagine this:

> You come back from holiday and encounter a near-silent room – full of previously sociable colleagues all avoiding eye contact – 'too damned quiet' still applies. You move to your desk, which is cleared, but there is an envelope on it marked 'Personal and confidential'. What is your heart rate? How much hyper-vigilance, how much clamminess, is present?

We have seen that conditioned reflexes provide different forms of reliable early warning for the organism. They allow the body to gear itself up to cope with potentially advantageous or potentially threatening situations. Our state of constant readiness in this respect is governed by the autonomic nervous system, which acts through the glands and the smooth muscles, to help us gain an *edge* over our potentially hostile environment. Thus we do not have to wait until the burglar whom we suspect we have heard downstairs actually hits us over the head before we begin to react to the out-of-normal-context sounds downstairs. Our pulses are set racing, our muscles will stiffen ready for action, our pores will open, sweating will begin so that we can cool our body efficiently if strenuous activity follows, our pupils will dilate so that we can make best use of what light there is, the blood-clotting mechanism goes to def. con. II in case we are injured, and so forth. Similarly, we do not have to wait to be told that because we have failed adequately to prepare for an unexpectedly important meeting, we have entered a sequence of events where we stand at risk of losing the esteem of our colleagues and our employers, possibly of losing our livelihood, of being discredited socially, and so on. As far as our bodies are concerned, we might be getting ready to take on a medium-sized bear. The fact that under modern social conditions, to run away from a threat, or to punch it in the eye, is seldom an adaptive response (though some meetings do give rise to satisfying thoughts in this direction) is neither here nor there. Evolution has not yet caught up with this fact, and so conditionability has its side-effects. Case example 4.4 demonstrates this point.

CASE EXAMPLE 4.4

Mrs Wood, aged 40, was referred to the Social Services Department for 'support' by her somewhat exasperated family doctor. In his view Mrs Wood suffered from agoraphobia (fear of going out of doors), a 'dependent personality' and a number of (unspecified) 'psychiatric difficulties'. Knowing how to motivate social workers, the doctor also said that he had some worries about Mrs Wood's young son, because not only had Mrs Wood not left the house in the previous three years, very little had been seen of the child – a stimulus which is reliably associated with being grilled before a child abuse enquiry and having your photo on the front of the *Daily Mail* (*close* to a UCS).

Background

During the first interview Mrs Wood was wary of discussing her problems, and was still reacting to her doctor 'washing his hands' – an interesting phrase, because she did lots of that too – of her case and passing her on to Social Services and the outpatient department of the local hospital – which, of course, she could not possibly reach. During the second home visit Mrs Wood was more forthcoming, and the following patterns in her problems emerged:

- ☐ She described herself as 'always having been a nervous person'. She recounted stories about dismounting from her bicycle as a child whenever a car came up behind her; going some distance out of her way to avoid a barking dog in a garden near her home, feeling *very* shy and conspicuous as a teenager and so forth – a range of normal-enough fears, but noteworthy in their combination and extent.
- ☐ She reported a strong and persistent fear of hospitals and of all medical encounters, stemming from her mother's blood-curdling account of the birth of her younger sister. Her mother had apparently nearly died in childbirth, and had filled the early years of her children's lives with graphic stories of medical mismanagement.
- ☐ Mrs Wood became pregnant 'by accident' comparatively late in life. In order to persuade her to have the baby in hospital, the doctor had played up the dangers of a home confinement, raising her already high level of anxiety.

☐ One hot summer's day when she was seven months' pregnant, Mrs Wood had fainted while crossing a footbridge spanning a small river near her home. 'I was sure I was going to fall in, and when I came round, people said an ambulance was on the way and I panicked. People were trying to hold me down, covering me with clothing.' She fought to get free: 'I knew I had to get away, I got very upset, and eventually I persuaded someone to take me home. When I got in I was shaking all over. I shut and bolted the doors, back and front. . . . I was sure that the ambulance was going to call at the house. . . . I hid out of sight of the windows . . . and eventually (it took about an hour) I calmed down, and sat waiting for my husband to come home from work.' 'Catastrophic' or even 'paranoid' thoughts of this type are an important feature of panic reactions. Mrs Wood knew that there was a compulsory dimension to the psychiatric help she had been advised to seek.

☐ Mrs Wood had her baby at home against medical advice, painfully, but without major complications. She tried to go out several times after that but never got further than the front garden, or, if at night, as far as the back gate.

She reported the following feelings at each attempt: 'Shivering; awful feelings in the pit of my stomach; pounding heart; light-headedness.' In the daytime everywhere seemed 'very bright'. She felt conspicuous out in the open, 'almost as if I might be struck down'. Her breathing felt loud in her ears and her biggest fear was that she would collapse again or 'go mad'.

☐ Mrs Wood eventually gave up these attempts and remained indoors for the next four years. For the first two years she reported that she didn't really miss going out: 'The family and the next door neighbour were very good, they take the baby out; get the shopping, they are marvellous.' Later, however, Mrs Wood began to experience feelings of frustration with her confined existence and was ashamed when she felt unable to attend her mother's funeral.

☐ When Mrs Wood felt she *had* to go out, for example, to peg out washing, she reported making a quick dash, hoping no one would see her or try to talk to her, and 'great relief' when she got back inside. 'I think there must be something seriously wrong with me . . . in my mind' was initially her best idea as to the causes of all this.

If we examine this case in the light of classical conditioning theory, the following pattern is evident:

1 Mrs Wood may have possessed a predisposing personality for strong fear-reactions (see Claridge 1985; McGuffin *et al.* 2005). Certainly her accounts of her previous life showed her to be eminently conditionable to a range of not objectively threatening circumstances.

2 Against a background of heightened anxiety about pregnancy, dreading the thought of the possibility of having to go into hospital, Mrs Wood experiences a traumatic incident (UCS) which arouses in her a powerful fear reaction or panic attack (UCR).

3 This incident, when paired with the previously neutral stimulus of the footbridge and other stimuli associated with being out of doors (CSs), produced a conditioned

response to these stimuli. Even after the incident itself had passed, the pregnancy was over, she was perfectly well, and the crowd was no longer in sight, she still experienced fears associated with this context.

4   Mrs Wood reported that her emotional state was made worse by the attempts of would-be helpers to restrain her until the ambulance came. Natural escape behaviour was prevented, thus intensifying her fear, as it always does.

5   This conditioned fear response quickly generalised to virtually all outdoor circumstances, even though objectively they barely resembled the circumstances of her collapse. Furthermore, every time Mrs Wood tried to go out of doors she was punished for the attempt by her powerful emotions (setting up a 'fear of fear' reaction) – even though, on reflection, she saw such feelings as irrational.

6   Every time Mrs Wood managed to escape from the outdoor circumstances that elicited the conditioned fear response, her strongly aversive feelings were reduced via negative reinforcement. This strengthened avoidance behaviour and made future experiments less likely.

7   Mrs Wood's sister and friends unwittingly reinforced her long-term maladaption to her phobia by relieving her of many of her responsibilities regarding her child, and by reassuring her that they did not mind her staying behind. The impression grew, strengthened by early non-cooperation with the treatment scheme (see p. 246), that Mr Wood rather liked having his wife at home and dependent upon him.

It will not have escaped the reader's attention that as we move from the laboratory to examples of conditioning in the natural environment, it has become more difficult to specify the key stimuli combinations with the same precision. Was it the already-learned fear of hospitals which became connected with particular outdoor circumstances? Or was it, perhaps, loss of consciousness, embarrassment at this, or fear of loss of control? Or was it, perhaps, a fear of falling helplessly into the water? All of these fears were mentioned during interviews. To what extent did fears for the unborn baby play a part? To what extent did the unsympathetic words of the family doctor and the daft hospital referral predispose Mrs Wood to what happened? It is likely that all these factors were influential in triggering the panic response.

In the natural environment, stimuli tend to come in untidy bundles, as do responses, and it is often difficult to tease out their different origins and effects. Mrs Wood remembers particularly the idea of being 'a prisoner of the crowd'; the fear of hospitals, and the narrowness of the footbridge (though it was made of iron, and quite sound). She also had a vivid recollection of the brightness of the day (pupil dilation effect?), of being helpless out in the open, of wearing an overcoat on a hot day because she didn't like the idea that passers-by could see she was pregnant. *Therapist*: 'What was wrong about signs of pregnancy – which is where we all come from?' *Client*: 'I hated the idea of people being able to see [laughter] what I'd been up to.' Mrs Wood had strong associations between sin and sex put into her head by her mother, and through her close membership of a Christian sect (which, rather against the views of its founder) was strong on sin and not very forthcoming on aspects of love and redemption. The preserve in this case of religious 'Stockholm syndrome' was immune to rational discussion – hence the largely behavioural emphasis with a picking up on cognitive factors when the opportunity arose (sometimes this happens in reverse order). Her memories cover the key stimuli but we have only a limited idea of their relative importance. The analysis is not as neat as the one provided by Pavlov in his controlled experiments, but it is one made within the framework he constructed, and is dependent upon exactly the same general principles (the therapeutic programme used in this case was systematic desensitisation; see Chapter 7).

Now we must turn to some other dimensions of classical conditioning process.

Classical extinction

In Pavlov's experiments, if the bell was rung repeatedly without any food ever appearing, the conditioned salivary response eventually disappeared. This too is biologically advantageous since there is no survival value in responding forever to only temporarily reliable associations. The process is called *extinction*, and it is an important feature of operant conditioning too (see p. 109). However, well-conditioned responses such as the phobia discussed above are very resistant to extinction; they take a considerable time to 'unlearn'. This may be because of a repeated pairing of key stimuli; because, as in the present case, of one very dramatic conjugation (as in cases of PTSD); or because, as in Case example 4.4, the new behaviour can acquire 'positive' secondary consequences not readily apparent to outside observers; or because the fear-association is kept alive by mental rehearsal or cognitive or behavioural avoidance behaviour conditioned by worry and negative reinforcement (see p. 110).

Here are some brief examples (vignettes) of how aspects of respondent conditioning have operated in cases known to me:

☐ An 8-year-old child physically abused at the hands of her alcoholic father, who once in care responded to virtually any situation of routine dependence on an adult (particularly a male adult) with fear and aggression, disrupting her placement thereby (see p. 241).

☐ A young man, who had been trapped in an overcrowded high-rise office lift for twenty minutes who panicked and had to be restrained, and who then regarded all confined spaces as threatening, walked up and down the fire exit stairs of his tower-block (and so was slow at his job but felt he could not explain the reason for this since he felt ashamed), could not use the underground, and often hopped off buses before his stop due to shortness of breath, sweating, palpitations, etc.

☐ A man who frequently exposed himself in public places (mainly underpasses) who learned to associate expressions of disgust from women with power and greater sexual arousal.

☐ A young man who, as a child, had been ridiculed by a teacher for feeling queasy following a routine immunisation procedure for polio. This was after seeing scare stories in the press with pictures of children encased in 'iron lungs'. For a time he developed a somewhat self-fulfilling fear of fainting in formal situations where a plausible exit would be difficult (e.g. concert halls, lectures, etc.).

☐ A learning-disabled young man whose mother was physically disabled, whose school bus was involved in an accident. He was shaken up but not physically hurt. However, he subsequently refused to travel on any form of transport, resulting in reclusiveness for the whole family.

☐ A borderline anorectic young woman who, after a troubled childhood, began to associate ritual self-injury (cutting and burning) with (negatively reinforced) feelings of relief and expiation for (almost wholly imagined) sins and failures, and subsequently with sexual arousal.

All of these cases were treated by a mixture of psycho-education, cognitive therapy (focused in particular on the feedback loop between catastrophic thinking and arousal), but most tellingly, by exposure therapy – apart from the third case! – and counter-conditioning. The fourth case is me, but I did go on to train as a nurse – which was a version of ungraded exposure therapy (flooding).

Experimental neurosis and learned helplessness

Following his work on classical conditioning, Pavlov and his co-workers conducted a series of experiments to investigate how animals cope with being conditioned to contradictory or ambiguous stimuli. Such situations are prevalent in nature and especially so in the complex social environments of human beings.

The experimenters conditioned animals to anticipate food on the presentation of a particular visual cue. For example, the animal was taught to salivate to a circle of light but not to an ellipse (see Shenger-Kristovnikova 1921). It was then made increasingly difficult for the animal to distinguish between these stimuli by arranging for the circle to become narrowed at the sides and for the ellipse to flatten out. Another variation in such (rather cruel) experiments involved the random substitution of consequences – so that the animal was unable accurately to predict whether food or an electric shock would follow a given stimulus (see Masserman 1943). The effects of these studies were that the animal's behaviour became agitated and very uncharacteristic – hence the term 'experimental neurosis'. Later (and this is the important point), when the original stimulus conditions were reinstated, the animals lost their ability to make even crude discriminations, and the experimenters began to use words such as 'depression' and 'catatonia' to describe their immobile state. In other experiments animals just accepted shocks rather than taking an easy and obvious escape route because they had been unpredictably shocked in the past for so doing.

This work has given rise to research aimed at the parallels between the artificial environments of these animals, and those found in human society. Some of the most fruitful work was that of Seligman (1975) whose *Learned Helplessness* theory is of great interest to cognitive-behavioural therapists. Seligman's view, based on analogue studies with humans, is that when an individual learns through experience that there is little or no reliable connection between stimuli, and that his or her behaviour has little effect in modifying the environment of consequences (reducing painful effects and boosting pleasant ones) their behaviour first becomes erratic as they cast about trying to re-establish some control, but if this fails, then, just as in animal experiments, they gradually withdraw, since the environment no longer supports attempts positively to adapt to it. Neither conditioned emotional reactions, nor the anticipation of pleasure, nor the arousal states useful in combating threats, serve any useful, predictive or strategic purpose and so they die away, leaving the individual in a state of apathy. The historical material on 'shell-shock' during the First World War (see Rivers 1922) supports this model.

Learned helplessness formulations will also have a ring of truth to anyone familiar with the case histories of some psychiatric patients under treatment for clinical depression, or to anyone familiar with the backgrounds of clients labelled as 'inadequate personalities', or of those said to belong to 'problem families' and so forth. Cognitive-behavioural approaches help to combat such states by attempting to re-establish some order and predictability in the circumstances of clients by helping them to understand their experiences, and, in a sympathetic, step-by-step way, by teaching the skills necessary for the reassertion of *some* control over unpredictable, or non-positively reinforcing, environments.

Operant conditioning

The term *operant conditioning* (together with its synonym, *instrumental conditioning*) refers to the way in which organisms *operate* on their environment, which in turn selectively increases, strengthens or *reinforces* certain patterns of behaviour at the expense of others. This can happen either haphazardly, or because the environment has been specifically programmed to support certain behaviours and discourage others, as in the workings of families, organisations, or through the rules of the classroom. (*Operant* is not a jargon term, by the way; it can be found in *Hamlet*, Act III.) But if you are thinking about rats, do remember that this is a Pavlovian reaction.

The root principle of operant conditioning is that *behaviour is a function of its consequences*. Parents who respond favourably, first to the random gurglings of their infant, then to specific noises, then to approximations of words, are making use of this principle and helping along the acquisition of spoken language – for which the biological facilities already exist (see Pinker 1996). Similarly, the school child who notices that an unplanned act of disruption produces a level of peer approval previously unknown, will be more likely to repeat the behaviour in future.

An operant, then, is a sequence of behaviour, often exploratory in nature, and not under the direct control of anyone else, that produces an environmental consequence. A useful analogy here is that of sonar or radar. Individuals manoeuvre themselves through their physical and social environments according to the 'return signals' they receive from it in the form of consequences and symbols of impending consequences. The more (or less) pleasurable the environmental feedback, the more (or less) likely they are to engage in the behaviour again in similar circumstances.

The groundwork for this deceptively simple theory of stimulus–response learning was carried out by E.L. Thorndike (1898). However, the extension and detailed investigation of the theory was the life work of B.F. Skinner (1953, 1974). Skinner's contribution was to investigate with great precision the large number of variables that influence the course of learning through experience of consequences; to formulate this into a comprehensive theory; and to apply the theory very successfully to human behaviour. A description of Skinner's basic animal experiments will be useful in clarifying first principles.

A pigeon or a rat (not both) that, let us say, has missed its breakfast, is placed in a glass-sided box (now called a 'Skinner Box') equipped with a food dispenser which, once discovered, is capable of being operated from inside by means of a disc or a lever, or from outside by the experimenter. The advantage of this device (from the point of view of the experimenter) is that the ratio of the delivery of food to the animal's rate of correct responding (called the *schedule*: see p. 115) is, unlike in everyday life, readily controllable. Therefore, the experimenter has power over the main environmental contingencies that affect the behaviour of the animal. These can thus be systematically varied and any resultant shifts in the pattern of responding accurately recorded. The results of these experiments are recounted below and we don't need to trouble animals with them any more since they are all on video.

Types of reinforcement

There are two main types of reinforcement: *positive* and *negative*. Both processes *increase* the frequency, and/or magnitude, and/or speed of a response. Another way of putting it is to say that positive and negative reinforcers increase the probability of a response, or that they 'accelerate' certain sequences of behaviour.

Positive reinforcement

In Skinner's famous experiments a rat was placed in a special box and left to its own devices. Eventually, through random exploratory activity (operant behaviour) the food release lever is nudged and a food pellet drops. The release-operating behaviour then occurs more frequently, and is said to be positively reinforced by the food consequence. The term 'reinforced' simply means strengthened, and refers to the fact that, as a result of a certain consequence, the particular sequence of behaviour leading up to it is demonstrably more likely to occur under similar circumstances in future. Therefore *a positive reinforcer is a stimulus which increases the frequency of the response that it follows.*

Reinforcers are defined exclusively in terms of their effects. Corn is unlikely to strengthen the disc-pecking behaviour of a bloated pigeon, and so it is not a positive reinforcer in that instance. The everyday term 'reward' is too vague to describe this process, since it is derived mainly from the apparent intentions of the would-be rewarder, or is used because the stimulus belongs to some general class of things or happenings *usually* experienced as pleasant by *most* people, or usually responded to predictably by an animal. In fact, there is hardly such a thing as a universal reward. This has long been recognised in the old adage: 'One man's meat is another man's poison.' Appetites also change markedly over time and from setting to setting. Praise given by the schoolteacher with limited corridor cred for a certain style of dress, although intended to reward the behaviour, will often have the opposite effect. The police officer who ticks off an unruly youth in front of his pals is intending to inhibit rowdy behaviour, but may well positively reinforce it by conferring hero status (antisocial behaviour orders are a source of pride for some).

The following quotation from Richard Cobb (historian of French culture) regarding his commanding officer in the Second World War makes the point nicely:

> He displayed a watchful and petty hostility to all university graduates under his command, and a positive loathing for those who had been to Oxford or Cambridge, as if they had gone there on purpose, in some mysterious foreknowledge that they would be meeting him at some point later in life. From the start, I could not help feeling rather flattered that he should have taken such an active, vigilant dislike to myself; I thought it did me credit, it was a sort of tribute. There is something very satisfying about being disliked by the right sort of people.
>
> (Cobb 1997: 86)

So, regarding reinforcers, whatever the intentions, however they come packaged, 'by their effects shall ye know them'.

Negative reinforcement

This is a clumsy term and in my experience causes students more trouble than anything else, so let us start with a simple, everyday example. Sometimes when I am writing, my dog (*The Archers* fan) paces back and forth beside me, emitting panting and occasional coughing noises. He has been shaped into this unwholesome behaviour by previous experience. Having tried all kinds of stimuli to get me to give him access to the great outdoors, he hit upon this. Perhaps on some previous occasion of genuine throat-clearing, fearing for my rugs, I had jumped up and opened the door for him. But aetiology aside, the lesson has been well learned, and the deal is that he paces and pants until I let him out for a sniff around the garden. In *his* case such behaviour has been *positively* reinforced by me. He gets his way much of the time and so the behaviour is established in his repertoire. In *my* case, the behaviour of leaving my writing table, just in case he isn't fooling this time, and to get rid of the distracting noise is *negatively reinforced*. Contingent on certain behaviour from me, an unpleasant set of stimuli (noise and anxiety) is terminated and I am also given a little avoidance break. So dogs condition people too.

Here is another example of the negative reinforcement of behaviour. A man with a drink problem wakes up feeling awful. He feels anxious, low, with a craving for more alcohol. His family eye him suspiciously and take him to task over the condition in which he came home the night before. He goes into the garage, pours himself a tumbler of vodka from his secret store, and starts to feel better. The craving subsides, the world is a brighter place and takes on a pleasantly out-of-focus aspect which anaesthetises him to the pain of everyday living. He takes another swig to intensify this effect. This man's initial drinking behaviour was negatively reinforced. In the short term, alcohol had the effect of reducing aversive stimulation (withdrawal symptoms, sensitivity to disapproval); in the long term its effects on others will probably lead to an intensification of aversive interaction, and so the vicious circle continues.

A useful way of clarifying the difference between positive and negative reinforcement is to imagine a Skinner Box equipped with a loudspeaker or an electrified floor. To turn off an unpleasant sound or irritating electric shock for a while, the animal operates a lever. On this occasion the behaviour is negatively reinforced since it *removes* a negative stimulus rather than *providing* a positive one. Any sequence of behaviour that reduces the effects of aversive stimuli will be readily repeated when the person/organism is faced with similar circumstances in the future. The learning that results is acquired through a kind of 'relief-conditioning' process and a surprising amount of our daily behaviour is predicated upon it.

To sum up: *a negative reinforcer is a stimulus which, if removed or lessened contingent upon a certain response, results in an increase in the probability of that response in similar circumstances in future*. This is the case with obsessional behaviour where lining up the furniture, or repeatedly scrubbing one's hands, reduces high levels of anxiety, usually within the context of a 'superstitious' cognitive rationale about contamination.

At a less threatening level, the influence of negative reinforcement patterns is visible in much of the *avoidance behaviour* that people exhibit when confronted by a challenging task. When working at home I am prone to make large pots of complicated soup which need lots of seasoning and stirring – 'avoidance soup' as it is known to members of my family.

Conditioned reinforcers

Conditioned reinforcers provide an important point of connection between the classical and operant models. This term describes the process whereby anything which is regularly associated with the reinforcement of an operant will eventually acquire an independent reinforcement value of its own. If then we were to switch on a flashing light every time we positively reinforced the disc-pecking behaviour of a pigeon, we would expect that the pigeon would eventually respond to the light alone. The light becomes a *conditioned reinforcer*, since eventually it itself reinforces the disc-pecking behaviour. The extent to which the pigeon's behaviour can be maintained in this way depends upon a number of factors. The first is contiguity: the proximity of the light and the interval of time that elapses between delivery of the goods and the light. The second concerns the number of times the light and the food are paired – the more often this happens (up to a point) the more reinforcing the light becomes. However, this power of 'reinforcement by proxy' is lost relatively quickly when all food is withheld (extinction).

I will provide one further animal example to make this clear. Animal trainers have a problem in trying to reinforce items of behaviour at a distance. They cannot constantly be popping eatables into the mouths of their charges after every piece of apparently clever behaviour, and there is a limit to the extent to which behaviours can be linked together so that reinforcement need only occur at the end of the sequence. In the training of dolphins for public performance (the really interesting question here being why performing animals reinforce the zoo-attending interest of humans) the trainer needs something to stand 'in lieu' of fish when the dolphin is doing tricks in the middle of the pool. He (silly ass) uses the sound of a whistle which has been repeatedly paired with feeding. This sound eventually becomes a reinforcer in its own right. In turn, certain attending, emotional and motor responses in the crowd are reinforced by the relative absence of controls. Skinner (1974) has proposed that the less conspicuous the controlling features of complex behaviour, the more interesting and credit-worthy it becomes; hence the attraction of apparently non-directive dolphin training. It represents a high degree of control over a usually-hard-to-manipulate part of the environment (a basic human drive) and we find this vicariously pleasurable: 'Look no hands; look no fish!'

These highly controlled examples give us a clue to the much underestimated function of conditioned reinforcers in everyday life. Stimuli, in the form of attention, praise, grades and so forth, maintain responding when larger scale positive consequences are long-delayed, as when someone is studying for a diploma or working with a difficult case, where outcomes lie well into the future. These symbols or tokens are secondary events associated through learning with a more basic pay-off, such as greater prestige (itself a conditioned reinforcer) or more money. However, the reader may like to consider just how close to being 'primary' reinforcers are. There is nothing *intrinsically* satisfying in any of the above examples. They are each a link in a chain leading back to genuinely primary, biologically based reinforcers: warmth, shelter, food, sex and so on. But then men and women sometimes forgo these basic needs and drives to obtain dignity, justice, prestige, or even diplomas. It was not always thus.

There is, however, another aspect to this process. A situation where particular conditioned reinforcers were linked only to particular primary deprivation states, or primary needs, would limit responsiveness dramatically, and produce stereotyped and ultimately not very adaptive behaviour. Where this happens the result can appear bizarre and not very creditworthy: 'Everything Bill does is with an eye to the main chance'; 'Fred thinks of nothing but his stomach', and so on. But in the natural environment, in most cases, conditioned reinforcers *generalise*. That is, they become associated with more than one primary reinforcer. A wide range of responsiveness is maintained thereby owing to the increased likelihood that one or other of the primary deprivation states, or something close to it, is likely to be present at any given time.

Money is a good example of a generalised reinforcer. We associate it with, and can procure with it, a wide range of goods and benefits, and therefore whatever deprivation state we happen to be in, or whatever sources of stimulation happen to be near us at the time, there is a chance that money will enhance the possibilities of satisfaction. For this reason tokens were once used in certain behaviour modification programmes; for example, those aimed at shaping the pro-social behaviour of institutionalised psychiatric patients. The tokens could then be exchanged for a wide range of goods and services. A better approach, which we eventually got around to, and which, in my view, has been a major policy success, was to remove clients from the institutionalising contingencies (see Sheldon & Macdonald 2009: ch. 13). If you think all this is rather artificial and mechanistic, feel in your pocket and consider the purpose of the tokens you will find there.

Skinner also cites sensory feedback, and the successful manipulation of the environment as examples of generalised reinforcers.

In cases of disruptive children referred to me, inappropriate attention is undoubtedly the commonest source of unwitting generalised reinforcement of bad behaviour and inattention to good behaviour. Attention usually precedes, and is concurrent with, primary reinforcement in a social setting, and because of this it acquires its own behaviour-strengthening effects. It becomes worth having even when mixed in with irregular amounts of other stimuli intended to deter. Because these contingencies operate in only a vaguely reliable way, the behavioural connection of attention with pleasure is eventually quite difficult to remove see (p. 194).

To sum up: a generalised reinforcer is a conditioned reinforcer which strengthens several types of behaviour in several situations.

Some further general points about reinforcement

☐ The reinforcement status of a stimulus is established by observing the *effect* that this has on behaviour through experiments: whether through the controlled experiments of researchers, or through the less well-controlled assessment procedures employed by therapists. The principles, at least, are the same.

☐ We are not surrounded by stimuli which it is possible to classify on an a priori basis as reinforcers. These potential properties are not of the stimuli so much as of the organism on which they impinge and its previous learning experience.

☐ Behaviour is reinforced, not people. To say that Ms A is trying to reinforce Freda is sloppy except as a form of shorthand, where all concerned know that it is Freda's low-level assertive behaviour that is the target.

☐ Reinforced responses may be thought of as 'semi-automatic', in the sense that sometimes we behave in a very stereotyped way in response to contingencies, and think about it afterwards. Sometimes we think about the reasons for our behaviour *as* we behave. At other times stimuli give rise to memories, thoughts and feelings about potential actions which we perform later, and which are affected by these feelings. In any case the consequences produced play an important role in determining how often, and in what circumstances these responses are used in future.

☐ 'Unconscious' learning can occur; that is, we may not always be able to specify the precise nature of the reinforcement contingencies that elicit certain responses from us – as when we find ourselves repeating patterns of behaviour which are against our interests without understanding why.

The shaping of behaviour

By selectively reinforcing features of a behavioural performance, or by reinforcing only those responses that occur at a certain level, we can gradually alter the nature of responses. Skinner worked with pigeons in this way to produce unusual neck-stretching movements and eventually a repertoire that included playing ping-pong with their beaks! Using the same basic principles, Isaacs *et al.* (1966) shaped the behaviour of a chronically withdrawn schizophrenic patient whose typical behaviour consisted of sitting silently and staring into space. During a ward meeting the therapist pulled out a piece of gum, and noticed that the patient's eyes moved slightly in his direction. The patient was given the gum and, once the response was established, performance levels were gradually increased. The stages in this were: head turning; eye contact; holding out a hand; then responding with more complex speech. At each stage only slightly exceptional behaviour was reinforced, and this is the key feature of operant shaping. Keeping it going is the challenge. Lovaas and colleagues performed wonders with largely silent, self-injuring, socially disconnected children ('psychotic', he originally called them, but autistic is more likely). By the end of his project they were talking, telling stories from imagination, not head banging or otherwise hurting themselves. However, when they were sent home, only those parents and carers who were willing to reinforce these gains quarter-hourly, day by day, reported maintained results (see Lovaas 1967, 1987). Referring to the shaping power of the natural environment, Skinner had this to say:

> Operant conditioning shapes behaviour as a sculptor shapes a lump of clay. Although at some point the sculptor seems to have produced an exclusively novel object, we can always follow the process back to the original undifferentiated lump, and we can make the successive stages by which we return to this condition as small as we wish. At no point does anything emerge which is very different from what preceded it. The final product seems to have a special unity and integrity of design but we cannot find the point at which this suddenly appears. In the same sense an operant is not something which appears full grown in the behaviour of the organism. It is the result of a continuous shaping process.
> (Skinner 1953: 91)

Shaping, when systematically applied, is a therapeutic technique with considerable impact (see Chapter 7) as when a health visitor selectively congratulates a parent for responding more matter-of-factly and calmly to an over-demanding child and then, over time, such reinforcement becomes conditional on longer and/or more complex sequences of behaviour.

Sometimes the shaping of *verbal behaviour* is important for therapeutic purposes. For example, in the case of an excessively shy and unassertive individual, speech containing personal references, expressions of opinion or statements of intention might be selectively strengthened by increased attention and small signs of approval. A little increased attention to a client considering something in his or her life less irrationally, goes a long way in interviews, so long as the process never becomes artificial.

Fading

Fading is the process whereby control of a sequence of behaviour is gradually shifted from one set of reinforcers to another. This process is central to socialisation, where, for example, parents (once) gradually faded out the regular positive reinforcement of sitting at the table for meals, until the behaviour was maintained by purely non-verbal signs of approval, and by conversation, plus the signalled threat of disapproval for breaking social rules. Similarly, a reinforcement programme that begins by encouraging adaptive behaviour in a child with the use of treats can hardly continue in that vein forever. The aim of behavioural programmes is to bring adaptive behaviour under the control of 'naturally occurring' (i.e. culturally consonant) social influences. Fading in this type of programme can, if necessary, be accomplished by the use, alongside material reinforcers, of attention, praise, affection and so on, so that material rewards can be given less often or in smaller quantities as the behaviour comes to be maintained by CRs.

Although fading is a common enough feature of daily life and of childhood experience, my impression is that far too little attention is given to it in therapeutic settings. Perhaps it is the fault of the medical model which tempts us to think in terms of 'cure' rather than adaptation. Or perhaps it is the *setting up* of cognitive-behavioural programmes that reinforces our own therapeutic behaviour because it is the most optimistic part. The relatively mundane business of ensuring that any useful effects can be maintained in natural settings smacks a little of 'after-care' and is (mistakenly) seen as a less important activity. 'Talk and hope' programmes, as they are called, have resulted in wastefully high levels of relapse in the past.

Discriminative stimuli

Discriminative stimuli (S^ds) are stimuli which (as a result of learning) signal to us that reinforcement (positive or negative) may be available for particular forms of behaviour. In the animal laboratory, a coloured light might readily come to signal that the food lever mechanism is live (a positive CS) or that the floor grid will soon be live unless some action is taken. S^ds are especially important in complex social settings and much of the process of human socialisation is taken up with establishing finely tuned responses in relation to such cues.

These stimuli are important in our work with clients, in that, if we learn what signals tend to precede particular behaviours, we may be able to intervene at this early point to sensitise clients to their warning potential so that they can institute pre-rehearsed self-control procedures (see p. 231). If feelings of boredom reliably trigger excessive eating, or a partic- ular sort of conversation within a peer group reliably predicts aggression, then action can sometimes be taken to divert behaviour into another channel. Attention to these antecedent factors can allow us to interrupt a sequence of problematic behaviour *before* it becomes fully developed.

Stimuli can also acquire a negative signalling value. These have the subtitle *delta stimuli* (S^Δs) and come to indicate by regular association that no pleasurable consequences are likely to occur or that something unpleasant is on the cards.

In cases where a client's behaviour is 'overgeneralised', where, for example, he or she fails to discriminate between those people who are out to punish for previous misdeeds, and those who wish to help, an extra emphasis on identifying the differences in settings, behaviour, probable intentions, demeanour, function and so on may aid future discrimination. But not all is benign here, as S^Δs can also trigger patterns of negative cognition ('it's not safe in here, where's the nearest exit'; 'my chest feels tight, am I having a heart attack?'; 'this person looks bored, or is it tired?'). These thought sequences (which need not be accurate appraisals) then trigger emotional reactions, which in turn trigger more negative thoughts, more emotion, and so on until not always adaptive behaviour is triggered, which in its turn [. . .]. Teaching clients to recognise these sequences, to try out relaxation techniques in the face of them, or to talk to themselves differently, are useful therapeutic applications.

Let us now turn to some effects that different *patterns* or *schedules* of reinforcement have on behaviour.

Schedules of reinforcement

This next set of considerations stems from the fact that stimuli impinge, or can be deliberately presented, in different *sequences*. This can have a marked effect: (1) on the rate and level of acquisition of responses; (2) on the way responding is maintained; and (3) on the resistance the behaviour shows to extinction (see Ferster and Skinner 1957). Therefore, such factors are of clinical importance.

The following factors are the most potent: (1) the number and ratio of responses receiving reinforcement in a sequence; (2) whether this pattern is regular or irregular; (3) the interval between responses. Each of these factors will now be discussed in turn.

Fixed ratio schedules

Descriptions of this type of schedule are usually abbreviated to FR, with an index number following giving the number of responses which have to occur before reinforcement takes place. Thus FR6 equals six responses of a particular kind before reinforcement occurs. Natural environment contingencies rarely provide such a regular pattern, but a piece-worker who receives payment according to the number of items of work produced is on an FR schedule, as is the school child who gets a star rating (CR) for every three marks of B+ and above.

FR schedules have the effect of speeding up responses: the more items of designated appropriate behaviour performed, the greater the level of reinforcement supplied. Thus their chief characteristics are high and stable levels of responding, and (as with continuous reinforcement schedules – see below) the fact that their effects are relatively easily extinguished if contingencies are not reliable. Secondary features are that the accuracy of the responses monitored on this schedule need be no more than adequate to obtain reinforcement (think some 'target' regimes); that the number rather than quality of outputs is what is being reinforced (think of the universities' obsession with publication *rates*). Indeed, if the ratio of response to reinforcement is high, then a certain amount of 'trimming' occurs; that is, embellishments (which might provide opportunities for shaping) are dropped in the interests of speed, and following reinforcement for a long sequence the frequency of responding may well drop temporarily as another long series looms. Obviously, if the ratio is too large then the behaviour extinguishes altogether.

Fixed ratio schedules are used in practice when a high, fast and regular rate of discrete and easily definable responses is required. The rate can be varied so that it is easily manageable to start with and then increased later by gradual steps.

Continuous reinforcement

This is said to be occurring when every occurrence of a target behaviour is reinforced and is the way in which treatment programmes with a behavioural component start off. The aim is to establish and strengthen a particular sequence as quickly and effectively as possible, and it is worth knowing that experimental evidence shows clearly that reinforcement on a continuous schedule works fastest and best in this regard. If a client only rarely engages in eye contact, then every single appearance of this behaviour should be positively reinforced with whatever works – perhaps increased attention, perhaps a smile, perhaps a favourable comment. Once the new behaviour is established, a different approach is required to maintain it – to avoid the therapist turning into a nodding dog mascot.

Behaviour monitored on a continuous reinforcement schedule is easily extinguished. That is, if reinforcement stops, apart from the possibility of a brief 'spurt' to test out the contingencies (as in work with disruptive children), the response rate drops like a stone. This fact has obvious implications for practice, and in particular for the question of how to maintain desirable behaviours without *artificial* reinforcement after the professional has left the scene. Anyone concerned with advising on therapeutic programmes will be familiar with this 'straight up and straight down' phenomenon present in case data, where adequate behaviour is maintained on a continuous schedule until the client has 'improved'; then the case is closed. Three months later it is re-referred with the client in virtually the same or a worse state, and the therapeutic approach is said 'not to have worked' or to have produced only short-term, 'symptomatic' benefits. The real point is that no thought has been given to 'immunising' new behaviour against extinction by exposing it to short, irregular periods of non-reinforcement. To resist the onslaught of natural environment contingencies, behaviour is best *developed* on a continuous schedule and *maintained* on a variable schedule.

Differential reinforcement of other behaviour (DRO schedules)

Another way to speed up acquisition is through providing a set of contingencies which 'contrast' one particular behaviour with others in the repertoire. To do this we continuously reinforce the desired sequence while placing nearby competing, less desirable behaviours on extinction (as in the case discussed on p. 194).

Intermittent and variable schedules

There are two categories of intermittent schedules: (1) ratio schedules; and (2) interval schedules. In the case of a ratio schedule, reinforcement occurs after a certain number of responses. In the case of an interval schedule, reinforcement occurs after a given amount of time has elapsed; that is, it might be given for every twenty minutes spent in the rehabilitation unit, or for every half hour of cooperative play without incident. The next important influence is whether the ratios and the elapsed intervals of time determining reinforcement in the two cases above are fixed or variable.

Variable-ratio (VR) schedules have very powerful behaviour-maintenance effects and provide built-in resistance to extinction (referred to above). With VR schedules, reinforcement occurs for an average number of responses, but the important point is that the precise ratio of reinforcement to responses alters over time. Thus, reinforcement alterations may be made for every sixth, tenth or fourteenth response – in sequence. This schedule would be called VR10 since the mean is ten. A good example of a VR schedule in everyday life is the 'fruit machine' where excitement and persistence are derived from the unpredictability of reinforcement and small 'superstitious' changes to how the buttons and levers are pushed and pulled. Lab rats do this too.

With complex versions of this schedule the individual cannot easily predict when the next 'score' will occur, and so not only is the response maintained at a high and stable rate, but the quality of response is good since there is often experimentation to 'perfect' it and so bring on the reward; the response can thus be shaped. Thus the organism/person guesses at the contingencies associated with certain consequences, and tries out variations in behaviour to see whether this makes a difference or changes its luck. The little rituals displayed by examination candidates (four pens, three pencils, two sharpeners, etc.) provide another example. The investment of effort is small, it reduces temporary anxiety, and the potential gains or losses are high – an inverted lottery effect: '*someone has to lose*'.

If VR reinforcement is terminated completely the rate of responding tends to stay level for a considerable period just in case the next sequence produces the long-awaited pay-off. However, while resistance to extinction is a considerable advantage when the issue is how to maintain new behaviour acquired in therapy, it is an equally considerable disadvantage when trying to remove maladaptive behaviour from the repertoire. Most behaviours acquired in the natural environment are reinforced on variable-interval schedules. Thus Jamie's mother does not respond with cuddles *every time* he has a tantrum; she did so at first (continuous reinforcement), then she decided against this mollycoddling and ignored the next two upsets. The third was a really bad one and she felt that she couldn't ignore it, and that something must be the matter. The next tantrum was ignored completely. During the one after that

Jamie was shouted at. In the one after that Jamie's mother tried pleasant diversionary tactics. When the health visitor called a month later she advised Jamie's mother to ignore tantrums from now on so that they would extinguish. Nineteen sad experiences later the mother gave up on the scheme entirely.

Punishment

Punishment requires discussion, not because it has a prominent place in our repertoire of techniques, but because of its controversial nature. First, it is important to distinguish punishment from negative reinforcement. It is commonly believed that negative reinforcement is just a fancy term for punishment; it is not. Punishment is the effect of applying an aversive stimulus or set of stimuli, contingent upon a certain response, thus *decreasing* the probability that the response will be made in similar circumstances in future. Imagine a Skinner Box where the pressing of a lever always resulted in a shock or a loud noise. This would result in a *reduction* in the performance of this response, or more likely, its complete suppression.

The aversive stimuli may also take the form of contingent removal of positive reinforcement – as in the deprivation punishments of childhood. Two terms which the reader may encounter in the literature are: 'positive punishment', for the *presentation* of an aversive stimulus; and 'negative punishment', for the *withdrawal* of a positive stimulus. The important points here are: (1) that in both cases the effect of the stimulus is to weaken the response that it follows; and (2) negative punishment (deprivation) is less likely to produce unwanted escape or avoidance behaviour.

Thus the use of the word *punishment* in the behavioural psychology literature is somewhat different from our everyday understanding of the idea. First, it does not necessarily imply that anyone is deliberately setting out to inhibit certain behaviour. Second, there is no implication that the subject was necessarily doing anything 'wrong', or that the aversive event was retributive in character. Through trial and error, or accident, certain environmental or internal physiological consequences occur that inhibit the behaviour with which they are associated. In other words, punishment is a naturally occurring phenomenon as well as something people do to each other on purpose.

Many of our clients live in extremely punishing environments, which is why so many of them withdraw from the constructive problem-solving attempts that often look to those not directly involved (e.g. tabloid journalists) like *obvious* solutions to their and our difficulties. An example of this kind of suppression of adaptive responses is the familiar situation of the 'multi-problem family', who, on balance, experience fewer aversive consequences by 'muddling through' than by attempting to get to grips with their difficulties (a syndrome also not unknown to social workers and health staff with unmanageably large case loads). When choice-making behaviour, or self-assertion in any direction, leads to punishment, apathy results.

Punishment (in the technical sense) is a popular idea, except in child care, where perfect parents are always expected to have done something previously to obviate the need for it. The reasons for this are:

☐   It is easy to formulate punishment contingencies – much easier than trying to discover precise deficits in social skills which result in inadequate performance, and easier still than trying to find reinforceable behaviour incompatible or competitive with maladaptive behaviour. Interestingly, and perhaps for this reason, when students in my psychology classes are presented with case material describing deviant behaviour they usually spring immediately into discussions about ways of suppressing it, not deflecting it.

☐ Rewarding low-level adaptive behaviour in the context of a serious maladaptive performance calls for clear discriminations – not only on the client's part, but on the part of outside observers. Often the community and its representatives are unable, or unwilling, to make such fine distinctions; to do so would look too much like condoning the bad behaviour that happens to occur nearby. It is safer and more comfortable to attribute behaviour entirely to durable, internal predispositions which might be susceptible to 'short, sharp shock approaches'. Therefore, however ineffective the results, nothing nice can be allowed to happen to juvenile delinquents; somehow they must be reformed through controlled suffering.

☐ Another reason for the popularity of punishment is that it is believed to act as a source of vicarious suppression for similar behaviours in others, as in 'making an example' of offenders – so long as they think they will ever be caught, that is.

But there are many problems associated with the use of aversive stimuli.

☐ Naturally enough, it induces escape behaviours in those on whom it is used. These can be at least as maladaptive as the original problematic behaviour, and the negative reinforcement of successful responses in this class can give rise to a new generation of difficulties. For example, a child may learn that he can escape punishment by lying really convincingly.

☐ Punishment gives rise to revenge motives. A good way of avoiding its unpleasant effects is to remove, or act against, the source of these effects. If this is the professional, however benign his or her intentions, he or she may be left either with no one to work with, or with a client who will regard every suggestion as a signal to do the opposite.

☐ Punishment alone, whether arranged or accidental, gives no guidance as to what alternative behaviours might be more effective than the response that is being discouraged.

☐ Punishment acts as a *general* suppressant. It tends to have a 'blanket effect', removing wanted as well as unwanted responses from the repertoire, sometimes leaving nothing much for the therapist to work with.

☐ Punishment has only short-term effects, and influence based on visible coercion is influence easily disregarded once the heat is off.

☐ Punishment can easily generalise to its users. Someone who makes regular use of it will find it hard to use positive reinforcement effectively with the same client in the future. Think back to being smiled at by the teacher who has twice put you on report – it could go either way.

These problems need to be kept in view when the therapist in a statutory setting is putting together programmes that have a necessary control element, particularly when they involve children. These points do not add up to a case for the complete abandonment of punishment as an engineered consequence; rather they are intended to serve as a reminder that many of our clients already inhabit environments rich in aversive stimuli, and only rarely will it help artificially to add to these.

Therapists cannot have their heads in the clouds about punishment. It is not a very large feature of the repertoire of the behavioural element of CBT, but as an *effect* it is all around us. Some clients may even see the very presence of a would-be helper in their homes as a punishment (Case example 4.5).

CASE EXAMPLE 4.5

Mark, aged 10, was referred to Social Services via the Education Social Work Service (the department already held a supervision order on an elder brother following three instances of theft). His teachers were greatly concerned about Mark's disruptive behaviour in class and were beginning to use psychiatric terminology to account for this. Exclusion (potentially his third) was likely unless something could be done, and there was official concern regarding the amount and type of punishment used at home following these incidents.

In common with that of his brother, Mark's childhood had been somewhat troubled. A history of marital difficulties between parents, and two lengthy periods of separation from them while in the care of relatives, were the most distinctive features.

Family life seemed to have settled down of late and the case file contained optimistic reports about this. However, it was known that the parents had often disagreed to the point of violence about disciplinary practices in the home – the mother favouring the strict enforcement of rules, but the father, when present, following a 'boys will be boys' philosophy, this, perhaps, to excuse some of his own wayward behaviour. The father, a jobbing builder, drank quite heavily, and was always a person of interest to the Inland Revenue.

Mark was not a bright child and had reading difficulties requiring remedial teaching – with which he rarely cooperated.

With the hesitant cooperation of the school authorities, an investigation of Mark's disruptive behaviour began in its natural setting. The student social workers took it in turns to observe lessons (they were introduced as 'students' and spent periods sitting unobtrusively at the rear of the classroom to observe and record Mark's behaviour). Data recorded by these observers revealed the following. (1) 'Disruptive behaviour' usually meant: 'Mark leaving his desk or group activity'; but then after that he would occasionally make loud noises, slamming down objects, teasing, pushing and pinching other pupils, and generally interfering with their work. (2) Some teachers had more difficulty with Mark than others. (3) The most common methods of dealing with Mark were: reasoning with him or speaking sharply to him, both of which seemed to have only a marginal and temporary effect; trying to distract him, which only worked in the short term; placing him outside the door – to which he did not seem to object at all, and which again had no effect on his subsequent behaviour. By and large teachers tried to ignore him, most operating what the headteacher referred to as: a 'sleeping dogs policy'.

The working hypothesis developed in this case was that Mark's classroom behaviour was largely a product of the following contingencies. (1) When Mark was at all well behaved (which records showed was a fair proportion of the time) he was ignored. Most teachers were wary of him and left him alone. (2) Conversely, whenever Mark caused or threatened a disturbance he received immediate attention from his teacher on virtually every occasion. (3) Attempts to punish Mark were ineffective, not only because the teachers were admirably half-hearted about this, but because of his immunising exposure to much more serious forms of it at home. (4) Mark's reading difficulties sometimes made it hard for him to join in lessons even with the help of a teaching assistant. He was bored and a little embarrassed by this, and escaped from these conditions by amusing himself with other, more dubious pursuits.

The reinforcement patterns thought to be operating in this case are as follows.

Mark was *positively reinforced* with attention for bad behaviour (a commodity in short supply at home for *any* behaviour). A further contrast between consequences of good and bad behaviour was provided by the fact that the teachers would stay away from him when he was not being difficult, and in any case saw all too little to reward in what they called 'his attitude to school work'. Thus the teachers were only persuaded to reward *extended* runs of good behaviour, and these occurred rarely.

Mark's tendency to get out of his seat, and his disruptive behaviour, were also *negatively reinforced*. The work was difficult for him to succeed at because he did not possess the skills required, and so he became bored. If called upon to contribute to class work, he usually tried, but made a mess of things. Thus leaving his seat and disruptive behaviour had the effect of terminating or reducing his boredom and embarrassment about failing. On one occasion, Mark automatically placed *himself* by the door after a confrontation with a teacher.

Developmental, cognitive and family problems also came into this case. Discussions with Mark himself showed a high level of impulsive, revenge-tinged interpretations; and since he often knew exactly where a classroom problem would eventually lead, he felt an urge to 'short-circuit' it: he 'got his retaliation in first', in other words. Pausing and thinking things through were not really in his repertoire. His mother felt that having been 'shamed' previously – having to go to court re Mark's older brother and seeing Mark 'inevitably' heading in the same direction – she felt she needed to stamp out the behaviour as early as possible. She hated letters from the school, but really thought that it was all due to a failure of the teachers to control him, so why should she be blamed? She thus supported the idea of school-based problems belonging in the school. She was less cooperative with discussions of home life. Mark's father agreed to attend family meetings, but always absented himself – once, over the back fence – 'anyone with a briefcase and he's off', the mother explained.

Results from the attempt to reverse the reinforcement contingencies discussed above and to provide positive reinforcement for remaining seated and concentrating on school work, and none for disruptive behaviour, and the methods used to good effect will be discussed later. This approach is called *differential reinforcement* and the family, including Mark, at least understood it as an attempt to fend off unwanted consequences. The treatment approach is described on p. 193 onwards.

Modelling and vicarious learning

So far, we have examined (1) the means by which new responses are generated through stimulus association, often in chain-like fashion (classical conditioning); and (2) the way in which responses are established in the repertoire or lost from it as a result of the (intended and unintended) consequences they produce (operant conditioning). We turn now to a third process, derived in part from the other two, and called variously *observational learning, vicarious learning, modelling* or *imitation*.

These processes are the means by which new responses are acquired, reinforced or extinguished, *at a distance* (vicariously), through observation of the behaviour of others and by imputing to them patterns of cognitive appraisal and emotion. A large proportion of the behavioural repertoire of each of us is developed in this way, not through direct personal experience, but through watching what others do in particular circumstances and how they fare as a consequence. Its basis in simple imitation is visible in the biologically endowed, facial expression-copying of young babies (see Figure 4.3). Mothers have known this for thousands of years, but as you can see from the hairstyles, psychology only caught up in the 1970s.

Modelling is the process through which we learn the speech patterns of our parents and the accents of our peers; learn to act a little like our favourite TV star; pick up the rudiments of a dance style; learn how to behave in unfamiliar surroundings; learn how to approach strangers for amorous purposes; learn how to intimidate opponents; come to approach decision-making in as neurotic a way as our parents; and learn how being aggressive gets people their way, or the opposite.

Modelling is a powerful influence in human socialisation and its importance has been enhanced considerably by the arrival of the mass media. Through modelling we select, observe and learn to imitate in approximate form elements of the behavioural performances of others (inferring the cognitive and emotional concomitants) most days of our lives. When we are in promising or demanding circumstances, under threat or in strange surroundings, we become avid modellers, searching in the behaviour of others for clues as to how to behave.

At certain stages in socialisation, during adolescence in particular, models are actively sought and copied as the young person experiments with different styles of behaviour, trying

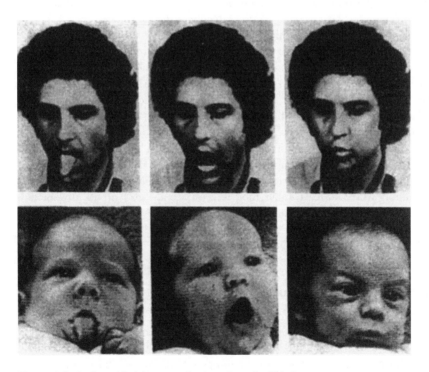

Figure 4.3 Imitation of facial gestures by 2- to 3-week-old infants
Source: Harris (1972).

them on like clothes and discarding them later; learning how to walk again. Paradoxically, this copying is done as a way of establishing a *distinct* identity – this is only achieved later when judicious editing, fluency and the combining of different performances produces a genuinely unique style of behaviour. Most psychology classes will pretend that this didn't happen much to them, but it did.

As in the case of the other forms of learning reviewed above, we can acquire both useful or destructive, good or bad, self-enhancing or self-defeating, confident or fearful, responses through observational learning. The process is exactly the same. Albert Bandura (the foremost researcher in this field) makes the point that were operant conditioning the only means by which human beings could acquire a behavioural repertoire, the planet would be littered with the mangled corpses of those whose responses had been ineffective:

> Thus, in laboratory investigations of learning processes experimenters usually arrange comparatively benign environments in which errors will not produce dangerous conse-quences. In contrast, natural settings are loaded with potentially lethal consequences that unmercifully befall anyone who makes hazardous errors. For this reason, it would be exceedingly injudicious to rely primarily upon trial and error learning and successive-approximation methods in teaching children to swim, adolescents to drive stick shifts, or adults to master complex occupational and social tasks. If rodents, pigeons or rodents toiling in contrived situations could likewise get electrocuted, dismembered or bruised, for errors that inevitably occur during early phases of learning, few of these venturesome subjects would ever survive the shaping process.
>
> (Bandura 1969: 143)

Skinner's analysis of what happens when we observe the behaviour of someone else and then perform it ourselves takes the standard operant view outlined in Figure 4.4.

In Figure 4.4 S^d represents the discriminative stimuli present in the modelled performance, R denotes an overt matching response, and S^r the reinforcing stimulus which follows this performance.

It will be immediately apparent that although this explanation may approach suffi-ciency in very controlled conditions, where considerable prior learning has taken place (e.g. a dancing class), for many everyday modelling situations it is inadequate. First, there is the problem of acquisition; that is, how the observer comes to acquire the new set of responses in the first place. Second, there is the problem of the retention of a modelled behaviour pattern for days and weeks before it is performed overtly. We may go to the cinema and observe a particularly cool, collected performance by an actor and not try to re-enact aspects of this until we are next confronted with a departmental panic-monger.

An experiment to demonstrate the role of reinforcement in modelling was performed by Bandura (1965). Children watched a film of an actor displaying aggression towards blow-up dolls. The conditions under which this behaviour was performed were systematically varied. In one sequence the actor was reprimanded; in another, rewarded with praise and sweets, and in another, no particular consequences were seen to result from the battering behaviour. Immediate post-exposure observations of children from the audience, in another setting, showed high levels of aggression. The highest and most varied levels of aggressive behaviour

S^d ——————— R ——————— S^r

Figure 4.4 Observed behaviour: the operant view

came from the groups who had seen the model's aggression reinforced or to attract no negative consequences. For them the surrogate violence was seen to pay off, so they imitated it at the next opportunity. This experiment has been repeated many times since, with the same results.

Post-performance reinforcement undoubtedly plays a part in the modelling process as this classic experiment demonstrates, but as a complete explanation it is inadequate. Paying attention to what other people do in interesting or demanding situations is likely to be reinforcing in itself. (Bandura's argument that modelling can occur in the absence of external reinforcement seems a little thin, since it depends on an absence of CRs from previous live experience.) There is also a key role here for the *anticipated* reinforcement (S^ds) of any imitation which will add new response options to the stock. Individuals have a wide range of possible responses according to the circumstances in which they might happen to find themselves in the future, are more likely so to be able to obtain satisfaction and more likely to avoid adversity. In this sense, the knowledge that novel response-options are being stored in memory as behavioural 'capital' for later, might itself reinforce attentional and response-matching behaviour.

The rest of the modelling process occurs in symbolic, that is, in cognitive form. We *think* ourselves into the role of the performer, imagine and, to some extent, experience the emotional accompaniments that he or she might be experiencing (easy in the cinema and on television because of the cues provided by the accompanying music). Next we anticipate how successful we would be in performing this behaviour (efficacy expectations) and what the probable outcome would be for us in given circumstances (outcome expectations). A child who watches others breaking down a fence with consummate skill need not perform similar behaviour on the next fence he comes across. A variety of different conditions (S^As), some of them social in origin, will determine when the behaviour 're-emerges'.

Another form of modelling where covert factors (feelings this time) play a large part in the acquisition process has been called *empathetic learning*. The fact that we tend to 'feel along' with the performances of a model (as a result of a lengthy process of classical conditioning) tends to make us want to re-perform the behaviour to obtain internal, emotional reinforcement from the various states of arousal previously known or thought to accompany it (Case example 4.6).

CASE EXAMPLE 4.6

Years ago I went to see the film *Grand Prix* (no particular interest, but free tickets), a banal motor-racing film with action scenes shot from car-mounted cameras. Walking out of the cinema my girlfriend and I were met with a wall of sound. The night air was thick with blue smoke as hundreds of teenagers revved up their ageing cars and raced each other down the Bristol Road, seats all the way back, arms straight, windows down. When my girlfriend asked, 'Why are you driving like a maniac?' I replied that I had always driven fast, and that anyway it was skill that mattered. This behaviour lasted for about ten miles (when I remembered that I was supposed to be practising being cool and impervious to external influence, after James Dean).

The current status of this theory as an explanation of modelling is viewed by Bandura as similar to that of the operant conditioning model. Such factors may well be at work, and may play a relatively large part in modelling under certain conditions, but they are background rather than central features in most cases:

> Sensory-feedback theories of imitation may therefore be primarily relevant to instances in which the modelled responses incur relatively potent reinforcement consequences capable of endowing response-correlated stimuli with motivational properties. Affective conditioning should therefore be regarded as a facilitative rather than as a necessary condition for modelling.
>
> (Bandura 1969: 132)

In other words, the cognitive, problem-solving content of modelled performances can be sufficient to secure imitation.

Research in this field has had a considerable impact on practice in the form of programmes to teach child management skills to parents with children at risk (see Macdonald & Kakavelakis 2004), and to equip psychiatric patients with the social and other skills necessary for survival in the community (see Emmelkamp 2004).

Cognitive-mediational theories of modelling

Theories of observational learning which emphasise the importance of the mental representation of the sequence to be re-performed are called *cognitive-mediational theories* (see Eysenck & Keane 1990). They concentrate on the hidden stages that occur between observation and performance. Two systems are said to be at work here to represent a performance in our heads for later retrieval: a process of imagination and a verbal process. Performances are encoded into particular image sequences and word symbols, and stored in the memory.

Let us look at an experiment that demonstrates the role of such symbolic representation in modelling (Bandura 1965). In this study children were asked to pay attention to filmed sequences of complex behaviour. One group of children was instructed to watch carefully; another group was asked, as well as paying attention, to speak along with the models on the screen and describe and label the models' behaviour out loud; a further group was instructed to watch attentively, but to count rapidly at the same time (this to prevent the encoding of information). When asked to re-create the sequences they had seen, the children in the 'verbal-labelling' group were much more effective in their performances than the watch-silently group) and produced yet more accurate responses than the group that had had to engage in a competing activity. Thus training children to attend to current circumstances and thinking about responses to them is an important aspect of CBT in such cases.

Most of us will have had the experience of talking ourselves through a difficult or unfamiliar task – either out loud, as in childhood, or subliminally ('under our breath'): 'Right now, that's the support on, and now I put the *large* locating screws on the *left* so as not to mix them up with these *smaller* ones over *here*' (IKEA stress syndrome, not yet in DSM). The point here is that it is the encoding and organising of complex modelling stimuli by the brain that ensures accurate reproduction. Similarly, the more complex and unfamiliar the test the more likely we are to open an extra channel of sensory input to guide our actions.

So far we have seen that offshoots of both classical and operant conditioning procedures play a part in getting us to attend to, and reproduce for ourselves, the behaviour of others. However, neither of these processes fully accounts for this form of learning, which is made possible only through cognition. This allows us to re-enact, in symbolic form, the little dramatic performances we have selected from the behaviour of others and that we anticipate

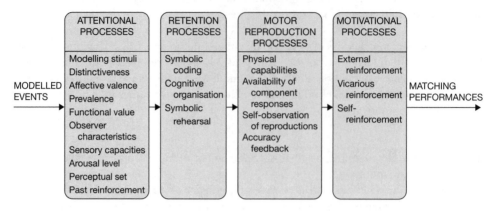

Figure 4.5 Component factors governing observational learning in the social learning process
Source: Adapted from Bandura (1977).

(sometimes wrongly) will be useful to us. Figure 4.5 provides a summary of the various stages of the modelling process. The reader will see that the first list of factors is associated with the characteristics of the modelled stimulus, and what it is about it that we selectively perceive and attend to ('attentional process'). The second list relates to the coding, organisation and storage of a 'mental script' of the performance. The third set concerns the rehearsal of modelled performances, and the fourth the factors that decide the place of the performance in the repertoire: how often it is likely to be performed, whether it will be developed further, or lost, and so on.

Therapeutic applications

Modelling procedures are useful in a wide range of circumstances, particularly the following.

☐   To remedy behavioural deficits. Clients often just do not have the behaviours or the thinking strategies necessary to solve their problems in repertoire. They may simply never have learned them, or they may have lost them owing to intervening experiences. In this case there may be little or nothing for therapists to shape or reinterpret. Some of the most heart-rending problems ever to confront us are the result of a failure to learn basic human characteristics because no examples were available nearby:

> That girls are raped, that two boys knife a third,
> Were axioms to him, who'd never heard
> Of any world where promises were kept,
> Or one could weep, because another wept.
>
> (W.H. Auden, 'The Shield of Achilles')

☐   To reduce interfering anxiety. When individuals are forced to cope despite considerable social and behavioural deficits, their actions usually become stereotyped and awkward. Knowing this, they tend to avoid any circumstances (where they are unlikely to perform well or will experience anxiety. Anxiety (anticipated punishment) can enhance a performance up to a certain level, but beyond this optimum level it interferes progressively with performance (see Hebb 1972; also p. 220), resulting in increasingly inadequate and poorly discriminated behaviour. This, in turn, sets up a vicious circle leading to greater anxiety and more generalised avoidance. Modelling techniques may be used to demonstrate and teach better coping skills that are more likely to lead to reinforcement. The rehearsal of these new behaviours, to a point of reasonable competency, usually carries with it a 'desensitisation' component. Fears are lessened both by vicarious extinction and by operant extinction – that is, by watching someone else perform the target behaviours without apparent anxiety, feeling sympathetically relaxed thereby, then practising under relatively benign conditions and with increasing competency.

☐   Modelling and social skills training can also be used to re-establish behaviours which were once in the repertoire of the individual but which have been lost or suppressed owing to lack of available reinforcement or through adverse experiences. If these are present at a very low level, then shaping is likely to be a lengthy and labour-intensive process. Sometimes short cuts can be attempted by modelling appropriate behaviour and showing it obtaining reinforcement – as in programmes to re-establish social skills after periods in psychiatric care.

We have now passed the point where largely behavioural conceptions of learning can account (without undue contortion) for the phenomena under review.

Cognitive influences

Several writers have argued that there is a type of learning – leading to the acquisition of new and visible responses – which is substantially independent of (distinguish from uninfluenced by) the different associative mechanisms on which classical and operant conditioning depend, and on which modelling effects have been seen partly to depend. There are various labels for this: *cognitive learning, insight learning, latent learning* and so forth. Each of these terms refers to an overlapping set of concepts that lay stress on the importance (particularly in complex learning tasks) of selective perception, understanding, prior knowledge, attribution, imagination, memory factors, concept formation and creative intelligence – the results of various forms of 'cognitive structures'.

Skinner's Box analyses, though economical and often persuasive, equally often leave one with the feeling that they are too 'pat'. Creative problem-solving and artistry are surely something entirely different. Indeed, investigators of the origins of complex learning argue that crude and uncoordinated stimuli affecting an individual ought to result in crude and uncoordinated responses – unless, that is, something extra is added inside the 'black box'. The extra 'something' must be the effect of complex cognitive structures; that is, symbolic, mental 'maps' stored in memory, from which, and to which, items are added and subtracted, and between which interchanges can take place to create new orderings of information, and hence new response options. The 'machinery' of thinking, when examined in cognitive experiments, is surprisingly dedicated to 'the usual output'. We often think first in stereotypes, and then reconsider them later. Thus, ask a psychology class to consider the word 'Frenchman'; then ask what in the reflex mental image is this person wearing? (stripy jumper!); headgear? (beret); any vegetables in the picture? (onions!). Then try 'Desert Island' – how many trees in the picture? (one) how many figures? (one). The audience knows that these images are cultural stereotypes and hardly exist in nature, but somehow they suffice for routine information-processing purposes until reconsidered later. There are many examples of this: thus the road sign for a level crossing shows a steam train (even though they have not been around for fifty years in this country), and for a speed camera it is of a 1920s bellows/plate camera. Thus we often think in iconographs to start with.

Take virtually any two words and conjoin them, and an entirely new image with entirely new meaning and implications arises. Try 'Golden' and 'Mountain'. Few if any of us has seen such a thing (at dawn, in the desert, something close perhaps), yet we have no difficulty conjuring up the image, or even a newly created folktale to match. Indeed, we have to work very hard to produce grammatical word sequences with no apparent meaning: 'Colourless green ideas sleep furiously' is the standard example from philosophy, but note (1) the *quest* for meaning that this sequence triggers, and (2) that to anyone brought up on Bob Dylan songs, or interested in conservation politics, even this comes close to metaphorical sense.

In case I am giving you cause for concern, consider that much of our daily mental activity when we are not 'on task' is taken up with divergent speculation at least as unusual as this. In the longer term it pays off; it generates novel, humorous and creative insights and solutions once in a while. We are probably all intuitively aware of something like this going on when we come across a new idea that functions, at both a conceptual and an emotional level, as a key piece of an incomplete jigsaw puzzle enabling us to see a new 'picture'. We also have inside our heads the facilities to put items of information derived from incoming stimuli on 'hold'; dredge up concordant information from memory; run a series of simulations vaguely akin to computer models; select the best one (that is, the best match and the one we think from experience is most likely to lead to reinforcement), and then behave according to this programme, changing course in the light of feedback from environmental effects.

The main idea here is that of *anticipated reinforcement*, gauged through the setting up in systematic form of 'thought experiments': 'Now what would happen if I did x rather than y?' The answer is likely to be based on prior experience of similar situations. Cognitive postulates of this type have given rise to the notion of *covert conditioning* (Homme 1965) where 'operant thoughts' derived from prior experience are reinforced or extinguished according to whether they add constructively to a problem-solving formula (via CRs) and are likely to pay off for the individual when it is translated into behaviour. Thus, when we think of solving our financial problems by robbing a bank, the thoughts are usually extinguished quite quickly by other associations about the possible consequences, except where, 'just for the fun of it' (that is, for the emotional feedback), we deliberately control the mental drama to make sure we get away undetected. I am now thinking of the final scene in *The Italian Job* and I *think* I know how [. . .]

Analyses of this type of problem-solving behaviour in traditional stimulus–response terms are also available (Skinner 1974), but they are exceedingly complex and cumbersome, and quite often the game is just not worth the candle.

The view that environmental influences do not simply enter the brain as stimuli and leave as responses in 'ping-pong' fashion is hard to resist. Just what kind of cognitive 'pinball machine' they do go through before they re-emerge over time as effects, and often quite divergent and unusual effects at that, is that growth area in psychological research and in neuroscience – which through imaging techniques can plot the interaction of brain sites: so much so that a new field of cognitive science is with us (Dennett 1991).

One can trace back this interest to the Greek philosophers – the introspection of Wilhelm Wundt (1907); the 'metabehaviourism' of Tolman (1932); the observations of Vygotsky (1962) that thinking in language follows from the social pressure to communicate with others about plans, play, work, things and actions, not the other way around; the work of Jean Piaget (1958) on stages in intellectual development – to modern preoccupations with the principles of artificial intelligence and attempts to apply them to the study of human behaviour. The complex models that are emerging have one thing in common: they all serve to refute Cartesian notions of a separate, internal, calculating system directed *sometimes* by the 'will' towards problem-solving activity in the exterior world. They all stress the incorporatedness of the dynamics of the external world, past and present, in consciousness.

For practical purposes the important question is: Can we successfully intervene through the medium of language to alter preferred but not necessarily accurate or useful cognitive patterns, beliefs, 'mental maps', attributions, ways of seeing and so on, so that more adaptive *behaviours* are generated? Let us address the problem through an analogy. If we think of cognitive structures as forming a proposed plan for a building project (future behaviour), could we alter the shape of the eventual building by changing the plan – or does it all still depend largely on how the builder has done things in the past (learning history); whether he has the skill to do anything different (repertoire); whether he could be bothered to work on a building of a different shape (motivation/reinforcement); whether such a building would 'work' or whether it would collapse in the face of environmental stresses (longer term reinforcement)? These questions need to be approached with caution. As we saw in Chapters 1 and 2 the automatic assumption that changing thinking readily changes behaviour has often led to ineffective clinical methods being used. In fact, we know rather more about the power of non-coercively induced behavioural change to alter thinking.

What then is the form of a 'cognitive structure' and what effects can these be seen to have on behaviour? It could be argued that once again we are in danger of reifying an activity and making it into a 'thing'. Certainly we have combinations of neurones programmed to fire in certain combinations rather than others, but this is hard for most of us to imagine. Even harder to imagine is that preferred patterns and preferred combinations of connections – like well-worn pathways across fields – are influenced by experience in early childhood while the brain is still developing. So the environment, particularly our early environment, gets inside us at a physical level, influencing subsequent learning.

The contents of the skull are dense. It is dark in there. But it is often imagined to be hollow, and filled with the light and sound of experience. So we heuristically infer that we have cognitive structures because the private processing of information about environmental contingencies tends to follow certain patterns. We quickly learn that stimuli are not always what they seem, that not all brightly coloured tablets are sweets and that not all 'sincere offers of help' are sincere offers of help, and that sometimes the absence of stimuli predicts much:

> 'Is there any other point to which you would wish to draw my attention?'
> 'To the curious incident of the dog in the night time.'
> 'The dog did nothing in the night time.'
> 'That was the curious incident', remarked Sherlock Holmes.
>
> (Conan Doyle, *Silver Blaze*)

Thus in some cases it is an *absence* of concern or fellow feeling that gives us clues as to the origins of problems (see the case example on p. 236).

Given the niche-filling pressures of natural selection (e.g. camouflage), responding to the surface features of stimuli would always have been dangerous for our primitive ancestors – as in different ways it still is – and so the behaviour of *interpreting* readily attracts reinforcement. As an activity, it contains the following elements:

☐ An examination of sensory data in great detail.

☐ The action of looking at the *context* of stimuli to establish their meaning (a pie cooling in the kitchen evokes quite a different set of responses from a pie cooling in a field).

☐ Responding to the images which stimuli evoke in our heads through classical conditioning. For example, if I write *red car* it is virtually impossible for you not to 'see' a red car. This image may be followed by an association with Redcar (the place), then with horse-racing, or with any other number of items linked with the image by prior knowledge or experience.

☐ Attempts to establish causality and intent (a hand placed unexpectedly on the shoulder can mean friendly support or the sack).

☐ The action of looking at relations between stimuli: two sets of stimuli are not just one set plus one set. Their conjunction can produce quite different implications. The client who assures us that things are getting better to the accompaniment of non-verbal signals of anxiety may be said to be 'adopting a strategy' (for any one of several different purposes). Only further interpretation of these conjoined events, perhaps followed by some careful encouragement, will discover the true meaning or intent contained in the behaviour; that is, the effect it is designed to have, or the internal state it is designed to conceal. In these cases, usually, 'believe the behaviour' is good advice.

☐ Stimuli produce a range of conditioned associations only partly stored in the memory. These are the raw materials on which future computations about how best to behave are made. In addition, they help trigger and sustain emotional reactions which then enter the equation as inhibitors or enhancers of particular behavioural options. Thus if we recall that last time we were in a particular kind of fix we 'stuck to our guns' and this image is accompanied by pleasant feelings of control, then unless there are powerful contra-indications present, we are unlikely to hesitate long before repeating this sort of sequence.

☐ We use the facility of language (inner speech) to talk to ourselves about contingencies: 'Now wait a minute [warily], someone must simply have *dropped* this pie, there's *bound* to be a logical explanation, bit surreal though, shades of Magritte [. . .]'.

☐ The use of previously reinforced and shaped problem-solving strategies. We manipulate data in pre-set ways. There are many possible variables here. For example, we may have learned that *speed* in decision-making is crucial, and so we select a course of action on the basis of little detailed evidence that this plan will 'pay off'. Or we may tend to 'weigh' such issues (scan and re-scan the data) because we have learned that precipitate action leads to regrets. Similarly, we may approach a problem (a complex set of contingencies) on the assumption that it provides yet further evidence that others are out to get us. Or, in the absence of any well-practised methods of computing likely outcome, that it provides yet further evidence that we are getting 'past it' and can no longer cope. These *thinking styles* give rise to 'self-concepts'; that is, to views of our likely efficacy in influencing the environment, our abilities in discriminating among complex stimuli and so on.

☐ 'Insight (cognitive) learning' may occur. The process here is one of scanning outer (environmental) stimuli, and inner (physical/emotional) stimuli, and by manipulating, or even deliberately suspending the rules by which such events are assessed, coming up with highly original responses. (I've just heard an actor in a radio play, on in the background, say, 'nothing is ever perfect'. Thought, automatically, about my manuscript, then about a few glitches; then said to myself: 'depends on the magnification level you are using', so conjuring a concept from somewhere else entirely.) In man, these creative responses often attract generalised reinforcement. They produce a satisfactory feeling of cleverness.

Together these factors give the experience of 'insight', or creative problem-solving, its unique 'Eureka!' feel. In addition, most kinds of problem-solving, however refined, take place against a background of negative reinforcement possibilities provided by worry and anxiety. We often experience relief when we reach a tenable solution to a problem which has been bothering us, or use our 'wits' to escape a seemingly unavoidable, troublesome, obligation.

☐ The development of rules. Human beings can produce what seem like entirely novel and spontaneous responses because they learn the abstract rules that govern the relation and succession of stimuli, and the likely effects of particular actions. This is particularly evident in language development where the rules are born in us, reflecting evolutionary influences about things, kinds of things, and kinds of action, yet lead to the point of view of an inferred, controlling I (see Pinker 2004 – do read this, its full of insights). Rule-following behaviour is sparked off by hosts of discriminative stimuli present in the environment, and the application of existing rules to new combinations of stimuli can lead to new combinations of responses. This kind of computation gives to human behaviour its special 'knight's move' characteristics.

It could be objected that not all thought processes are so consciously strategic as in the list given above. Cognitive patterns of these types give us important clues as to how clients develop problems, and why they are resistant to extinction (therefore they will be discussed in more detail in Part Three). For example, in the case of 'daydreaming' or contemplation, the thoughts we experience are not driven by an urgent need to come up with a quick behavioural policy; quite a lot goes on when we lie in a darkened room before sleep. The philosopher Gilbert Ryle had this to say about thinking of this kind:

> Not all pondering or musing is problem tackling. While some walking is exploring and some walking is trying to get to a destination, still some walking is merely strolling around. Similarly while some meditating or ruminating is exploratory, and some, like multiplying, is travelling on business, still some is just re-visiting familiar country and some is just cogitative strolling for cogitative strolling's sake.
>
> (Ryle 1979: 28)

But then you never know what you might encounter on a cogitative stroll – an until now unrealised danger, or a solution to a long-standing puzzle.

Ryle's is an important distinction, but not one which seriously threatens the analysis already developed. We have long known from studies in physiological psychology that the brain cannot easily do nothing, not even in sleep. It is just not 'wired up' that way. The system is at an optimal level of arousal when it is working away. Far below this level, strange things begin to happen. These are symptoms of 'stimulus hunger' which can even include hallucinations and depersonalisation. We all experience something a little like them on long motorway drives when we conjure up people walking in the road (so-called motorway ghosts); it is just the brain in 'what if?' mode.

Ruminative thoughts, although not about urgent behavioural decisions, nevertheless are likely to be connected to more distant general contingencies. Thus, even outside depressive illness, we ruminate about our long-term future, in this case without too much anxiety, and without feelings that a solution must necessarily be found quickly. External stimulation of even a slightly unusual kind disrupts this pattern and replaces it with thought patterns geared more directly to short-term problem-solving. There is undoubtedly a role for reinforcement here too, and it is likely that relatively non-specific thinking is maintained by conditioned reinforcers (see p. 111).

If these assumptions are roughly correct, then there is no reason to view private, cognitive events as in some way disconnected, non-physical phenomena which have little to do with behaviour, nor to assume that they obey principles markedly different from those contained in the various theories of learning reviewed above. That said, we are all aware of some sequences of complex thought in the form of object, event or picture *symbols* rather than in fully formed 'photographic' images or fully formed words and sentences. These bio-electrical flashes 'stand for' things and concepts allowing us to compute from sensory experience or memory with astonishing rapidity. Musical memory, for example, conjures up images (the Bach Cantata No. 140, black horses, banks and overdrafts now – curse them; the British Airways advert employs the gliding notes of *Lakme* to distract us from the usual airport and 'in-flight' experience). Abstract thought is a challenge to cognitive psychology's attempts to say what thoughts are a bit like – internal speech, pictures, sounds, smells. In the end, we may have to accommodate the view of the philosopher who, on being asked what he thought in, answered, 'I think in thoughts'; he may be as right as the psychology professor who defined IQ as 'what intelligence tests measure'.

If the phenomenon of interpreting and thinking about stimuli and their response connections complicates matters rather, then the fact that, in man, 'the environment' virtually always includes 'the social environment' multiplies these complications many times over. A response to a response to a response is a common-enough occurrence in everyday life. Sane people, other than games theory researchers, do not try to draw such complex inter-relationships schematically, but this is not to say that they completely defeat rigorous analysis.

Social learning theory

This is a formulation that rests heavily on theories of vicarious learning (see p. 121). This conceptualisation shares many of the assumptions of cognitive theorists, and yet in Bandura's view it is compatible with many of the basic tenets of behavioural psychology. As a theory, then, it has always been well placed to help integrate a number of current trends in this discipline.

Here are two quotations that should give you the flavour of social learning theory:

> Stimuli influence the likelihood of particular behaviors through their predictive function, not because they are automatically linked to responses by occurring together. In the social learning view, contingent experiences create expectations rather than stimulus-response connections. Environmental events can predict either other environmental occurrences, or serve as predictors of the relation between actions and outcomes.
>
> (Bandura 1977: 59)

And as to the question of determinism, and whether behaviour and the learning function is powered from inside or outside the individual:

> Environments have causes, as do behaviours. It is true that behavior is regulated by its contingencies but the contingencies are partly of a person's own making. By their actions, people play an active role in producing the reinforcing contingencies that impinge upon them (as with laws and academic awards). As was previously shown, behavior partly creates the environment, and the environment influences the behavior in a reciprocal fashion. To the oft repeated dictum, 'change contingencies and you change behavior',

should be added the reciprocal side, 'change behavior and you change contingencies'. In this regress of prior causes, for every chicken discovered by a unidirectional environmentalist, a social learning theorist can identify a prior egg.

(Bandura 1977: 203)

You will have gathered that questions of *ultimate* causality do not worry Bandura very much. The fact that man is above all things a social animal means that he both creates, and is created by, these special environments. It is Bandura's view that behaviour within this huge closed circuit is dominated by two sets of influences:

☐ *Outcome expectations:* the estimate of a person that given behaviour will lead to certain outcomes.
☐ *Efficacy expectations:* representing the conviction or otherwise that one can successfully execute the behaviour required to produce a specific outcome.

These two influences are differentiated because a person can believe that a particular course of action is likely to produce certain outcomes but retain serious doubts as to whether they are capable of making the against-the-grain changes necessary to bring about these outcomes. Alternatively, they may feel that a given objective is well within their grasp, but do not actually, genuinely, value it.

These are the constituent parts of Bandura's concept of *perceived self-efficacy*. According to him, all psychological change procedures, whatever their type, are mediated through this system of beliefs about the end result of an action and the level of skill required to perform it adequately (see Figure 4.6).

Of these two elements, efficacy expectations are the most important. Attempts to modify outcome expectations by verbal persuasion alone have relatively weak and temporary effects, particularly in the face of contradictory experiences. Similarly, so-called placebo effects, though they may have an enhancing effect on therapy, are unlikely to provide a sufficient basis for lasting change, and will rarely serve in place of a logically constructed programme of help. The main effect on outcome expectations is through the strengthening of efficacy expectations perhaps by setting up small experiments and then re-evaluating.

Bandura lists the following sources of efficacy expectations:

☐ Performance accomplishments: gained through participation, and desensitisation to perceived threats or failings which inhibit an approach to feared circumstances. (Bandura sees reinforcement as an *incentive-giving or regulating* influence, cognitively mediated and reflected upon.)

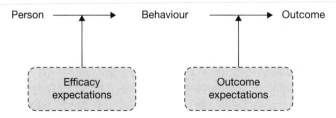

Figure 4.6 Efficacy and outcome expectations
Source: Adapted from Bandura (1977).

☐ Vicarious experience: gained through watching others perform tasks with an element of risk (modelling).
☐ Verbal persuasion: by suggestion, guided self-instruction, interpretations and so on.
☐ Reducing fears associated with particular performances by *imagining* oneself coping in a step-by-step manner. Other approaches include: relaxation techniques and graded exposure (imagining and discussing one's worst fears for lengthy periods as a way of mentally extinguishing them).

Bandura suggests that the main effort of the would-be helper should go into directly modifying thoughts and feelings which affect perceived self-efficacy. This is in line with many of the treatment procedures and styles already made use of by therapists. However (referring to research into pathological fears), he adds a word of caution – and this is the point where his theory is connected to mainstream cognitive-behavioural practice:

> Developments in the field of behavioural change reveal two major divergent trends. This difference is especially evident in the modification of dysfunctional inhibitions and defensive behaviour. On the one hand, explanations of change processes are becoming more cognitive. On the other hand, it is performance based treatments that have retained their power in effecting useful clinical changes. Regardless of the method involved, treatments implemented with an actual performance element achieve results consistently superior to those in which fears are eliminated via cognitive representations of threats. Symbolic procedures have much to contribute as components of multiform performance-oriented approach, but they are usually insufficient by themselves.
>
> (Bandura 1977: 78)

All this is in line with the review of early outcome studies contained in Chapter 1, but the situation has changed over the years. Predominantly cognitive approaches, but with *some* behavioural exposure and practice, do as well in depression and anxiety as behavioural approaches, with *some* examination of cognitive interpretations. However, the 'purer' forms of either, if they can ever be found, do less well than the amalgam. Objections to Bandura's theory fall into three groups. First, those which object to it on the grounds that it is less *parsimonious* (economical) than existing formulations, and that the predictions made by the theory can be adequately explained by existing knowledge (see e.g. Eysenck's cogent analysis: Eysenck 1978).

The argument here is that there is no need for Bandura's theory, since classical conditioning theory does the job in a more simple and more easily verifiable way. Second, there are objections that Bandura's theory contains ambiguities, particularly in the precise differences between outcome and efficacy expectations. However, in clinical practice, there is a growing body of research to show that modelling procedures and social skills training have useful if not unilaterally striking effects (see Heinssen *et al.* 2000; Emmelkamp 2004). Bandura's contention that behavioural change occurs mainly through a strengthening of perceived self-efficacy (as in motivational interviewing approaches) is as yet unproven.

At this stage then, cognitive-mediational theories of this type have made great gains in the research literature, and no longer need to be approached with caution. They offer the possibility of a meeting ground for therapists of different persuasions. In addition, they are attractive in that they deal in an ungrudging fashion with the private 'world within the skin' of which, however awkward in scientific terms, we all have personal, though not objectively accurate experience. Further, they are likely to be welcomed by those working outside controlled clinical settings, who have to rely to a considerable extent upon programmes that aim to develop a degree of *self*-control in clients.

I have already given some indication of the places where existing formulations are relatively inadequate and my own position is that existing theories provide an adequate explanation of the various problems that fall within their scope; a strong skeleton structure which provides a secure framework on which to base experiments in areas where the therapeutic implications of existing formulations are difficult to implement (for example, the hard-to-motivate families struggling with multiple problems at once, which make up a solid proportion of most social care and health case loads and in the psychoses). As long as the established standard of evidence, and the established ways of evaluating therapeutic outcomes are kept in sight, what is there to lose? Certainly there is much to gain, providing that we proceed according to the results of the kind of research reviewed in Chapters 1 and 2.

We have seen so far that the special nature of human behaviour is conferred on us through what Pavlov called 'the second signalling system' – language, and through it the facility for 'inner speech' and symbolic imagery, which enables us to act upon the environment in an extraordinarily strategic way by conducting mental experiments to see what might happen if we did A or B, *before* we actually do it (see Pinker's *Words and Rules* (1999) and *The Stuff of Thought* (2007)). On the face of it then, there is such a *prima facie* case for supposing that in some cases we may be able to intervene effectively in the causal chain at *this* point: (1) by suggesting an alternative evaluation of the data on which the client is basing decisions or lack of them; (2) by challenging actions based on negative self-concepts ('I'm bound to mess it up'; 'I'm just not good at . . .') which do not seem to us justified by the evidence or by any comprehensive view of the individual's potential; (3) by trying to substitute different imagery from that evoked by existing stimuli; (4) by trying to get the individual to consider new evidence on his or her existing view of personal efficacy; (5) by presenting a different interpretation of the likelihood of certain positive or negative consequences occurring; and (6) by trying to reinforce a different pattern of self-commentary to run alongside particular actions. To this list I would add the rider: that effectiveness is likely to be strongly influenced by the extent to which therapists can overcome any professional agoraphobia and abandon their computers and the office for a bit, which often means (gulp) going outside to where clients live (about 80 per cent of our time is now spent inside), visiting the school, or whatever job centres are called this year, enlisting the help of partners and families, etc. to ensure that the trial *behaviours* that occur as a result of such approaches are reinforced.

All these caveats aside, we now have intellectual riches to back our endeavours as never before. The *behavioural*, not the cognitive task remains; which is to extend these approaches to those who do not readily self-refer or initially cooperate.

5 Emotional reactions

Feelings let us catch a glimpse of the organism in full biological swing, a reflection of the mechanisms of life itself as they go about their business. Were it not for the possibility of sensing body states that are inherently ordained to be painful or pleasurable, there would be no suffering or bliss, no longing or mercy, no tragedy or glory in the human condition.

(Damassio 1994: xvii)

The nature of emotion

Although it is understandable that psychologists and neuroscientists concentrate upon the extremes of these stirred-up states of feeling, and clinicians upon severe exacerbations, it should not be forgotten that lower level expressions of emotion are with all of us throughout each day. Otherwise there would be no feelings of mild contentment; basic decency; no sense that we might just need to keep our eye on a problem, no worries in need of remediation one of these days; no warm glows, guardedness; no vicarious, everyday pity felt in front of the TV screen, in fact nothing much worth having at all.

Every single point about research on the nature of learning in Chapter 4 is dependent upon emotional arousal. Classical conditioning works mainly through this experience (CRs), but so does the operant model (S^ds and S^As) since external rewards and aversive events work through acquired associations. Modelling and vicarious learning also depend upon what we are motivated to copy or not. The cognitive factors, too, are strongly influenced by arousal for there are few thought sequences which are not coloured by an emotional 'backing track'. Some cognitions are *triggered* by emotion, 'A mysterious Alliance' as Damassio calls it (1994: 83). Whatever the emphases in favoured disciplinary diagrams (see p. 5) we are, make no mistake, dealing here with an inseparably *integrated* system of interaction between the external and internal environment, sometimes beneficially, sometimes not. Charles Darwin tried to get us to understand this in *The Descent of Man* (1871) when he wrote of 'the indelible stamp of lowly origins which humans bear in their bodily frame' and we would-be-helpers need to understand the patterns of these skeins of emotion, cognition and behaviour when we search for snags in them.

However, professionals often balk at the necessarily unemotional treatment of emotion when it becomes a subject of study, preferring to hear more subjective descriptions of its admittedly marvellous range and subtlety. This reflects a belief that it is better simply to experience emotion than to analyse it. Anyone who has had to take *As You Like It* apart, line by line, or to dissect a Mozart piano concerto note by note will allow that there is something to be said for this point of view. But if we wish to understand something as completely as possible – even something as intensely personal as emotion – then we have to analyse it thoroughly. This is certainly the case if we wish to use our knowledge to help someone with 'an emotional problem' – that undifferentiated catch-all of psycho-social assessments. We need to know what emotions are, what instigates them, whether they cause behaviour or are a concomitant upon it (I can give you the answer right now – both), what is their relationship to cognition and whether, or how, they can be changed. Sometimes this may even leave us with a greater respect for these experiences.

Certain basic forms of emotionally laden responding are inborn; for example, fear, crying, clutching, smiling and so on. This does not mean that they are unaffected by environment, which shapes these reactions from the moment of birth and teaches us how to cry so as to attract our parents' attention, and later when to suppress crying; what to fear and what not to fear. However, the idea that incoming stimuli automatically trigger emotions neglects the immediate modifying influence of learning – through which processes we are sensitised to some signals, or inured to others. Think about driving: two heavy metal objects, one with us in it, approach each other at a combined impact speed of, say, 100mph. A three-inch movement of the right hand means certain death, but we are calmly chatting or listening to the radio. However, it was not *always* so, was it?

For some, meeting a group of unfamiliar people is like taking a driving test, but then, in more complex situations, though we may be highly aroused or depressed, exactly *what* we are feeling and why involves cognition more. However, such appraisals and attributions are often inaccurate and self-deceiving.

More complicatedly, some emotional responses are (not in a Freudian way) unconsciously or semi-consciously handled by the back of the brain as routine 'seen this before, no need for the cortical department to get involved yet' events:

> When I say I'm angry, I may be, but I might also be wrong. I might really be afraid, or jealous, or some combination of all of these. Donald Hebb pointed out long ago that outside observers are far more accurate at judging a person's true emotional state than is the person himself . . . perhaps many of the things we do, including the appraisal of the emotional significance of events in our lives and the expression of emotional behaviours in response to those appraisals, do not depend on consciousness or even on processes that we have conscious access to.
>
> (Le Doux 2003: 65)

Another way of saying this is that the seat of evaluation in the brain (the hypothalamus, the amygdala, the limbic system) has often delivered the signalled raw implications of a set of stimuli (good, bad, threatening) well before the cognitive (cortical) appraisal systems have even registered *what* the stimuli are, let alone what they presage. This explains why many clients with anxiety disorders or phobias find it so difficult to talk about exactly *what* is feared and why and when: 'it just came over me' is a typical response.

The experience of basic emotions is largely dependent upon physiological changes that occur within the body predominantly as a result of external stimulation (but not entirely: remember colic). The relevant systems lie within the sympathetic nervous system – the site of fight/flight readiness – and within the parasympathetic nervous system (located in the cranial nerve nuclei and the lower spinal cord) which acts to moderate energy availability and hormonal secretions. (The relationship between the two is analogous to the dual control of limb movements by extensor and retractor muscles.)

When some aspect of the environment triggers either a primary physiological reflex, or a powerful conditioned reflex, a number of biologically functional (but not necessarily socially functional) things occur rapidly together.

☐   Heart rate increases, vasocontraction puts up the blood pressure, and hormonal release (e.g. adrenalin) maintains this.

☐   We start to breathe more rapidly.

☐   Skin pores dilate to aid cooling of the body in the face of potential exertion.

☐   The blood sugar level rises to meet the potential increase in energy demands from the muscles.

☐   The pupils of the eyes dilate to let in all available light.

☐   The salivary flow dries up and keeps our throats clear for rapid mouth breathing.

☐   Blood flow is directed to the vital centres (that is, the brain and large muscles).

☐   Movements in the gastro-intestinal system are greatly reduced, but in extreme cases the bladder and rectum contract (a common but little discussed aspect of combat situations).

☐   The capacity of the blood to clot is strengthened by chemical and enzymic action in case we are injured.

☐   Muscle tone increases.

As previously discussed, these mechanisms, derived from evolution, help to prepare the body for action (fight/flight) in the face of danger. Other stimuli evoke different combinations of effects – as in the case of sexual arousal where some of the above mechanisms are involved, but are accompanied by powerful sensations of pleasure and the release of different hormones – which reactions are conditioned to other previously neutral stimuli such as sights, sounds, objects, touch and other sensations.

Neuro-physiologists long ago located specialised centres deep within the brains of animals which seem to be responsible for producing pleasure and pain. Olds (1956) began the experimental study of this by inserting fine electrodes into the brains of laboratory rats. The animals in these studies operated a lever controlling a mild electric current, continually forgoing food, water and the opportunity to mate so as to stimulate themselves. They did this to the point of exhaustion. A small repositioning of the electrode produced equally strong pain-and-avoidance reactions. It has been found that similar, more interconnected, centres in the brains of humans provide the physiological basis for reinforcement (see Le Doux 2003).

There are several theories of emotion that build upon these basic physiological components. Let us discuss these in historical sequence.

Theories of emotion

'We do not run away because we feel fear, we feel fear because we run away' observed William James (1890). According to the James–Lange theory of emotion it is our perception of combinations of physiological changes of this type that we call 'emotion'. Fear is both the product and the precursor of the most obvious and effective types of action for bipeds to take. The cause of our behaviour here is the escape-behaviour-provoking stimulus, whether genetically programmed (as in the case of large, looming objects, loud noises, sudden movements) or learned by association. The bodily changes experienced are, in the first place, concomitant not causal (see Figure 5.1 clockwise).

However, this theory has long had its opponents. It fails, for example, to explain convincingly how we are able to appreciate the subtle differences between varieties of emotional experience. The bodily changes described above, though they may occur in slightly different combinations or at different levels of intensity, are relatively crude. One critic (Cannon 1927) pointed out that the nerve supply to some of these internal organs is insufficient to account for the tremendous speed and intensity of emotional reactions. Having tried (and failed) to induce replica emotions in individuals by chemical and other means (e.g. the injection of adrenalin)

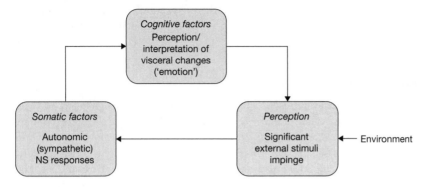

Figure 5.1 Emotional arousal (James–Lange theory)

he turned his attention to the role of the thalamus in the brain's central core. In association with the Danish physiologist Bard, he developed the view that this centre acted as a kind of 'telephone exchange' for incoming stimuli, rerouting 'messages' to both the cerebral cortex and (via the sympathetic 'trunk lines') to the other organs of the body concerned with emergency action. The key difference here is that (counter-intuitively, since we feel that emotions originate elsewhere in the body) the brain is the seat of emotion (see Figure 5.2 right to left).

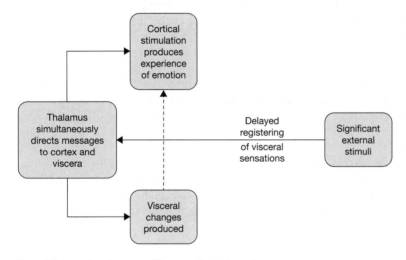

Figure 5.2 Emotional arousal (Cannon–Bard theory)

Source: Adapted from Hilgard *et al.* (1979).

More recent research has identified centres for the processing of emotion-arousing stimuli in the hypothalamus and the limbic system. One ingenious method of studying the relative part played by concomitant visceral responses and by higher centres is to study people with high spinal cord lesions placed in emotion-arousing circumstances, or volunteer subjects given temporarily paralysing drugs. In this way the dimension of visceral stimulation is controlled out. There is no doubt that people affected in this way, either by accident or by experimental design, experience *something* similar to ordinary emotion, which they are disposed to act upon. But it seems from their descriptions to be qualitatively different from what most of us feel. Here are the comments made by a quadriplegic clinical subject in one such study:

It's a sort of cold anger. Sometimes I get angry when I see some injustice. I yell and cuss and raise hell . . . but it doesn't seem to have the heat. It's a mental kind of anger.

(Hilgard *et al.* 1979: 336)

Cognition and emotion

The dominant theme in present-day research is that of the role of cognition, appraisal and memory in emotion. It may be (in line with the James–Lange theory) that the visceral changes we experience as emotion are relatively undifferentiated (in line also with the Cannon–Bard conclusion; see Figure 5.3) but that an 'overlay' of cognitive factors gives them added subtlety. The current consensus is that cognitions alter and direct emotional (visceral) experience, and that emotions strongly influence cognitions – all in reciprocal fashion (see Damassio 1994; Le Doux 2003). It is in the middle of this complex set of interactions plus chemical effects (e.g. by serotonin levels) that CBT approaches have their influence. This via a rational reinterpretation regarding the prospect of control of emotions, or experimenting with emotions and their behavioural manifestations (as in exposure therapy).

There is common sense in the view that waiting for an important exam to begin or going out on a first date produce, objectively, if not subjectively, rather similar sets of feelings: a tightening of the abdominal muscles, mild palpitations, an inability to think straight and so on. An increasingly accepted view is that fine gradations of emotion are the result of the cognitive labelling and attribution of visceral experience according to the nature of the evoking stimulus and our memories of similar past experiences. This view opens the way to an amalgamation of the various themes discussed so far (see Figure 5.3).

In some cases of mild arousal, cognitive variables will be predominant: in other cases of strong arousal, physiological variables will largely control behaviour, and thinking will merely reflect upon this or attempt to 'steer' us on a careering course.

Where clients have learned that a particular collection of stimuli is hazardous and respond with a high level of physiological involvement (experienced as fear or, if arousal is less strong, future-oriented and continuous, as with anxiety), this is certain to inhibit cognitive information processing about how best to respond. Whether the perceived threat, say, of being the only female in a group of male strangers has special properties in itself for the individual based on myth, knowledge or hearsay, or because of a prior learning experience, or because the situation is associated with other feared happenings, makes little difference. The vicious circle of high emotional involvement, thought-of escape behaviour and/or faulty and inhibited adaptive performance increases the likelihood of an adverse reaction and of confirmation of the original association. Phrases such as 'cognitive restructuring' or 'cognitive appraisal' – used to indicate how crude physiological reactions are turned into more subtle and specific emotional experience – remain somewhat global, but can, as we shall see in Part Three, be further broken down.

What mechanisms are at work? In a series of classic experiments, Schacter and his co-workers (Schacter & Singer 1962; Schacter 1964) sought to implicate causal attribution. Figure 5.4 gives a summary of the key factors.

In usual, everyday circumstances Schacter believed cognitions and physical arousal to be highly interrelated, one leading to the other and vice versa. Sometimes, however, they are interdependent. This is exemplified by the early work of Maranon (1924). He injected 210 patients with Epinephrine, which is sympathetic-like in its effects, and recorded their introspections. Seventy-one per cent reported only physical effects and 29 per cent reported in terms of emotion, but the labels which they applied to their feelings were of the 'as if' kind.

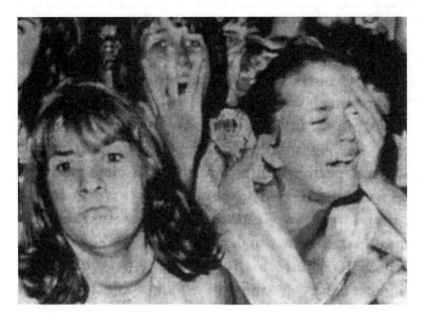

Figure 5.3 Young women in a state of ecstasy at a rock concert, not showing shock or grief

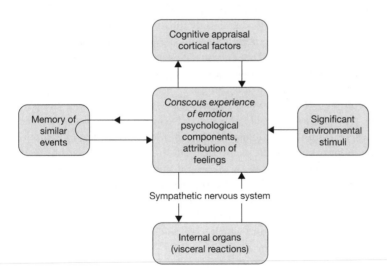

Figure 5.4 The elements of emotional arousal (right to left)

They said they felt 'as if' they were afraid or excited. Maranon could only produce 'genuine' emotional reactions by providing them with appropriate cognitive labels. Schacter suggests that the 71 per cent who did not show this effect in Maranon's study had a perfectly appropriate cognition to explain their altered state: the injection. This point led Schacter on to the question which guided much of his subsequent research: What would be the result of a state induced by a covert (non-explicable) injection of Epinephrine? (see Strongman 1987).

Schacter's volunteer subjects, who knew they were to be given a drug under medical supervision, were led to believe that this was 'Suproxin' – allegedly a vitamin-based compound. In fact they were injected with either Epinephrine or a saline placebo (imagine trying to get this past an ethics review these days). This experiment exposed subjects to three different conditions: (1) 'Epinephrine-informed', where subjects were told of possible 'side-effects' such as arousal, palpitations, flushing, faster respiration, etc.; (2) 'Epinephrine-ignorant', where nothing was said to prepare subjects for the effects; and (3) 'Epinephrine-misinformed', where subjects were misled into expecting unlikely 'side-effects', such as itching or headaches.

It was then contrived that subjects would wait in a room to allow the 'Suproxin' to become absorbed, and then they would be asked to complete certain 'vision tests'. In fact, the rooms contained experimental confederates who exhibited two types of behaviour: (1) anger, supposedly in response to the increasingly demanding and personal nature of a questionnaire which subjects were asked to fill out; (2) euphoria, where the confederate behaved in an outgoing, excited way and played basketball with paper balls. The responses of the subjects were recorded through a two-way mirror.

Outcome measures in this experiment were (1) a self-report questionnaire, embedded in which were two scaled questions about mood states: 'How irritated, angry or annoyed do you feel now?'; (2) covert observations as to the extent to which the behaviour of naive subjects came to match that of confederates (admittedly somewhat 'soft' measures). The results showed that when subjects had no explanation for their induced emotional states they made sense of them in line with the local environmental conditions – modelled anger and euphoria – in which they were placed. Subjects who had an explanation (the injection, and a true expectation of its effects) did not – though they felt exactly the same bodily reactions.

These fascinating if ethically unsettling experiments lend support to the proposition that cognition – more precisely interpretation and attribution – play a major part in colouring our relatively crude physiological 'surges' their unique sense of origins and implication.

Current research suggests a continuum, from strong feelings with little cognitive justification – 'I do not like thee Dr Fell, the reason why I cannot tell' – to the more usual interplay of cognition and emotion typical of everyday life, through to background moods such as mild anxiety or uneasiness where ruminative cognitions play the dominant role. This model suggests that therapeutic opportunities exist in the extinction of arousal which has been conditioned to certain objects, social situations or places, and in reviewing with clients any unlikely or self-damaging patterns of thinking – 'No one would be able to understand or forgive me if I gagged over my food and spoiled everyone's evening' (as in the Case example on p. 104). Given the continuum discussed above, it makes most sense to construct programmes which contain both elements, and which to some degree educate clients about the origins and the biological functions of emotions.

There are more complicated and detailed flow charts to be had which resemble benefit entitlement-charts, but I am not sure what actual benefit they have for practitioners or for increasing our understanding (see Le Doux 2003).

Anxiety

Anxiety is anticipated punishment. It is a strong motivational force in our lives, acting through the negative reinforcement opportunities it provides to propel us into early, pro-active, precautionary modes of behaviour. It is easy to see how it was selected by evolution process on 'better safe than sorry' principles. Indeed, a measure of background arousal, a tingle of

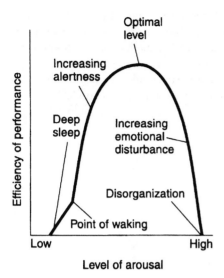

Figure 5.5 *Figure 5.5* Emotional arousal and performance
Source: Hilgard *et al.* (1979) (after Hebb 1972).

anticipation or a frisson of danger helps us to engage effectively with problems, both at a cognitive and a behavioural level – that 'firing on all four cylinders', 'mid-season form' feeling which we learn to associate with competence and mastery. The problems associated with arousal are demonstrated in Figure 5.5.

The relationships on this graph are: performance accomplishment as measured in different studies of task efficiency in the psychological laboratory; and measured level of arousal (via the GSR). The most important dimension is the rapid fall-off of performance efficiency which follows optimal arousal. Only modest additional increments are required before emotions begin seriously to interfere with, and thus disrupt efficiency. (Proponents of the new 'goading' schools of management and 'total quality assurance', please note.)

'Anxiety', whether as one more source of unhappiness; as something that leads to mal-adaptive associations (e.g. social phobias); as a basis for self-defeating avoidance, or in the form of generalised anxiety states (see p. 44), is a constant feature of our work with clients. Cognitive-behavioural techniques for dealing with excesses of this everyday phenomenon are based on the following aims:

☐   Greater understanding of the nature and origins of anxiety – why it is useful in some situations and maladaptive in others.
☐   Accurate attribution of sources of anxiety, which tend quickly to generalise.
☐   Clear identification and evaluation of the origins of perceived threat, from most to least provocative, and from most to least rational, so that priorities can be assigned to dealing with the sources of current reactions.
☐   Counselling to encourage the client in a rational, step-by-step approach to problem-solving, and coping mechanisms for keeping catastrophic thoughts at bay.
☐   Relaxation, exposure and desensitisation approaches, environmental experimentation.
☐   Reinforcement (self or extraneous) for attempts to gain more control of the environment of provocative stimuli, particularly in the face of unreasonable demands.

Some clients are trapped between competing emotional states. In certain neurotic conditions, for example, clients, as a result of vulnerable personalities (see Eysenck 1965; Claridge 1985; Sheldon & Macdonald 2009) and adverse life experiences, set off in pursuit of contradictory, unattainable, self-defeating life goals (e.g. to be as good a person as my mother's sacrifices require) and so hover between anxiety-avoidance on the approach trajectory, and guilt-driven behaviour on the withdrawal trajectory (see Figure 5.6).

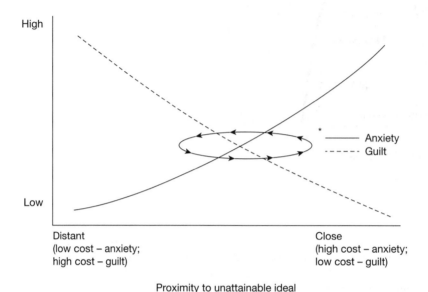

Figure 5.6 A model of neurotic decision-making: approach/avoidance conflicts

Note
• Typical pattern of approach/avoidance behaviour.

But remember that not all strong emotions, or even feelings of hopelessness, are inappropriate given the circumstances in which they arise. In cases of bereavement and profound loss, one may have more concern for clients who are *not* (one hopes temporarily) swamped by strong feelings of loss, anger and doubt regarding the impracticality of any future, independent existence. Such emotions need to be acknowledged, absorbed and confirmed as normal – 'the price we pay for loving' and usually worth it. In other cases (e.g. in some juvenile cases, in child welfare or child abuse work), we may occasionally feel that clients are not anxious *enough* in the face of the consequences which lie in wait, and measured doses of motivating anxiety may have to be introduced.

The main point of the foregoing discussion is to alert the reader to the fact that there is an 'internal environment' (our bodies and its visceral sensations) as well as an external environment. Both are replete with opportunities for conditioning; both are the subject of cognitive appraisal and attribution exercises, but again, not always accurately carried out.

Thus far in this book we have been considering the contextual and theoretical factors which we need to understand, change or draw upon to be effective practitioners of this approach. The emphasis now changes to consideration of skills and techniques, beginning with assessment.

Part Three

Intervention techniques including assessment

6   Assessment, monitoring and evaluation

Truth itself, however unpleasant, is interesting always. But the conditions of storytelling are harsh; they demand that scene shall follow scene.

(Virginia Woolf)

Everything is what it is because it got that way.

(d'Arcy Thompson)

These three themes/strategies are being taken together, so interrelated are they. For what can be claimed at the end of an intervention depends substantially on the quality, i.e. the validity and reliability, of the original assessment, the goals which this leads to and how progress regarding their achievement is tracked. Working the other way, the quality and accuracy of assessments, which often in our field include measures of risk to self or to others (I am annually astonished to see that I need at least £6.5 million professional insurance cover, and that, not being a banker, I could possibly do this much damage in a given hour). Such factors can only be judged against indicators of progress or lack of it and against the outcomes which follow. Thus there is a question, important for the development of our skills, as to how confident we can be that any progress is due to the approach we have taken, and not to background, collateral factors.

Before we get into procedures of assessment there are some general points to make about the process.

1   First, we should make sure that there is one. This is less of a problem in private practice, but in the NHS and Social Services there are many competing demands on our time and clients are often referred at short notice, in urgent circumstances, and have waited a long time for treatment. This is particularly the case with depression where medication has failed to have its expected impact. A recent survey by the Royal College of General Practitioners shows: (a) that since the NICE guidelines, most GPs would like to be able to make referrals to CBT practitioners; but also (b) only 15 per cent of patients receive help within two months, and two months is quite a long time in cases of severe depression. The point being that, having already been medically assessed and placed on a disorderly waiting list, the clients/patients who we eventually get to see are often not disposed to go through their life histories again, or to fill in psychological assessment forms; they feel they need help *now*. In this they are probably wrong, but understandably wrong.

The issue of this lack of a comprehensive assessment (distinguish from a collection of reports of episodes or events in the client's past life) is a common conclusion in inquiry reports into the deaths of children or of people with serious mental illnesses over the past few decades (see Sheldon & Macdonald 2009: chs 10 and 13). I was once co-chairman of an inquiry into the death of a psychiatric outpatient. The files showed an array of letters from Social Services to the client asking him to get in touch with them again, and to his GP expressing concern that he had broken off contact and was off medication and on crack cocaine. The only problem was that: (a) he couldn't read(!); (b) that a standard letter a day was sent without noticing that no one was replying or telephoning; (c) that the GP on the file had retired three years earlier, and (d) that no one *noticed* that he hadn't replied. Thus the purpose of all this was defensive, like bookies laying off risky bets. Before he died, possibly aided by the effects of past large doses of neuroleptic medication on his heart, he, it turned out, spent most of *his* days in a cafe 100 yards away from the building where his designated helpers spent *their* days. Only the housing officer, who noticed that he had (untypically) stopped paying his rent, actually walked out of her office and went looking for him. The paperwork, the assessment of his needs, the risk assessment, were all fine, but these were effectively placed on the file for storage purposes, and as a defence against future blame. This is not what assessments should be about, otherwise we get therapeutic paralysis, which is all too common under the influence of meddling, risk-averse political initiatives which almost always make things worse in most of these sad circumstances. So what, typically, throws us off course?

2   Increasingly, the approach to assessment in CBT has been to collect together scores on standardised instruments (e.g. the Beck or Hamilton scales for depression, the Social Situations Questionnaire, the Behaviour Rating Index for Children; The Self-esteem Rating Scale) (see Fischer & Corcoran (2007) for a helpful collection of instruments with research data on their validity and reliability). This approach has now largely replaced unaided clinical judgement. It is to be recommended as an aid to accurate assessment, providing (a) that the results are shared with clients and their implications for the present plan discussed, and (b) they form part of a dynamic, regularly reviewed, person-centred assessment rather than just being lodged in files. All results require professional interpretation of their significance in *individual* cases, not just as statistical likelihoods. When things go wrong inquiry reports in both mental health and child care are almost guaranteed to recommend greater sharing of information between agencies; rarely is the *quality* of professional *judgement* examined forensically; it is as if the recorded information had the power automatically to signal its importance inductively to us (see Thiele 2006). In reality we tend to operate deductively, interrogating data against hypotheses or concerns (see Popper 1963; Sheldon 1987).

3   Assessments are often delayed (particularly in the statutory sector) by the very urgency which triggers the referral in the first place. We need to have the confidence to explain to clients that, whatever 'first aid' measures are required, there has to be an assessment not only for the client's benefit, but for our own technical purposes, so that we can accurately devise a treatment strategy. As consumers ourselves, say, of the NHS, we expect to receive one in all but the most dire circumstances. When we do not, as in the case of 'reflex prescribing' by GPs, or repeat prescriptions without obvious benefit, we feel uneasy. Most clients will accept this idea even if they have told their stories before – because they haven't told them to *you* and so you haven't been able to enquire into events, thoughts, feelings and actions.

4   There is a beguiling idea, long in circulation, particularly in social care, that 'assessment is an ongoing process'. True, but it cannot be never-ending. It needs to be thought of as a definite, concentrated, diagnostic stage near the beginning of contact, focusing on the aetiology of problems and getting clients to, as it were, rewind the videotapes of their lives and take stock.

5   A good assessment should end in a formulation, agreed as far as possible with the client, as to what went wrong and why, and a set of goals, which are logically connected to undoing or replacing this pattern. These are formal statements having some of the qualities of hypotheses, i.e. they need to be tightly phrased and so placed at risk by subsequent events. In other words, if no, or slower than expected progress is being made, then we need to be able to tell that this is the case. Revision or fine tuning can always take place or a new formulation agreed. The enemy of this process is 'flexible goals'; though democratic sounding, they can always be adapted retrospectively to what actually happens.

Distinguishing features of cognitive-behavioural assessments

The following discussion provides an outline of cognitive-behavioural assessment and distinguishes it from other approaches with which the reader may be more familiar.

☐   This form of assessment is concerned with *who does what, where, when, how often*, with *whom*, with *what* perceptions and calculations are influential along the way. It is also concerned to identify the absence or withholding of behaviours which it would normally be useful and reasonable to perform. lt deals also with the consequences which actions have for all the parties involved in them – those who are said to *have* the problem and those for whom someone else's behaviour is said to *be* a problem. The emphasis here is on both *visible*, problematic behaviour, and on the *absence* or the inadequacy of adaptive behaviour – where this could be used to reduce negative consequences for the client. Thus, early on in assessment, decisions need to be taken about (1) what behaviours are in *excess*: that is, what does the client or the people influencing him or her do *too much of* ? For example, aggressive behaviour well above what may be regarded as an unguarded response to everyday frustrations. (2) What behaviours are in *deficit*: what does the client or others do *too little of* ? For example: 'Mary has not spoken a word to any other resident of the hostel since she came here four weeks ago.' (3) What behaviours occur in the wrong place or at the wrong time? For example: 'Fred approaches people in the street and tells them about his personal problems, which reinforces their idea that he is an odd person.' To some extent this is an artificial distinction, since in the first example it could (tautologically) be said that the client *lacked* self-control or adequate means for dealing with frustration. However, it is useful in practice, and serves to remind the assessor to look out for what behaviour is and is *not* there.

☐   CBT assessment is concerned also with private sensations, such as doubts, worries, fears, frustrations and depression. It was noted in Chapter 4 that evolution has released humans from purely reflexive reactions to contemporary stimuli. Classical conditioning ensures that yesterday's learning environments exert a contemporary influence from inside us, through fears, anxieties and selective perceptions – sometimes profitably, sometimes self-defeatingly. We are driven to look for *meaning* in stimuli and we plan ahead, behaving a little like amateur scientists. By these cognitive processes we sometimes achieve breakthroughs in understanding and in preparing for the uncertain future, but we are equally capable of misreading evidence, taking undue note of limited data, and seeing what we expect or want to see (Sheldon 1987; Sutherland 1992; Gigerenzer 2007). The key concept here is *attribution* which means the assignment of causes and motives to the behaviour of others or ourselves (Heider (1958) and Bem (1972) were the pioneers). Clients talking about their problems often reveal patterns of either unconvincingly *internal* attributions or of unconvincingly *external* attributions; for example, a depressed person who feels that he has let his family down badly but can give only a few minor examples as to how, based largely on hindsight; or conversely, a child with a history of aggression and delinquency whose explanations reveal an unlikely pattern of irresistible provocation from peers, and criminal carelessness by shopkeepers. Cognitive-behavioural assessment seeks to investigate such sequences of thoughts and interpretations: 'I am unlovable'; 'I am bound to fail'; 'I can take better precautions and not get caught'; 'I am the victim of a conspiracy', which strongly influence how people respond to stimuli from the environment. However, it should be noted that all of the internal conditions referred to give rise to behavioural excesses or deficits: self-preoccupation, ineffective or ritual activity in the case of worrying; motionlessness, fixed expression, lack of social response, lack of attention to dress and hygiene in the cases of depression. People either *do* or *do not do* things as a result of emotional states and mixed-up patterns of thinking, and before-and-after comparisons of these observable things provide the acid test of whether what clients *say* they feel as a result of therapy is reliable. Having both kinds of information helps to reduce the influence of the 'demand effects' mentioned above – clients trying to please or to deceive by living up to expectations. However uncomfortable the idea may be, such distortions are a fact of therapeutic life.

☐ Considerable emphasis is placed on contemporary behaviour and the thoughts and feelings which accompany it. The search for the long-lost causes of problems is, in the absence of major trauma, regarded with suspicion. This is for the following reasons: (1) there is no guarantee that they will ever be found; (2) because the exercise is costly in time and resources; (3) when views as to the original causes of problems *can* be elicited they are not always agreed upon by the protagonists, nor are they necessarily valid; (4) dwelling on the history of problems can sometimes serve to intensify bad feeling and can distract from the necessity of doing something positive in the here and now. That said, the therapist must balance the above with the need for clients to understand the nature and development of their problems and the ways in which the various parties involved might have come to view things differently. One solution is to limit history-taking to brief accounts of the *aetiology* of the problem (the history of specific causes) and to emphasise to clients that problems are often reactivated every day by what people do or fail to do, and by self-fulfilling expectations. A crucial question here is: What maintains problematic behaviour in force, long after the original factors eliciting it have passed into history? Frequently Mr Smith scowls at Mrs Smith and decides to drink the rent money because of what happened yesterday and what he expects to happen today, not because of what allegedly happened on Boxing Day in 1997. However, if problems seem to be tied up closely with 'personality factors', that is, with typical, well-established and predictable ways of responding which vary little across circumstances, then it may be useful to investigate the *learning history* of the client. This includes identifying behavioural excesses, deficits and failures of discrimination as in item 1 above; trying to find out how particular reactions have come about; looking at patterns of reinforcement and secondary gain; and, concomitantly, why obviously ineffective responses have proved resistant to reinterpretation, extinction or change. This can help us to formulate a more accurate treatment plan, but it still leaves us in the position of having to work with the contemporary manifestations of problems.

☐ At some stage clear decisions have to be made with clients about what sequences of behaviour need to be increased in frequency and/or strength and direction, and what sequences decreased in these ways. Further questions include: What new *skills* (e.g. arguing or negotiating without threats) would be required in order for the client to perform other, more adaptive sequences?

☐ This concern over contemporary events is part of a wider attempt to establish the *controlling conditions* that surround a given problem. This part of the assessment may be thought of as 'topographical' in that it is concerned with the surface layout of the problem, and the aim is, metaphorically, to produce a 'map' of specified daily activities. Thus, we are concerned here with such things as *where* episodes tend to happen and not to happen; what happens around the client or to him or her just *before* a sequence of the unwanted behaviour occurs; what happens around the client or to him or her *during* the performance of the behaviour; and what happens *after* the performance of the behaviour. This emphasis reflects our knowledge about the way in which opportunities for certain sequences of behaviour are 'signalled' by prior events (S^ds) and how these are maintained by certain patterns of thoughts and expectations, and by prior knowledge of reinforcing consequences (see Bandura 1977). Any natural correlation or variance in these factors provides useful extra information. A simple example would be when John wets the bed every night *except* when he sleeps with his brother or *except* when he stays at his grandmother's. Or, when it can be seen that Mr Turner's bouts of excessive drinking and exhibitionism always result in his daughter coming to care for him until he 'feels better'.

☐ Cognitive-behavioural assessments are somewhat independent of the definitions and labels that others place on troubling and troublesome behaviour, but are not indifferent to them. However, we are concerned to find out what people who are said to have 'inadequate personalities' do and think; what 'hysterics' and other allegedly attention-seeking people do, don't do and think; what it is that Mark says to make his parents describe him as 'insolent'; how someone with 'antisocial tendencies' actually behaves, and so on. There are good ethical reasons for building such a label-examining stage into our assessments, but it is also necessary if we are to keep the element of subjective attribution present in most assessments of problematic behaviour to a minimum. *Naming is not explaining*, however much we intuitively feel that it is. In arguing that Mr Williams' 'manipulative' behaviour is due to his 'personality disorder' (which we suspect he has because of his dissembling behaviour) we are guilty of the same tautological and worst-case-confirming thinking that we often seek to change in our clients.

☐ The need for flexibility is always stressed in texts on assessment. While it is a matter of common sense that assessment procedures that are rigid and forced will probably be self-defeating, there is an equal need to make assessments as clear and specific as possible. Our main concerns should be as follows: (1) To produce clear *formulations* of problems (see p. 184); that is, to put together a concise account of how problems have developed and what might be maintaining them. These do not have to contain 'established truth' – just a coherent, 'best-available' view that is testable in practice. A good formulation leads to (2) *clear hypotheses* about what might affect the problems under review; that is, it should be the sort of statement that can be easily checked. The statement 'Mr Brown's low level of self-esteem is due to poor ego development' is a poor hypothesis since there is little or nothing that could ever happen to disprove it. 'Mary's avoidance of people is likely to reduce if she learns how to start conversations' is better. If Mary receives help on how to start conversations, begins to mix with others, and yet still does not talk to them for long and does not stay in their company, then the hypothesis as it stands is probably *wrong* and so the therapist knows something more about the problem. (3) Hypotheses lead to both long-term and short-term goals. These too have ideal characteristics and are similar to those listed above. The clear goal is one which provides definite feedback on progress towards some specific, and at least partially predefined, end-state. Thus we need to tell from the goals we set with our clients whether our assessment policy is on the right track or not. The objective 'to improve communication in the family' has little real meaning of its own. What will family members do more of, less of, do differently, do in different combinations, or in different places, as a result of family communication being improved? Obviously, 'circumstances alters cases'; the point is that some pre-described state – representing whatever behavioural, cognitive and emotional factors are held to be involved – should be the target of intervention.

Now that we have gained an overview of this approach we can start to examine the stages of assessment in more detail (see Figure 6.1).

Monitoring and evaluation: the use of single case experimental designs (SCEDs)

This is the point at which assessment joins progress monitoring and evaluation, and the first task is to decide how often behaviours or indicators relevant to the problem occur *prior* to active intervention. This is called the *baseline stage*. It is not a measure of the problem before *any* help has been given (see below). Baselines record the *pre-specific or pre-active* intervention level of a problem. They provide a standard against which the specific problem-countering policy may be assessed. Baseline data can exist in two forms: quantitative, i.e. measures of the *incidence* of overt behaviour; or qualitative, i.e. standardised measures of the *kinds* of cognitive and emotional factors we think are implicated in problems. As already proposed, the sensible approach is to combine both sets of factors into one record.

   Discussion of SCEDs is placed here in the assessment sequence and not (as is usual) at the end of it, because they are as much about monitoring and feedback as evaluation *per se*.

Baseline effects

Sometimes when clients set about measuring the extent of their current problems the situation improves. This so-called *baseline effect* is probably the result of focusing attention on specifics rather than generalities, and of the improvement in morale that a businesslike approach to problem-solving can bring. They are good news in therapeutic terms and a cross to bear for evaluators.

Records and recording

There is a variety of ways in which such records can be kept. The graph is probably the best method since it provides information at a glance, and patterns and trends show up quite readily. However, graphs frighten some clients, and therapists need to adapt the presentation of data to suit. That said, they do provide powerful visual feedback on progress. If they are introduced in a matter-of-fact way, and explained in simple terms, they pose few insurmountable problems in the majority of cases. But if graphs or similar paper exercises are not suitable, then a little ingenuity is required. Students of mine, working with youngsters with learning disabilities have used recording devices such as 'posting' tiddly-wink counters into a money box, and pasting favourite cartoon cut-outs on to a board as recording methods. Only a few clients refuse to keep records if their purpose is explained and they are adapted to their needs and capacities.

   On this issue of recording, it is my experience that clients respond favourably to the following: (1) the clearly demonstrated assumption on the therapist's part that effective

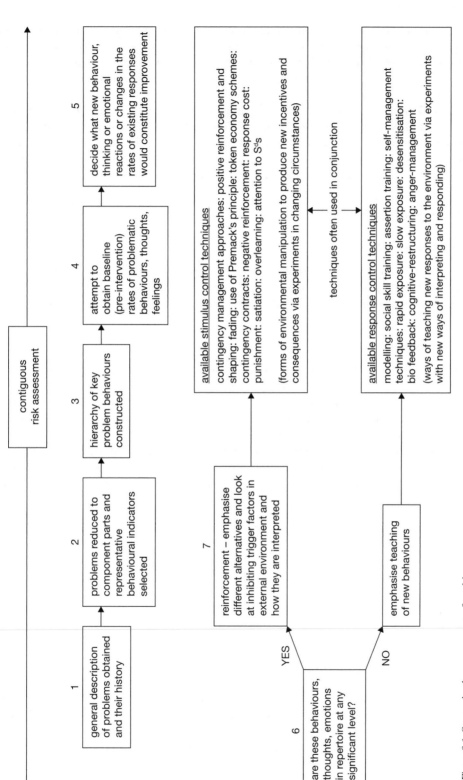

Figure 6.1 Stages in the assessment of problems

helping requires careful assessment and monitoring; (2) a sympathetic but matter-of-fact approach and time spent explaining how best to keep records and what problems might arise; (3) the social-reinforcement of record-keeping; (4) simple, well-produced pro formas with clear instructions written on them; (5) using records in front of clients and going over the data with them.

Record entries need to be made as soon as possible after the event in which we are interested has occurred. Clients often try to remember numbers until a single 'totting-up' session at the end of the day, but this is full of pitfalls and should be discouraged. Sometimes a recording device needs to be portable. A variety of methods may be used, including diaries, postcards, golf-score counters, marks on sticky tape around the wrist, and so on.

Methods of gathering data

Direct observation

This method is applicable where the problem events occur at a high frequency and so a relatively short period of observation gives a good idea of current rates. It may be used only where the presence of a non-participatory observer will not be a distracting influence.

Time sampling

Time sampling is used where it is impractical or undesirable for an observer to spend long periods of time with the client. Instead, ten five-minute observations, for instance, can be made at intervals throughout the day, perhaps by a mediator. This method is particularly useful in residential and hospital settings, but it can deal only with high-frequency behaviours which are relatively independent of time and circumstances.

Some problems occur only at particular times or under given conditions (e.g. mealtimes, or whenever clients find themselves in situations from which it is difficult to escape without embarrassment). In these cases data need only be gathered at these points of known vulnerability.

Participant observation

Essentially the same as direct observation, this method may be used where the presence of an outsider is less intrusive if he or she joins in whatever is going on. The behaviour under review needs to be somewhat independent of observer-effects, or a few dummy runs need to be made so that the observer 'blends' into the background. A stranger with a pad sitting in a day-room stands out like a sore thumb.

Mechanical, electronic and other aids to observation

Tape recorders, video sets, one-way screens and other such aids are increasingly available in child and family clinics and other specialist centres. Once clients become familiar with such devices their influence becomes stable and predictable and can be allowed for. However, it is rarely true to say that their presence is completely forgotten.

Self-observation

Again, this method is very useful in field settings. The success of self-recording depends on: (1) a well-organised scheme; (2) a clear definition of what is to be counted so that the client is in no doubt; (3) whether the behaviours or accompaniments under review are of a character to make deliberate distortion likely. It is a brave client who will report frankly on his or her own antisocial activities, and a foolhardy helper who offers an amnesty on such behaviour for recording purposes and so runs the risk of appearing to condone it (see p. 205). One alternative is to monitor the occurrence of positive (generally acceptable) behaviour which is incompatible with the problematic behaviours under review. Decisions of this kind, and decisions about whether to use mediators instead, depend largely on the amount of cooperation we can expect to receive from clients.

Self-observation is used to assess behaviours that occur largely privately – specific thought patterns, ruminations, inhibitions, feelings of panic – at low frequency and/or beyond the range of mediators. There can be a problem with cognitions in that noting when particular thoughts occur can increase their level. It is better therefore to use the ABC method; that is, to make entries on columns headed 'antecedents', 'behaviour', 'consequent thoughts' and 'feelings' plus 'consequences'. On the whole the method works well, and a client who will not cooperate with self-recording is unlikely to cooperate much with the therapeutic scheme that follows.

Reliability checks

It is possible to use these different methods in combination, thus adding greatly to their reliability. Where self-reports, reports of mediators, our own, and those of clients agree substantially with each other, greater confidence can be placed in findings.

Interpretation of baseline data

All data require interpretation; only rarely will a self-evident conclusion jump out. This is especially true of the kinds of data gathered in natural settings, which are at best a compromise between rigour and relevance.

The first consideration is the length and stability of the baseline measure. The aim in baseline recording is to obtain a typical *sample* of behaviour and so recording must continue long enough for odd fluctuations and recurring patterns to be seen in context. It may be that a pattern of aggressive behaviour on Mondays, or in the presence of another particular group of people, will emerge. It may be that the last two days just happen to have been particularly difficult or particularly good, giving an artificial impression. Over a longer period such effects will show up and can provide much valuable information (examples of SCEDs with both stable and unstable baselines may be found in Figures 6.2 to 6.13 below). But the ideal length for a baseline depends on several different factors:

☐ Some behaviours, for instance, eye-contact patterns, obsessions, or periods of detached silence, are likely to occur with *high frequency*, and so observation over a period of two or three days will give some idea of the stable frequency. We must use our judgement here. If different things happen on different days then it may be useful to see how this affects the data. A daily time-sampling approach may be the answer.
☐ Where behaviours occur with *low frequency*, for example, conversation in a withdrawn schizophrenic patient, enuresis, or stealing, baseline data must be collected over a longer period.

☐ In all cases the ideal is a *stable* measure where there are no great or untypical swings in the rate of performance. This is not to say that there must be no fluctuations, just that these must be typical and so roughly cancel each other out, or cluster closely around the median, with only one or two exceptions well outside the range. In cases where data are very difficult to interpret, simple statistical techniques are available. However, except in very intractable cases where we are grasping at straws, if we find ourselves having to do sums on baseline/outcome differences it is unlikely that we are achieving much of practical value.

☐ Ideally, the more recorded observations of the behaviours being monitored the better. In practice this usually means the longer the baseline period the better. However, a sensible balance has to be struck here between therapeutic considerations and the need for careful assessment. Although clients will sometimes suffer problems stoically for months or years, the arrival of professional help can make further delay difficult to bear.

Figure 6.2 is an example of the simplest kind of SCED, the AB design, which makes a straightforward 'before-and-after' comparison. A comparison between this example and Figure 6.3 should illustrate the difference between stability and instability at the baseline stage.

Setting target levels

The next stage in the assessment sequence is that of setting target levels. The client and the therapist have to decide what would constitute a significant improvement to the problem, remembering that in some cases it is not behaviour per se that is the problem, but the *rate* at which it is performed, or the *setting* in which it occurs. We all lose our temper occasionally, but some people lose it every day and do not feel that they should try to contain it just because they are in company. It is a useful check on the usefulness of a programme, and often a spur to everyone concerned with it, if target levels are written in next to goals as soon as these have been formulated. A simple statement will suffice, such as 'Mr and Mrs A. will consider that

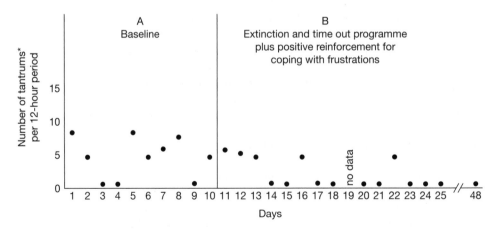

Figure 6.2 Example of an AB design with an unstable baseline: uncontrollable temper tantrums in a 5-year-old child

Note
* Operationally defined with parents.

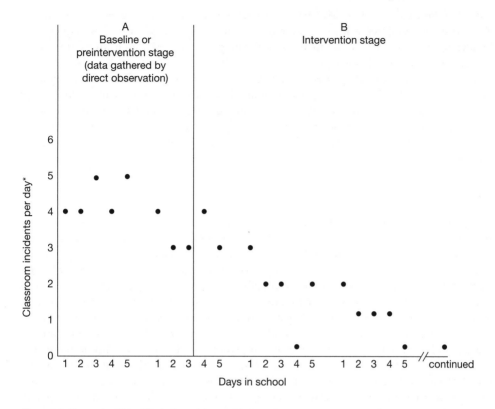

Figure 6.3 Example of an AB design with a stable baseline

Notes
Baseline data from classroom management scheme for a 'disturbed' 9-year-old boy under threat of exclusion from school.

* Predefined with teachers as any combination of: interfering with the work of others; hitting others; leaving his seat and failing to return within one minute of first being asked; making loud noises, or noises continuing long enough to distract other pupils.

their relationship has significantly improved if rows and prolonged silences fall to half the present level'.

We next have to decide whether the behaviours which will constitute an improvement are already *in repertoire* at any significant level (see Figure 6.1, p. 153). Decisions as to which group of cognitive-behavioural approaches we are likely to select depends upon the answer to this question. We need to know whether the person whose behaviour we are seeking to change *ever* engages in behaviours *anything like* the target behaviours, whether there are *any* social situations in which self-deprecating thoughts do not occur or occur less irresistibly or less frequently. If so, then these patterns might be reinforceable. If not, or if such events are at a very low level, it makes more sense to concentrate on teaching and developing new behaviours and alternative patterns of thinking. From this distinction is drawn the twofold classification of behavioural approaches used in this book: *stimulus control* techniques (designed to change behaviour through changing the environment and the consequences it produces), and *response control* techniques (designed to alter the range, type or level of responses that clients have in their repertoire, or to equip them with completely new ones (after Bandura 1969)). Obviously there are close connections between these two groupings, and many programmes will include elements from both – as when a new sequence of behaviour is first modelled and then approximate performances are positively reinforced during rehearsals (see Chapter 8).

The remainder of this chapter is concerned with the various methods by which cognitive-behavioural programmes can be monitored and evaluated and in particular with further examples of single case experimental designs. This approach to evaluation is not dependent upon the use of formal behavioural techniques. So long as the user is willing to link expected outcome to behaviour in some form, then, subject to the strictures put forward in Chapter 1, any method could be used.

AB designs

The reader will see from Figures 6.2 and 6.3 that the recording of the target behaviour (or some reliable indicator of it) is continued after the start of the programme designed to alter it. AB designs are a considerable advance on impressionistic case studies, but they are still *quasi-experimental*. That is, they offer correlational evidence of outcome; but we cannot be sure from them which of the many variables introduced into a case were the potent ones, or indeed whether the approach itself was responsible at all. lt could be the therapist's own behaviour; 'attention placebo effects' of various kinds; particular structural elements in the programme, or the passage of time. In the short term, this may not appear to matter much because the main job of helping is to help, not to research psychological techniques. But in the longer term, if we are to develop better 'recipes' for this, we need to think about sifting and refining the different ingredients of our approaches. Patterns do emerge between workers and between problem and client groups in a series of AB designs, but there is need for caution in interpreting data gathered in this way, as the hypothetical example given in Figure 6.4 demonstrates.

The centre graph gives all the appearance of a successful therapeutic encounter, but the larger graph reveals a 'natural' pattern in the course of the problem, under the control of other variables.

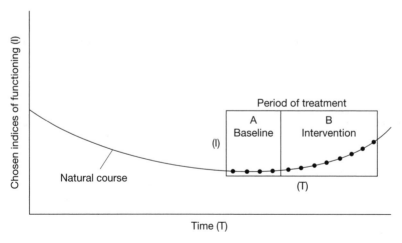

Figure 6.4 Diagram showing misleading interpretation of an AB design given hypothetical natural course of problems

If we happen to sample behaviour at a particularly fortuitous point in the natural development of a problem, then we can be easily misled. Although this is a hypothetical illustration, it is not a hypothetical problem. Patterns of this type do occur (e.g. in bipolar conditions). Manic-depressive illness follows a cyclical pattern, and a wide range of other problems are known to remit spontaneously. There are several things we can do to guard against such distortions in our data.

- ☐ We can get to know something about available research regarding the difficulties with which we are concerned. If the literature suggests that a particular problem is resistant to treatment (e.g. generalised anxiety states) yet we are managing quite respectable gains, then, with due caution, we may feel justified in concluding that this is not a quirk in the development of the problem.
- ☐ We can monitor over a longer period; that is, extend the baseline period and watch for trends of this kind which are seemingly independent of what we are doing.
- ☐ We can arrange follow-up contacts or visits. Clients are reassured by the prospect of these too, and they cost little.
- ☐ We can look very carefully at the differences between baseline phase and intervention phase rates. The ideal is for a clear and fairly rapid distinction to emerge between the two phases. Figure 6.2 proves little about effectiveness, whereas Figure 6.3 is rather more suggestive of it. In Figure 6.4 the 'trajectory' of the behaviours under review is already well established, and the *probability* is that such a well-established upward trend would continue if it represents genuine benefits for the client. In Figure 6.5 the difference between the two stages is well marked.
- ☐ We can employ a more sophisticated design (see below).

Follow-up data

A follow-up visit can solve many of the problems associated with simple AB designs. The fact that there is not always an established tradition (perhaps we would rather not know) is regrettable. Follow-up assessment is straightforward when a particular group of problematic behaviours has been reduced to nil (or virtually nil) prior to closure, since it requires only a brief visit, a telephone call or a prepaid letter to establish whether or not the position is still the same three months later. Similarly, when clients have experienced no great difficulties in recording items of behaviour they may be advised to continue to do this until the follow-up contact. But not all cases fall into these categories and so another strategy is required if we are to improve upon the client's subjective impressions of change.

I have found the following approach useful.

- ☐ The follow-up visit is fixed in advance at the time of closure.
- ☐ The client is encouraged to repeat the original measurements (or some other suitable person can do it) for a defined period before the follow-up contact is made.
- ☐ Rates at closure are compared with the average rate recorded immediately prior to follow-up. This is not foolproof; clients occasionally report that things have been untypically better during the pre-follow-up phase – perhaps because of the impending contact. This is particularly true of cases involving children. But then this tells us something about what is effective in controlling the behaviour in question, and brief, intermittent, maintenance visits may be indicated for a time. Certainly it makes little sense to squander our investment in a case for the want of them.

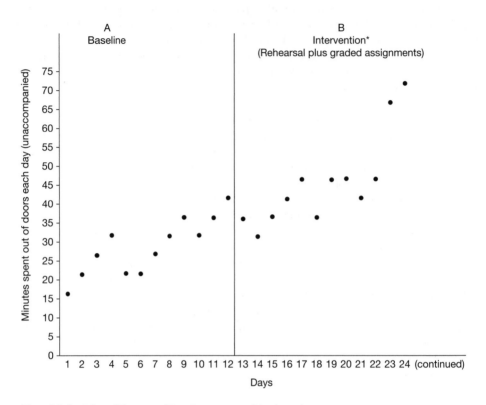

Figure 6.5 Social confidence problem in an ex-psychiatric patient

Note
* A CBT approach comprising attempts to change malign attributions regarding the intentions of others, plus modelling exercises and social skills training.

Figure 6.6 is an example of an AB design with a follow-up period built into it. The AB design with follow up (technically ABA, see p. 161), probably represents the best compromise between evaluative rigour and therapeutic reality available to us.

BA designs

Figure 6.7 provides an example of a BA scheme designed to produce clear feedback on expenditure for a family with chronic financial problems and resultant depression and drinking to excess. In this family, budgeting and rudimentary financial record-keeping were known to be virtually non-existent. Therefore there was no point in a detailed baseline phase. In this example we see that although the behaviours established by the budgeting programme were still in existence following the main effort to establish them, they were in gradual decline thereafter, and so some sort of 'topping-up' attention was required. In this example we are recording compliance with *means* thought to be related to the problem. The only worthwhile outcome indicator in such a case is reduced indebtedness. In cases of anorexia, whatever the causes, target weight maintenance must be the primary indicator.

The problem with BA designs is that if the target rate falls in the A phase then we have to add a further B (intervention phase); if it does not, then we assume that learning has taken

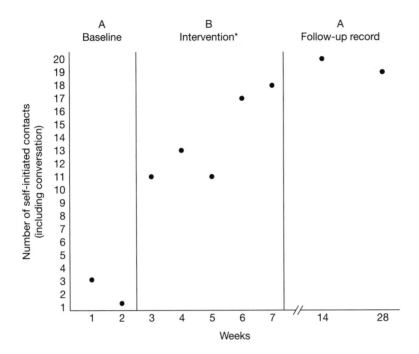

Figure 6.6 Assertion training with a withdrawn psychiatric client (ABA)

Note
* The cognitive elements in this case were buttressed by a programme of modelling and rehearsal, graded assignments, plus a back-up reinforcement scheme.

place – good news therapeutically, but we are left with no evaluation (see BAB and BABA designs, below).

ABA designs

The ABA design is an advance on the simple AB approach, since it includes a complete return-to-baseline phase at the end. Figure 6.8 is an example from a child guidance setting. In this case the item of behaviour being measured (night-time fractiousness/interruptions) is an *indicator*, since the child psychiatrist thought that the problem might really be a sexual and marital one (it came with an 'Oedipal problems' label on it originally). The prevailing hypothesis was that despite her concern mother and child were in unwitting collusion and that the mother was quite pleased to have her son in the marital bed since it removed the threat of unwelcome sexual advances from her husband. The couple were eventually referred for sexual counselling (they did have problems), but, although this was successful, the problem of the child's behaviour remained. It started as an indicator of another related problem but became a problem in its own right, requiring direct attention.

Whatever happens after this medical intervention (which was effective, but could not be said to have solved the problem in the longer term) should not be used as evidence in the evaluation of the programme *per se*: this is messy, but typical.

The next case illustration (Figure 6.9) concerns a 9-year-old boy who caused concern to his (single) mother and to his schoolteachers owing to his aggressive behaviour and swearing.

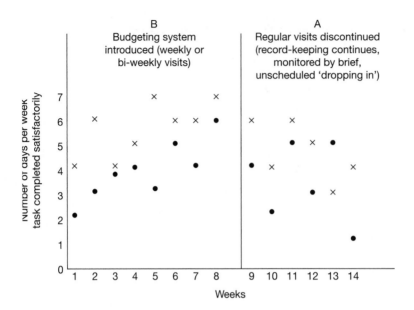

Figure 6.7 Chronic budgetary problems and stress

Notes

✕ Task involved conversion of electricity units into approximate daily costs.

● Sessions on stress inoculation and budgetary management training – tasks involved keeping daily spending within budget, including small payments against arrears (separately monitored).

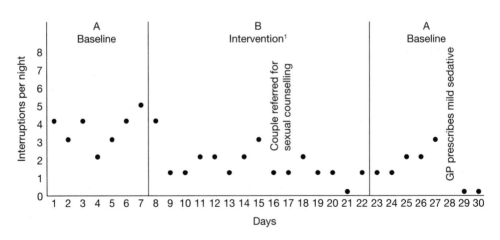

Figure 6.8 Sleep problems in a 4-year-old child, and waking of mother (ABA)

Note

1 Reinforcement programme used model farm animals, stories and a star chart.

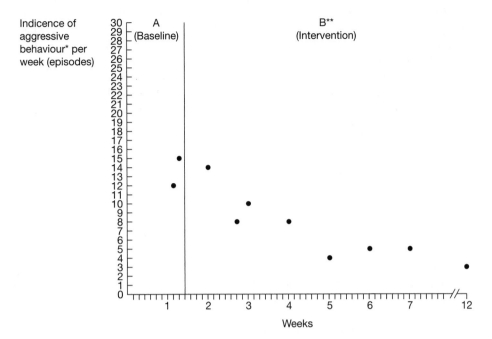

Figure 6.9 A differential reinforcement for other behaviour, plus response-cost scheme to control aggressive behaviour in a 9-year-old boy (AB + fading)

Notes

* Operationally defined as: shouting at mother or passers-by in the street; threatening mother or members of the public; swearing, pushing or throwing objects.

** Plus cognitive restructuring and modelling child management approaches with mother.

An operant scheme rewarding absence of this behaviour and reinforcing certain incompatible activities was used (see p. 193).

The ABA design has the following problems associated with it.

☐   If the B phase is exceptionally long, then some of the criticisms of the AB approach apply; that is, we can be less confident about whether it is the therapeutic input or something else that is responsible for the changes recorded.

☐   Similarly, where a lengthy intervention phase is used, one would expect, even hope (as may be seen from Figure 6.9), that learning would occur. In operant programmes where the therapist has tried to change the contingencies in the client's environment, confusion can arise as a result of learning effects. Let us suppose that relatives of a psychiatric patient first respond to and enquire into the content of delusional talk as usual, recording its occurrence (A phase); then, on advice, they withhold attention from delusional talk and reinforce non-delusional conversation (B phase); then they stop this programme and, under encouragement, do something close to what they always used to do; how are we to interpret the result from a case-research point of view if the delusional talk remains at a low level in the second A phase? Has some learning (in this case, operant conditioning) taken place? Or is this behaviour quite independent of the strategy being applied? The only answer to this question is to wait and see whether the behaviour returns. If not, then new behaviour has been acquired (see p. 167 for further details of this case). In such cases a return to baseline amounts to a reversal rather than a suspension of the programme. In this example, relatives were advised to start doing something again which they had learned not to do; that is, respond to delusional talk and keep a diary of its content. This kind of reversal procedure can be useful to check whether the treatment policy is the correct one, and whether the behaviour varies regularly under its influence. However, it then needs to be succeeded by a further treatment phase (ABAB; see below).

☐   Where two different treatment methods are introduced sequentially, perhaps owing to changes in the assessment, or lack of success, then specific results are easily confounded. The correct name for this type of approach is ABCA – in other words, baseline – intervention strategy 1 – strategy 2 – return to baseline. If a new treatment approach is introduced at the *end* of the first treatment phase, perhaps to supplement it, then this is called an ABCA design. The sequence is: baseline – treatment 1 – treatments 1 and 2 combined – baseline. The example shown in Figure 6.8 is technically an ABCA design since, although sexual counselling had only just begun by the end of the first treatment phase, it might have had a rapid effect, which could have combined with the long-term effects of the initial B phase and resulted in the modest gains of the second baseline phase. The point is that in these more complicated variations of ABA the *relative* potency of the different approaches is very difficult to establish. Each new phase which is added could be helped along by what has gone before.

Two methods in combination, superseding one or both of these methods applied separately, can have very different effects. This is not a serious problem from the therapeutic point of view since it is the treatment 'package' which we want to evaluate. However, if we are trying to find out which type of approach is likely to be more effective – perhaps with an eye to future work – then, ideally, a separate return to baseline must follow each separate treatment phase. Ideal, but not very practical.

ABAB designs

This is undoubtedly the most satisfactory procedure from a case evaluation point of view, although widespread application may be hindered by practical and ethical considerations. ABAB designs may be used in those cases where (1) it is possible clearly to define and separate out the target behaviour; and (2) the behaviour is likely to respond markedly to pre-planned environmental changes (contingency management). Therefore the widest application of this evaluation method has been in operant work.

In this sequence the problematic behaviour (or its chosen indicators) is recorded prior to intervention in the usual way (A). The main treatment programme is started (B). If this shows a positive effect it is halted for a period while monitoring continues (A). A comparison between the two phases is made, then the treatment programme is restarted (B) and further comparisons are made at the end of this phase (see Figures 6.10 and 6.11). Results obtained by this method are extremely reliable, since there are two points at which the behavioural effects of intervention and no intervention may be compared. This fact does away with the criticisms which, strictly speaking, can be made of AB, and (to a lesser extent) ABA designs from the case research point of view. However (the point is worth reiterating), even these comparatively simple designs represent a considerable advance on what has passed for evaluation hitherto, and in field settings they are likely to be the optimum method of evaluation.

The idea of halting a successful programme just as it is getting into gear is often viewed with misgivings, and obviously there are cases where it would be dangerous and unethical to suspend help in order to make an independent check on its efficacy. But safety considerations aside, if a particular pattern of behaviour can be seen to vary with the contingencies applied to it, then this is very well worth knowing, and treatment procedures can always be re-established. Another consideration here is the very positive 'demonstration effect' that this type of design can have (it was particularly powerful in the case described in Figure 6.11). Where parents see that the problem goes away if they stop attending to particular antisocial behaviours in their children and concentrate on others, only to reappear when they temporarily reverse these conditions, then a powerful lesson has been learned. To prevent learning factors from interfering too much, suspension or reversal needs to follow quickly on the heels of the establishment of a stable trend towards improvement.

Two examples of ABAB designs are given below (see Figures 6.10 and 6.11). Figure 6.10 shows a clearly successful programme; Figure 6.11 is broadly successful, but the results are difficult to interpret.

Let us concentrate for a moment on Figure 6.11, since it demonstrates many of the problems of an attempt at rigorous evaluation in a field setting. The reader may be able to see several compromising features. The scheme starts off well: the first baseline period is of reasonable duration considering the state of tension in the family, and is just about stable, with the rate hovering between four and eight items per day in a range from two to ten with a clustering around four and five items per day.

However, the baseline shows a downward trend (regarded as untypical by the parents and probably a demand characteristic or 'baseline effect'). In addition, the intervention phase begins with a worsening of the problem, which continues for a while until the programme of ignoring delusional talk begins to take effect. In the second return to baseline (a reversal in this case, because parents were asked to keep a diary of the content of their daughter's delusional talk and whether it would respond to reason, and so their old practice of giving attention to these preoccupations was resumed) there is an upward trend which continued until near the end of the second A phase. Then the rate begins to fall again and so confounds somewhat the effect of restarting the programme – which produces a relatively stable and confidence-boosting downward trend.

This scheme, using parents as mediators, continued for another forty-six days, during which time the incidence of delusional talk (mainly the reporting of feelings of surveillance – her mother had once worked in an East European embassy during the Cold War) never surfaced again above two incidents per day. For twenty-two of these days it stood at nought. A brief follow-up at six months revealed a maintained level of improvement of approximately this order, punctuated here and there by the odd sharp increase which the mother was able to relate convincingly to various family episodes. In addition, the family and the client herself were able to report on and exemplify a number of worthwhile changes in the way in which family members related more positively to each other. The main effect came from providing attention for ordinary conversation, and little for delusional expressions.

Figure 6.10 represents a more complicated case (described on p. 196) but produces less complicated results. Here the return to baseline phase was abbreviated owing to the tensions within the family and the not inconsiderable fire risks involved in this case. Despite the misgivings of the client's father, the 'demonstration effect' of suspending treatment was very powerful indeed. It produced a 'shot in the arm' when the family saw that the behaviour was partly under their control and not caused by some junior form of mental illness. However, the requirement that a promising treatment phase should be temporarily suspended and reversed raises ethical problems, and this design needs to be used with caution and common sense. With hindsight, and a more confident knowledge of the research literature, I now believe that an ABA design would have been the best choice here. However, blanket

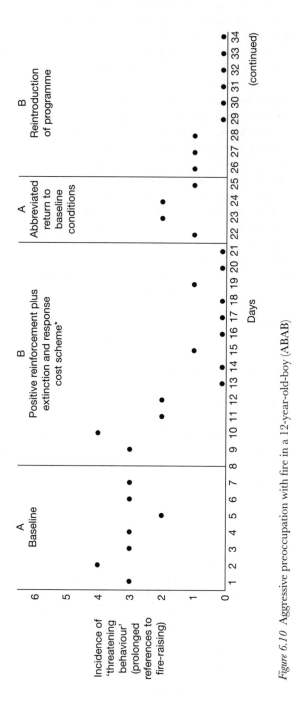

Figure 6.10 Aggressive preoccupation with fire in a 12-year-old-boy (ABAB)

Note
* Differential reinforcement scheme operated by parents, plus cognitive appraisal work with child.

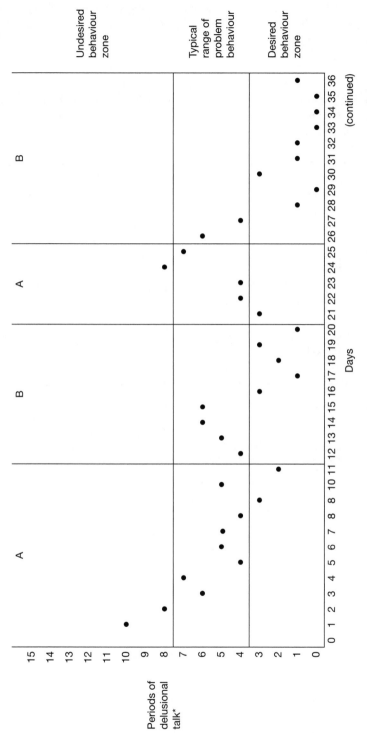

Figure 6.11 Contingency management plus cognitive restructuring and social skills training scheme for reducing delusional talk in a 24-year-old psychiatric outpatient (ABAB)

Note
* Operationally defined with relatives; largely paranoid in character.

objections to the use of such methods need to be seen in the context of the equally pressing ethical questions regarding whether the service being provided is effective, a waste of everyone's time, or even damaging.

BAB designs

BAB designs are ideal for operant work where, for various reasons, it would be unwise to delay treatment until a baseline can be established. This design may be used where target behaviours are clearly dependent on identifiable environmental contingencies, and these are subject to manipulation.

Figure 6.12 is an example of a BAB design. In this case the urgency which precluded baseline recording stemmed from the fact that the child was acquiring a reputation for being 'withdrawn' and 'troubled' among nursery school staff despite reassurances from mother and the health visitor that he was outgoing enough at home. The fact that he was the only black child in the class may have been a trigger, but the school staff had encouraged inclusion, just not very determinedly.

Multiple baseline designs

The multiple baseline design (see Figure 6.13) uses each defined element of a problem as a control for the others. There are two distinct advantages with this approach: (1) it does away with the need for a suspension or reversal phase; (2) in complex cases one method at a time may be tried out. The approach is really just a series of AB designs run in a particular sequence. The procedure is as follows.

First, the pre-intervention rate of each different target behaviour is recorded. When a stable rate appears in one behaviour, the treatment programme is applied first to that behaviour.

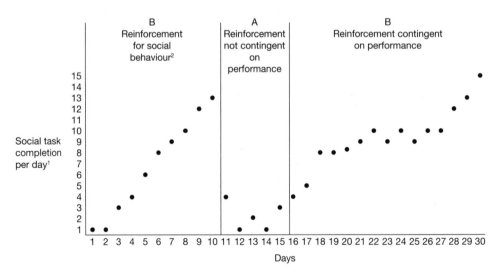

Figure 6.12 Shyness/isolation in a 4-year-old pre-school child (BAB)

Notes
1 Predefined tasks (behaviour shaping, ranging from showing interest in play of others, to solitary play nearby, to participatory play).
2 Approval plus small treats (given by nursery staff).

During the next stage two points need to be noted: (1) the difference that intervention is making (if any) to the first target behaviour; (2) whether the base-rates of the other behaviours (to which the treatment variable has not yet been applied) are changing substantially (covarying) with the target behaviour. If not, the programme is applied to the next behaviour, and, after a suitable interval, the procedures outlined above are applied again. This process continues until the scheme is in operation for all the target behaviours. Figure 6.13 gives an example of a multiple baseline design applied to a range of disciplinary problems experienced by a single mother and her children.

Multiple baseline designs have a wide range of uses with clients who experience a number of different problems. However, the approach has its drawbacks. The behaviours under investigation have to be fairly discrete; in other words, the occurrence of each must be assessed as substantially independent of the others. To the extent that the start of the first B phase produces a marked covariance in the other base rates, the experimental principle of using the other behaviours as a control is confounded. It may be that the procedure being used is particularly potent, or – later on – that generalisation is occurring. But this cannot just be assumed (however beneficial the result) and the sequence collapses into a concurrent series of AB designs – no great problem from a therapeutic point of view, little problem from a case-evaluation point of view, providing that a follow-up procedure is to be used.

Baselines across settings designs

Another multiple measurement approach is the 'baselines across settings' design. With this approach, problems in different settings are baselined and the treatment variable is applied to each in sequence according to the principles outlined above.

Other factors in the use of SCEDs

A wider range of single case evaluation procedures is available than there is space to discuss in this volume. However, the main approaches likely to be applicable to routine work have now been outlined. One or two general issues remain. First, assessment and evaluation procedures of this type do not have to be used in a 'mechanical' way. The question of balance between rigour and the intrusiveness of a particular approach must always be given careful consideration. This is not to say that at the first sign of difficulty the principle of rigorous case evaluation should be abandoned in favour of some vague notion of the need for general flexibility. However, where necessary, these procedures can be changed and reconstructed, as long as due care is given to their subsequent interpretation. They are widely used in clinical and social work settings in the United States in circumstances not *that* much more propitious than here.

Qualitative assessment of cognitions

At various points in this chapter I have argued for a combination of quantitative and qualitative information as the sensible basis of both assessment and evaluation. When considering qualitative change, we are interested in the character and in the general social effects of new behaviour, rather than in precise changes in the rate of its occurrence. However, we must avoid the trap of seeing these different types of assessment as completely different things. An increase in the level of self-assertion, though recorded as a quantitative change, can produce notable qualitative changes – perhaps in the way that the client views him or herself, or in the enjoyment they now get out of life. Sometimes the changes produced by treatment seem (at

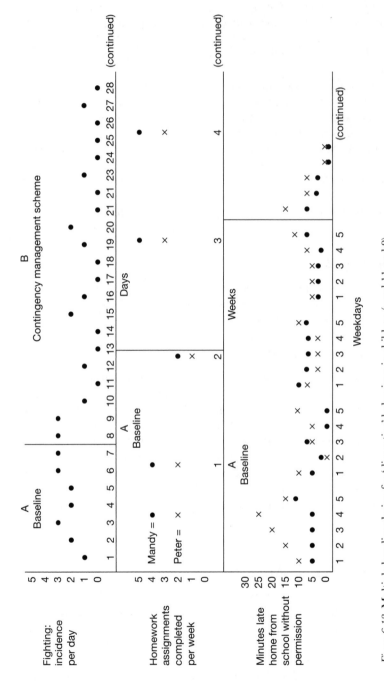

Figure 6.13 Multiple baseline design for 'disruptive' behaviour in children (aged 11 and 8)

Note

Programme equals: reinforcement of cooperative behaviour with star chart, small treats, comics, plus extra TV time and bonus outings, determined on a sliding scale, as well as agreed rates for deprivation of privileges.

a qualitative level) artificial or stilted because new behaviours are initially being grudgingly or mechanically performed. It should be remembered here that the availability of new sources of reinforcement produced by the behaviour can, given time, change the way these things look and feel.

Assessment of cognitive factors

As assessors, we are concerned to know about the patterns of selective attention, mental imagery, beliefs, thinking styles and constructs which clients have developed regarding their problems and the circumstances in which they arise. In other words, we need to know what their model of this part of their reality looks and feels like. We have to hypothesise about their hypotheses. Here is a list of mental events on which we might concentrate such investigations.

Perceptions

Logically we should concern ourselves first with the types and classes of stimuli and events to which the client appears to respond or appears to emphasise, and those which he or she ignores, or is relatively insensitive. Examples are: people who in the early stages of panic attacks focus on small, perhaps random, visceral changes (breathing, heart rate, swallowing) and by this concentration change them, setting up the bodily equivalent of microphone feedback – the greater the cognitive-attention the greater the change; the greater the emotional reaction – the greater the change; the greater risk of catastrophic thinking and so on. This is the first function of anxiety in the absence of manifest physical or well-conditioned threat (which produce the 'hard-wired' responses referred to in Chapter 4) – to induce a state of internal hyper-vigilance to small harbingers of danger (see Beck & Emery 1985). People with low self-esteem whose 'social radars' are tuned to provide early warning of rejection, for whom a knitting of the brows by another always spells disapproval and never concentration, exhibit this problem in comparable external form. These effects may be short term (they do not necessarily feature strongly in later memories of events) but they develop a contemporary 'cognitive-processing bias' often leading to self-defeating behaviour or social paralysis. Then there are stranger people, who interpret the playful and socially undeveloped behaviour of children as 'flirtatious', so justifying their sexual arousal towards them.

Note that each of these examples contains a *percept*, a preferential selection of stimuli, and consequent emotional arousal and interpretation. Indeed, as we saw in Chapters 4 and 5, so intertwined and rapid are these factors that it is difficult to separate sensory, cognitive and emotional factors. The sequence is automatic, it is conditioned, *it* happens to *us*. It can even occur pre-consciously; that is, without contemporary cognitive reflection, as in Dixon's (1981) concept of 'perception without awareness'. For example, words with sexual connotations flashed rapidly via a tachistoscope can trigger emotional reactions in subjects even when they cannot have 'registered' them, and cannot represent and recall them. Patients suffering from depression who are simultaneously presented with neutral and derogatory messages in dichotomous listening experiments tend to filter out the first and select the second, whereas controls do not (see Eysenck & Keane 1990). Therefore an important task in cognitive-behavioural assessment is to try to establish to which groups of stimuli clients are particularly sensitive. Clients give two kinds of evidence on these points.

1   They will admit to 'tracking for', 'scanning for' or 'tuning into' particular stimuli. Their attention is pre-focused, they are already interested in the possible presence of them.

2   They often describe how particular stimuli 'jumped out' at them, and acquired a sudden significance. We can all have this experience at noisy gatherings when we hear our name mentioned across the room.

By getting clients to think carefully about their first inklings of a problematic episode we can gather useful information as to the internal and external stimuli they are prone to discriminate; their problems of sensitivity and insensitivity; the degree of automaticity in their links between percept, cognition, emotion and behaviour; the resistibility or otherwise of these cued sequences, and what, if anything, works to suppress, interrupt or divert attention from them.

Thought patterns

Here we are concerned to assess what mental images or internal 'conversations' accompany given stimulus conditions. The former seem to us like pictures, though as we saw in Chapter 4, they are probably less complete before than after we talk to ourselves or other people about them. We 'join up the experiential dots', as it were, as with dreams. Getting clients to describe these images gives us clues as to their interpretation of events and their feelings about those events.

CASE EXAMPLE 6.1

I was once consulted by a young woman about a persistent fear of vomiting in public which was ruining her social life. She turned down most invitations from friends as a consequence and if she did go out she would carry a plastic carrier bag with her to avoid the worst. What was 'the worst'? The image (it had never actually happened) is of a crowded restaurant; she being eased into a chair at a table furthest away from the lavatory; friends looking at her, first with puzzlement as she begins to gag, then with embarrassment, then with horror as she throws up all over the food and covers everyone's clothing with vomit. This image was triggered by any social circumstance involving the consumption of food and was particularly prevalent if possible escape routes were blocked. Having this mental picture made things worse in that she would either concentrate on chewing and swallowing to the extent that someone would notice and ask if everything was all right, or she would overcompensate and bolt the food, which made her feel more nauseous (the approach used in this case is discussed on p. 229).

By asking clients to describe their thoughts in this way it is possible to gain an impression of the extent to which problems contain an element of 'catastrophic thinking', and whether their behaviour is being influenced by 'worst case' imagery. (Note how little possible control over social circumstances, or sympathetic understanding from others, the sufferer allows herself in the above description.)

Next we are concerned with inner-speech. What does the client typically say to him or herself about their circumstances and behaviour? '*What a fool I am, I shall never be able to carry this off, best get it over with quickly and get out*', perhaps. We 'talk' silently to ourselves about our behaviour, we appraise our actions and what we think we must look like as if we were third parties. These commentaries have a cueing function with respect to emotion and behaviour. We have all had the experience of a sub-vocal appeal to ourselves to stay calm, and many of us will have experienced bursts of self-condemnation expressed in something resembling speech inside our heads. However, for some clients these self-admonishing mantras are there most of the time, are inhibitory, intrusive and, together with the emotions (fear, shame, anger, etc.) which accompany them, block rational analysis and problem-solving. In this form of assessment we are concerned to know about the *quality* of these cognitive and emotional experiences, where they happen, and how long they last and how often they occur.

Beliefs

Working in a child and family guidance clinic, I was taken by surprise by the number of referrals received featuring young children allegedly manifesting behavioural problems or developmental delays which turned out to have more to do with unrealistic parental beliefs rather than with pathology, psycho- or otherwise, in the child. The belief systems of abusive parents are beginning to be taken more seriously in research and it is becoming clear that (given that child-rearing skills are not genetically endowed – though we often behave as if they were) many adults have beliefs about the supposedly malevolent intentions of babies and young children that are not only exaggerated, but implausible for developmental reasons; for example, that babies cry deliberately when parents are having a good time, or that they are trying to break up vulnerable relationships.

Beliefs are settled views of experience, and they condition us to seek information consonant with the little functional homeostases that we all expend considerable energy attempting to preserve. The chief task for the assessor is to elucidate the belief systems surrounding problems and clients' reactions to them, as a basis for comparing early descriptions with those given during and after intervention.

Attributions

The most important part of the search for meaning and valency in stimuli (i.e. experience) is the establishment of cause and effect and covariance. We conduct 'thought experiments' to establish what reliably goes with what, and where causes might lie; for example:

> 'Whenever I show my disappointment about being let down over the children he claims not to have realised the importance of the situation. So what would happen if I put this beyond doubt beforehand? Would he be there, and on time? Probably not. So what does this say about my level of real influence and my and their importance in his life?'

A further dimension of attribution is the direction of attributive judgements; that is, whether they are *predominantly external* – 'the bad things that happen to me are largely due to outside factors beyond my control', along a continuum to *predominantly internal* – 'the bad things that happen to me are mainly caused by me'. Remember that as assessors we are looking for patterns of unlikely predominance. Well-adjusted human beings are capable of blaming failures to meet deadlines on an (unappreciated) dedication and concern for quality, or, in moments of vulnerability, of blaming themselves for failing to live up to the unreasonable expectations of others. The question is: Do such patterns occur across a *wide range* of behaviour and circumstances – with delusions of omnipotence at one polarity and learned helplessness at the other?

In conducting thought experiments about our relationship with the environment we sometimes jump to conclusions on the basis of faulty or limited evidence. Many of our clients do this in an exaggerated and predictable way, and such patterns give important clues as to why they act in the way they do, or why they fail to respond (except passively or guiltily) to oppressive circumstances. The oddest behaviour can become 'logical' (distinguish from acceptable) when we come to see it in the context of its perceived justifications. Consider the following:

> *Bob*:
> There's been incidents where say I'm in a train going from Birmingham to Coventry with my family, and a woman got upset because I'd sat in a seat on the train that had been booked, but no one was going to be sitting on the seat. She was getting rather stuck up about it and I dragged her out of the chair and gobbed in her face. I said, 'Listen, my wife will sit wherever she wants. I'm not having you telling her where she's sitting.' My wife was carrying a baby at the time. I was rather upset about that as well, but then again it was crazy, you know, it was just over-reacting. There was no need for it. But she got up my nose and I just reacted violently, dragged her out of the chair.
>
> *Prof. Blackburn* (Forensic Psychologist, Liverpool University):
> How did she get up your nose?
>
> *Bob*:
> It was the way she was talking to me, the way she looked down at me. Just her general manner.
>
> *Prof. Blackburn*:
> How did you know she looked down at you?
>
> *Bob*:
> The way she was talking, like a stuck-up snob. I hated it. I ain't no different from anybody else. She might come from a posh house and a posh area, but she ain't no different from me. She got up my nose and I let her know about it and all.
>
> (BBC 1993)

Being at a safe distance from this dreadful situation allows us to take a cool look at it. Behavioural impulsivity is obviously present, but so probably is a faulty pattern of interpretation. Observations or requests from the victim trigger powerfully negative attributions from the perpetrator; she is out to put him down and belongs to a general class of people who have oppressed him in the past. The other passenger is not our client.

Attitudes

Once the dominant concept in social psychology, and still a major field of study, particularly regarding fixed, stereotypical orientations on such issues as race, age and gender, the whole idea of *attitude* came under attack from an earlier generation of behavioural psychologists as a redundant, circular, mentalistic concept (see Bem & Alan 1974; Rajecki 1982). Nevertheless, it has proved to be a very resilient idea. Here is Gordon Allport's classic definition:

> An attitude is a mental or neural state of readiness, organised through experience, exerting a directive or dynamic influence upon the individual's response to all objects and situations with which it is related.
>
> (Allport 1937: 9)

'Attitude' therefore (the term originally meant physical or spatial orientation towards some-thing) is a heuristic device for describing clusters of cognitive, affective and behavioural regularities which appear to transcend all but very strong differences in contemporary stimulus conditions. They represent the sum total of yesterday's learning environments which, through memory and conditioning, influence current behaviour. They are not an infallible guide to behaviour, but the concept of attitude maps on to something real, for it would never have been adaptive in our long evolutionary history, either biologically, socially or psychologically, for humans to respond to stimuli afresh each time. Analogously, under Deng Shao Ping, the *Peoples' Daily* typesetters stored pre-set-up blocks of metal type for a range of speeches knowing that only small adjustments would be necessary – saves effort. Hence we mentally develop, as it were, 'pre-taped' sets of responses for crucial sets of stimuli. Only rarely do we 'wipe' these; more often we record in new pieces of consonant information and edit out pieces of dissonance. When we do not, we tend to feel uneasy about inconsistency. This is something we learn through socialisation. Rough predictability is necessary for social interaction and so we are conditioned to feel anxious when we do not display it – which is why 'But I thought you always said that . . .?' is a somewhat threatening phrase to hear from anyone who matters.

Interaction of factors involved in assessment

Sometimes we catch ourselves responding to demanding stimulus conditions and agreeing with some doubtful proposition to please others. For example: 'these people have had a hard time, why make things worse?' (I'm being tactical and kind for their good). Sometimes a feeling arises in us (e.g. anger) which because of the context finds no overt expression. This too is uncomfortable unless we can say to ourselves something like, 'I hate your prejudice, but this isn't a safe place in which to say so' (I'll write a letter of complaint later).

Attitudes, then, result from the necessary economies of perception (knowing what best to search for in a complex field; from knowing what might give us an edge; knowing what might lead to gratification), all under the influence of previously conditioned and reinforcing emotions.

In assessment our main task is to try to elucidate the attitudes which lie behind trouble-some responses to problems, and tentatively to link together specific happenings, reports of emotional reactions and patterns of thought. These may take the form of general pre-dispositions: 'Give children an inch and they will take a mile', 'If you are really careful you won't be caught', 'Strong people look after you'. These will always have a previous history. Understanding problem-related attitudes provides us with therapeutic opportunities to inject controlled doses of dissonance: 'Yes your son *obeys* you while you are around Mr Adams, but what about when you are not – and does he *respect* you for what you are trying to teach him, or does he simply *fear* you?' When this was said to one of my clients, for whom 'respect' was all, but by which he usually meant 'compliance'; one could almost hear the crunching of mental cogwheels.

Problem-solving styles

Related to attitudes, and again based on experience, temperament and cognitive and behav-ioural deficits, these thinking patterns are inferable from regularly recurring approaches to problem-solving. For example, some clients faced with multiple challenges will pick the nearest one and exhaust their energies upon it. They have learned to feel better when they are taking action, *any* action. Debt counsellors are often confronted by clients who have paid off an insistent but by no means crucial creditor while allowing rent and tax arrears to accumulate. Conversely, some people can be exasperating in their 'wait and see, better the devil you know' approach to decisions. Case histories often reveal lost opportunities for, on the face of it, obvious alternative courses of action which are inhibited by previously reinforced ways of approaching difficulties. Such problems are seen in an extreme form in neurosis, when a self-defeating procrastination based upon anxious and over-inclusive perusal of *all* possibilities can be a feature (see Claridge 1985; Goldberg & Huxley 1992) but no one is completely immune to such influences. New approaches can be taught but first we must deduce something about current thinking and behaviour.

Many of the existing assessment aids employed in behavioural approaches may be adapted for the assessment of the cognitive accompaniments of behaviour. For example, clients may be asked to keep records of their thoughts in particular circumstances, either in diary form or on an 'ABC' chart. Or, in the initial stages of assessment, they may be asked to choose between various prepared statements about thinking patterns and how often they occur (see Fischer & Corcoran 2007).

Cognitive-behavioural therapists are interested in cognitive events for two reasons. (1) To test the hypothesis that if patterns of thinking (negative self-statements, inappropriate beliefs and attributions) can be modified, then the problematic behaviour which they accompany will also change. This, as we have seen, is to assign to thoughts the role of mediating variables. (2) To give us clues as to the type of consequences that maintain unwanted behaviour and prevent the emergence of more adaptive approaches. As with all types of assessment 'the proof of the pudding is in the eating', and we are most interested in how the client subsequently *behaves* as a result of intervention.

A good cognitive-behavioural assessment takes in three sets of factors influencing problems: cognitive patterns, emotional accompaniments, and behaviour itself. Each of the helping professions has had its preferences in the past, but there is now a considerable body of research suggesting that if we neglect any one of these components, then our attempts to help will be the less effective for it. Here are some further dimensions for your consideration.

The content of assessments

Referral and engagement

The ideal shape for any assessment procedure is, metaphorically, that of the funnel or tun dish; wide open to start with and then tapering off. A small experiment conducted with social work students learning communication and interviewing skills via closed-circuit television exercises (Sheldon and Baird 1982) demonstrated the need for such an approach quite well. Students (n = 30), were given identical information about clients, written on cards, but with referral and case information placed in different orders. The students were then asked to play the role of interviewer or client. What was fascinating was that if the first item presented involved concerns by teachers, the interviewer reflexively wanted to pursue education-related matters. If relationship problems between partners were placed first on the list the focus of the interview quickly became communication patterns.

People come forward or are impelled forward for help in often complex ways. Therefore the *route to referral* is the natural starting point for assessment. Sometimes clients have been to several agencies before receiving what they regard as useful assistance or none. This can mean that some feel they have already told their stories, and so may be reluctant to go through the whole process again. Getting hold of the back notes is not always straightforward either: sometimes for genuine reasons of confidentiality, sometimes owing to bureaucrat inertia.

Previous contacts can also result in a 'shaping' process whereby clients are persuaded that their difficulties are of a certain kind, with certain origins and with certain preferred solutions in prospect. There is also a large literature in social psychology on the subliminal power of initial impressions and of reputation (see Cohen 1964; Zimbardo 1992). Sometimes reputation and first impressions are more powerful influences than the *content* of what is said or done. Another aspect of pre-assessment experience is the way in which clients are received when they seek help. Rooms give messages. They may be welcoming and homely, or impersonal and threatening. On placement visits I have experienced the full spectrum of these impressions, from the bizarre – walls plastered with posters testifying to the idea that bed-wetting is largely a medical phenomenon (it isn't) because the receptionist's son had such a problem – to pictures everywhere of children in a hospice (creditably the receptionist was a volunteer in such a facility), but the overriding impression given was 'so you think *you've* got problems'.

There is no substitute for clinical staff taking an interest in the 'front-of-curtain' environment, since often this space simply does not seem to *belong* to those who work in the rooms behind it.

Dress and appearance are also important. Much of what follows may offend the free spirits among you, but it is frankly inappropriate to interview a troubled family or a bereaved elderly person in jeans and trainers, or a T-shirt bearing a slogan.

Staff should take notes during the conduct of an assessment because, as we have seen, memory is fallible; because clients' stories are full of dates, times and sequences which can easily get jumbled up, and because it is natural for listeners unconsciously to add in material to a narrative to round it off and make it 'coherent'. Yet sometimes it is the very 'incoherency' of accounts which makes for the most interesting starting point – which is why we started with the Virginia Woolf quote. But, in addition, imagine being interviewed by a financial adviser about your pension prospects, with him or her nodding sympathetically throughout but never writing anything down.

Family history

Patterns of unfolding interaction and their consequences for individual members and for the family as a whole are the stuff of a good family assessment. Tendencies to promote conflict or to sacrifice one's needs to avoid it; to seek dominance; to distance oneself; to play good person/child roles, or bad person/child roles are often played out as a matter of 'reflex'. Sometimes they are part of a 'game' which carries hidden reinforcement. Let us consider an example.

CASE EXAMPLE 6.2

Mr and Mrs D. got together in their late thirties via a contact agency; both had been divorced previously as a result of infidelity by their partners, and both were watchful in their later union. An unplanned pregnancy produced identical boy twins, and whether partly as a result of inborn temperamental factors (see Chapter 7) or largely as a result of their own, rather inconsistent parenting (both used the excuse of their age

---

and the 'unexpectedness of the boys' arrival'), both children were fractious, easily bored and mischievous at home and at school. However, one child was said to be the main offender, leading on the other. Thus Mrs D. referred one of her children (aged 6½) to a child and family guidance clinic saying that his behaviour was placing an intolerable strain on her marriage. Three main impressions dominated the assessment at this stage. (1) Both of the boys' behaviour was disruptive at home from time to time, but for longish periods one would lead off and the other would became a 'diplomat'. (2) The behaviour problems grew worse the more the parents tried to discipline the boys through threats and deprivations. (3) The behaviour problems – dogged disobedience, hurling parents' possessions around, low-level stealing – were not so challenging, but they were extensive.

Noting the rather negative nature of the parents' efforts at control, a simple positive reinforcement-based behavioural scheme was put into place (see Chapter 7). The referred child's behaviour improved steadily, and the case was quickly closed. Then a new referral was received for the other twin. When the therapist asked about his brother the mother said that he was 'good as gold' and that it was 'really' this other child whom she was worried about. More as a test than a treatment plan the behavioural scheme was then applied mainly to him. His behaviour quickly improved while the behaviour of his brother deteriorated sharply.

A series of more family-centred interviews were held, plus interviews with the children together and alone. This is what emerged. (1) The parents' somewhat obsessive attitudes towards their own 'rebound' marriage; their jealousy of each other and feelings that they were 'too late' having children, spilled over into family functioning much more than had been supposed. (2) Long sulks and frequent rows occurred which they tried to 'hide' from the children (children always know). Neither parent expected the relationship to survive long but were trying to stay together 'for the sake of the children'.

Interviews with the twins were fascinating. (1) They were worried about their parents splitting up knowing that they were unhappy (there were fears about homes and orphanages). (2) They talked together at length about what to do about this and had come up with a 'parent trap'-type scheme to deflect their mother and father towards concerns about them. They did this deliberately but felt 'very naughty' about it. They therefore managed this preoccupying disaffection by working shifts. One would give the adults something to occupy their minds while the other offered support, and then they would switch roles. It was almost as if, in these family circumstances, there was not enough love for two children at once.

A combination of CBT and conjoint family therapy, with the therapist concentrating on the unresolved feelings that the parents had brought to their marriage, had most effect in this case; second came getting the parents to talk to the children about their troubles in simple terms. The positive reinforcement scheme was reapplied alongside but quickly came to be used informally. Naming the 'family games' brought visible relief to all.

It will be seen that in this case taking a family history was no simple process of assembling facts and phases, but of establishing what events meant to the various actors involved. In this example, the history and its revisions, through adding in the separate psychological viewpoints from each member, and a few 'I didn't know, that you thought that I thought that . . .' breakthroughs, *was* the therapy. Histories are for *use*, not just for the file.

Current family relationships and circumstances

This part of the history is also concerned with qualitative issues (i.e. how relationships between family members have developed over time and what patterns of typical interaction have added to or subtracted from their problems), but it is mainly concerned with their current impact. Given certain situations, frustrations or dissatisfactions, which persons would typically intervene, how and why? Who would not, and why? This focus on contemporary manifestations recognises that although problems may have historical roots, they emerge in the here and now. What people did or did not do in the past may still be relevant, but so is the look of expected disappointment the parties give each other most mornings. If children are involved, family assessments need to be made against some template of parental functioning – I suggest against knowledge of empirical research from developmental psychology – which view leads one to bewilderment as to why such courses have been dropped from some training curricula and social work courses. However, while self-education should not be necessary, there are many good research-based texts available (e.g. Slater & Muir 1999; Berk 2005).

Tolstoy was right: well-functioning families exhibit a number of variables which render them resilient. (1) They provide opportunities for the expression of ideas and feelings in the expectation of being listened to. (2) No big family secrets exist which everyone pretends not to know. (3) There is a valuing of the different responsibilities and attributes of others. (4) There are rules that are flexible, explained, reinforced, but also enforced when necessary. (5) There are positive expectations of growth and change. (6) Good role models are available and discipline relies on these rather than ever more detailed instructions. (8) Love is shown and love returned; second chances are given. Writing this list is easy, but creating and maintaining these principles in adverse circumstances is quite hard.

Financial, material and housing circumstances

Our clients are often under heavy financial pressure due to chronically low income, debt, insecure and/or unsuitable housing, etc. Material problems of this kind add to the emotional problems of families, and in turn relationship problems can distract from sensible approaches to them. Clients (perhaps all of us at one time or another) are therefore often caught up in vicious circles; they often ignore financial problems, for example, rather than approaching them constructively and incrementally.

Health

Close attention to any physical or mental health problem is essential as these conditions can strongly affect social functioning even when they are not the main reason for referral. For example, one of the commonest causes of depression in elderly people is ill-health or worries about its prospect. These emotional factors can, in turn, lead to self-neglect, poor nutrition, self-imposed social isolation, and indeed to a worsening of the very physical health problems which started the cycle.

Education

If the family with which one is working has children of school age, then whether they present with problems or unexplained shortfalls in performance, or not, it is wise to enquire about their educational experiences since it is rare that this sphere does not affect the others. Bullying, for example, can have substantial effects on family life and often children disguise the fact that it is taking place. The child suicide, child depression and deliberate self-harm statistics hide thousands of such experiences.

Sometimes however, influences on family life are less dramatic, as when children are just 'not doing well', find certain subjects difficult, feel a failure, and so reject school and start truanting. Blunt consequences fall heavily on parents these days; cases have been given new attendance legislation, and this is particularly so where they have problems of their own. These may not seem like high-profile problems but they have manifold consequences. Recent systematic reviews of research show that although the commonest treatment for emotional problems in childhood is reduced doses of SSRIs intended for adults, some harmful effects have been noted, and combinations of CBT (see Chapter 7), advocacy with the school and family support schemes produce better outcomes (see Carr 2000; Macdonald 2001).

Reducing problems to their component parts

'What exactly is it in essence that is threatening, worrying or troublesome?' should be an early question. 'Where and how often do these events occur and what do clients do themselves to ameliorate them, and with what results?' should be the next one. Problems usually have cognitive, emotional and behavioural components. For example (from case notes of my own): '*I'll swear that child cries on purpose; he seems to know when I need a break*'; '*He* [partner] *makes me feel useless, he gets a kick out of it, and now I suppose I do feel useless*'; '*If someone takes you on you need to show them not to mess with you, so I never walk away from anything*'.

Another approach is to look at how and where problems begin and at what feeds them. Recurring difficulties often have identifiable 'triggers', are maintained by the reactions they get (e.g. 'You can stay out all night for me, it's your life.' 'Good, you said it.'), but sometimes these early precursors may yield to diversionary action.

Beginning with a list of problems is sensible, if clients have trouble helping to make one (e.g. by saying '*everything*'), then little thought experiments such as 'Imagine that it is a year from now and you are much happier, (1) what would have to have gone from your life? and (2) what would have to have come into it?' Or, 'If someone was able to record on CCTV everything that happened in your house/at work/at school on a typical day, what would they see/not see?' Or, 'If in six months things have improved for you and the exercise was repeated, what would we see and hear that is different?'

Sometimes single difficulties are central and give rise to satellite 'problems' (see Figure 6.14). Now it is quite likely that the father in the above illustration will see his alcohol dependency as a reaction to his distant, non-functioning partner; to his many worries; to the fact that he cannot get a job, and to the frustrations created by his 'out-of-control' children. But the more likely causal sequence lies in the opposite direction. Some problems are therefore symptomatic and due to underlying emotional difficulties. Some are based on self-doubt and self-defence. I have seen a number of children who have spent long periods in care who present with sharply different problems, showing, for example, aggression, self-centredness, and serious risk-taking behaviour once off the leash. Such children have learned

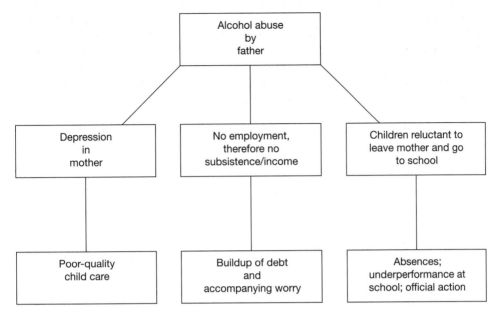

Figure 6.14 Interrelatedness of problems

to distrust the motives of others; they *expect* adults to let them down; they have few secure, counteractive relationships, and so they decide to look after themselves in whatever way seems safe or stimulating at the time. As W.H. Auden (1976, 1977) observed, '*Those to whom evil is done, do evil in return.*' The 'evil' does not have to have been intentional, by the way.

The trouble with the issue of presenting versus underlying problems, or of historical causes lying at the heart of current behaviour, is that it once got psychological therapists a bad press (see Brewer & Lait 1980). This is owing to the then quite widespread belief, derived from psychoanalytical theory, that 'surface' manifestations of problems – regularly drinking away the grocery money, neglecting children, stealing, etc. – were ubiquitously the result of some long-buried conflict. One can still come up against only slightly less evidence-immune behaviour from family therapists today, who seem always to be able to trace equally 'underlying' troubles to 'family system' pressures (see Chapter 8). Well, sometimes perhaps, but sometimes talking more openly about problems rather than in code, or avoiding them altogether, can influence matters positively. This is so even in cases where later evidence suggests that their problems were not directly due to 'family system' failures or twisted communication patterns (but then headache is not caused by lack of aspirin in the bloodstream).

Risk assessment

Once the therapist has achieved an overview of current problems, and has developed some ideas about their aetiology, it behoves her or him to undertake an assessment of any potentially serious risks posed. Given the high eligibility for service thresholds now in operation, most cases which come our way are likely to warrant this. We have to highlight this issue somewhere in the assessment sequence, but in reality it pervades all the stages under discussion. At the beginning we often have insufficient knowledge of the range and scope of problems to assess any risks that might attach to them or how these might be handled and so must return to the issue later. However, it is inadvisable to regard risk assessment either as a postponable phase, or as something that is done and dusted by a certain stage. In some cases we know at the point of referral that there is a real and present danger to self and/or to others and the circumstances giving rise to this perception will have to become the lead topic of conversation. In other cases, patterns of behaviour and/or circumstances may be deteriorating insidiously, and it is a mistake not to regularly review initial risk assessments.

Over the past few years a host of risk assessment instruments, national standards frameworks and departmental guidelines have been developed. However much comfort we allow ourselves to feel regarding these attempts, there are some provisos to enter about them.

1   As clinicians we inhabit an organisational and political culture which sees risks as virtually always foreseeable by someone; which sees the (as they turn out) mistaken priority accorded to certain *other* allegedly less risky cases (where nothing has yet happened) over the one where something *did* happen, as evidence of culpable misjudgement. In this fraught atmosphere we have – at a conceptual level – a difficulty in separating out risk; that is, *estimatable probabilities* from 'anyone's guess' *uncertainties*. This is an old problem:

> Uncertainties must be taken in a sense radically different from the familiar notion of Risk from which it has never been properly separated. If we do, it will appear that a *measurable* uncertainty or 'risk' proper . . . is so far different from an immeasurable one that it is not in effect an uncertainty at all.
>
> (Knight 1921: 205; original emphasis)

The tangible result of this confusion, and of the developing 'blame culture', is professional defensiveness; covert self-protection and 'going through the motions' behaviour by staff.

2   Many of the risk assessment schedules in use, which are intended to guide staff towards greater objectivity and consistency, are the products of a retrospective identification of factors present in cases where death or serious harm has already occurred. It is only recently that such guidelines have been subjected to validity and reliability tests. Validity raises the question as to whether an instrument actually measures what it purports to measure or just collateral factors. Reliability raises the question as to whether two or more different people (or one and the same person, at a different time) would come close as a result of using a given schedule.

3   There is another problem, this time regarding allegedly measurable uncertainties. Supposing we had a risk assessment schedule with an 84 per cent reputed reliability level (which because of a mental 'essay mark' effect looks first class in the prediction stakes), who would decline to use it? But collectively we are usually dealing with very large numbers of people who fall within a given orbit, namely millions of children, thousands of mentally ill people, etc., and we know very little about the base rates of 'suspicious' collateral circumstances in these populations.

The problem then with all but *massively* accurate screening instruments (we have none, nor does psychiatry, nor does education) is that when applied to large populations they yield discomforting numbers of false positives (not really a risk off paper) and false negatives (not a risk on paper but one in actuality). Therefore the risk of harm through hyper-vigilant good intentions should be as much to the forefront of our thinking as the risk of harm through lack of watchfulness.

It is important to distinguish between the general watchfulness that most staff adopt when working in risky areas and formal risk assessments undertaken at a particular point in time and designed to answer specific questions about the likelihood of harm. The former approach is an integral part of our responsibility for recognising, for example, children in need of protection as much as 'help'. The latter entails using a formalised approach designed to improve the quality of decision-making by providing a clear framework for the collection, organisation and interpretation of information. The most robust approaches are those based on established statistical associations between certain criteria and a s pecific outcome of interest (i.e. so-called *actuarial* models). These are the kinds of models that insurance companies use to assess risk and the subsequent cost of policies. As a general rule, these are better than those made on professional consensus (see Gambrill & Schlonsky 2001).

Given all these compromising factors, what then is the most secure way of approaching risk assessment?

☐ First, get to know the base-rates of the particular kinds of risk – risk assessment should therefore start in the library. For example, what is the recidivism rate for juvenile offenders with a record of certain types of criminal behaviour? What is the probability of someone who deliberately harms themselves, or attempts suicide, doing so again? The tendency for staff to focus on the uniqueness of individual cases means that we often rob ourselves of this appropriate challenge to our judgement and our (necessary) optimism. So, having been persuaded that someone who is remorseful and cooperative is not a serious risk regarding further violence, it is unlikely that we will pay much attention to statistics that tell us that 40 per cent of people with such a history are likely to do exactly the same thing again.

☐ Piece together the chronology of events, including contacts with other agencies. This 'picture-making' is routinely undertaken in circumstances when people have died, and typically leads to a good deal of information known to a variety of people never before put together in a way that allowed its significance to be appropriately assessed.

☐ Be explicit and transparent. Make it clear *what* information you have gathered, why you have gathered it, and what you think its significance is. Suggest what story you think it tells; estimate what it says about the likelihood of the risk you are concerned with happening, and over what sort of time period. Spell out the things you think might contain the risk, including those things which other agencies or other people can introduce. Ensure that they understand their role and its scope to avoid diffusion of responsibility which can be a side-effect of multi-disciplinary cooperation.

☐ Monitor the impact of particular forms of intervention and consider the length of time it is taking to bring about a given level of change. Is this in line with, or at odds with, the interventions literature for this approach? The latter point is particularly important when the risks one is dealing with are cumulative; for example, when children are routinely neglected but are not necessarily at a *specific* risk today or tomorrow, although their development and future life chances may be in longer term jeopardy.

☐ As new information comes to light, re-assess – preferably with a supervisor – your estimates of likely danger. Even though we can rarely estimate the absolute probability of something happening, we can, and should, be able to make a guess at estimates of relative probability. If someone is seriously depressed and at risk of suicide or self-harm, then learning that the same person has been left by their partner, or that they have lost their job, should alert us to heightened risk, and should prompt us to reconsider whether current services will be sufficient to contain it. For reasons of self-protection too, 'show your working out' regarding changing risk levels and anchor decisions in events as much as in conversations. *Invite* your supervisor to alert you to any logical 'jumps' or *non sequiturs* in your assessments. This process of active review is perhaps one of the most important aspects of risk assessment.

Case or problem formulations

Once *de rigueur*, they then fell out of fashion, but are now making a comeback in CBT. In the interregnum they were replaced by summaries of problems and the actions proposed which had few of the dynamic properties of formulations. In other words, the 'working out' was often not shown. A formulation is more than a summarising description. It should contain best guesses on the likely origins, patterns of development and present-day manifestations. Look at the following summarising statements from case records:

> This case contains many interactive problems to do with finances, inconsistent parenting, and pressures within the family system.

This statement gives *some* information, but leaves which? why? how? and so? questions largely unaddressed. It is difficult to get a clear idea of the therapist's thinking and plans from them. A good formulation is both a summary of main aetiological elements as seen by the social worker in negotiation with clients, but it has dynamic features too. That is, certain qualities should attach to problem formulations, the most important being clarity, unequivocality, and a sense that they could readily be overturned by subsequent information or experience – none the worse for that.

Here is an example of a good formulation (it was written by a student, incidentally). It concerns a case where the referral to Social Services came via the school, because teachers were worried that the children seemed tearful and fractious at going-home time:

> Because of his lack of experience with children and his anxieties about discipline, Mr A. tended, on joining the family, to crack down severely on minor infringements of rules – what he calls 'starting as you mean to go on'. However, the children's relationship with him is not sufficiently well developed that they are willing to accept this as his legitimate role. They see it instead as a rejection of them; as a desire to dominate them, and to replace their natural father. Discussion of this problem with the family and the drafting out of a simple agreement describing the obligations and expectations of both adults and children may be a useful temporary measure to reduce the present high level of conflict (rows and slaps) between Mr A. and the children. A separate series of meetings with Mr A. and Mrs L. aimed at teaching Mr A. how to express his positive feelings towards the children in a way that they can accept (including how to deal with rebuffs) should enable him to cope better in joint activities. It would be a good sign if these increased beyond their present low level.

Now of course, none of the above need be true; nor need the scheme outlined produce any worthwhile gains (although it did in this case). It may be that the social worker's encouragement that Mr A. should try to understand the children's apparent rejection of him and try to react differently *does not* result in him spending more time with them, or that it does, but that they continue to dislike it. It may be that the relationship with the natural father calls all tunes. It may be that the confrontations between adults and children continue at their present level, or that there are fewer of them but when they do occur they are *nastier*, in which case this formulation has proved inadequate and the helper will need to think again. However, having 'placed the bet' on the possible dynamics of this problem, he or she would have got to know about the need for revision quite readily.

Setting intermediate and longer term objectives

The word *goal* and the word *objective* tend to be used interchangeably; however, they do have subtly different meanings, namely :

> *Goal* N: Point marking the end of a race; objective, object of effort or ambition.
> (Oxford English Dictionary)

> *Objective* A or N: Belonging not to the conscious or the perceiving or thinking subject, but what is presented to this, external to the mind; dealing with outward things, exhibiting actual facts, uncoloured by feelings or opinions.
> (Oxford English Dictionary)

The word 'objective' thus emphasises the issue of how we will know when something has been achieved and what standards of non-subjective proof will be used. Thus, if a family 'seems happier these days', what it is that happens or no longer happens that leads one to the opinion that this partly qualitative, partly quantitative goal has been achieved? To concentrate only upon the qualitative (what *kind* of change) and ignore the quantitative (*how much*) or vice versa, is self-defeating.

In routine practice, intermediate and longer term objectives, and qualitative and quantitative factors tend to get mixed up together. This is partly due to the complexity of the cases with which we deal, but it also results from inadequate training in these matters, and from a stubborn occupational attachment to the heart-warmingly all-encompassing. Therefore, we think it wise to favour the second definition above and to take from it the question 'How will we know, and be able to show others we have achieved this?' That is, how will we know, over and above our subjective feelings, that something worthwhile has happened, other than through the subjective verbal commentaries of clients? Positive views from clients should by no means be neglected, but one should also expect to see tangible behavioural or circumstantial change to give these statements credibility.

Another problem is that the word *goals* is usually preceded in professional texts by the word *flexible*. This is to remind us that circumstances change and that we need to change with them. True, but in most studies of the process (see Sheldon 1977, 1985; Gibbs 1991) we find many more examples of vague, protean (i.e. anything that happens to happen can be wedged into the loose framework of goals) than of style-crampingly narrow objective setting. There is a balance to redress here. Our recommendations are to follow the advice of Karl Popper (1963) on finding out; namely, that conjectures and theorising can be as broad as one likes to start with, but then at some stage we must reduce opinions, hopes and expectations to statements *designed to be vulnerable to refutation*. Goals thus become self-administered challenges to good intentions. To switch metaphors, they are points to steer by, and the last thing that any navigator or those on board needs in a point is a *flexible* point.

CASE EXAMPLE 6.3

I once supervised an (able) student who was working on a demanding case involving a couple who were unremittingly at war with each other, but seemed in a strange way to enjoy this state of affairs. They had a 10-year-old son who was caught up in these games, which were vividly described by the student, who likened them to the couple in the play *Who's Afraid of Virginia Woolf?* The son was the main concern as he had long spells of something close to elective mutism. He was removed from home and placed in a specialist children's unit, with work continuing with the couple while options for his future were considered. Thirteen interviews were conducted but at the end of the contact there was little sign of change. Therefore the focus switched more firmly towards the welfare of the child and on the need to build a separate future for him. However, when the student had to compile case studies for submission with his placement report, he summed up this one in the following terms: 'At least all their hostility is out in the open now' (!) The view of the supervisor was that attempts to achieve certain goals in this case had failed. This did not constitute a failure on the student's part; nor was it evidence of a failure to select the approaches most likely to succeed according to the literature; it was a failure of influence. Better, surely, to admit this; to learn from the experience, and to realise that we cannot be of much help in the face of determined efforts to subvert. Later the couple split up; the child was successfully fostered; he regained his voice because silence was no longer the only safe course. See Kathryn Schulz's *Being Wrong* (2010) on the virtues of recognised error.

Now there is nothing wrong with the idea of a flexible *policy* in a case; it is just that when you come to goal-setting these need to be highly specific statements, that is, *inflexible*. There is nothing to prevent us, in the light of experience, from substituting one set of clear goals for another.

Monitoring

It *is* possible to weave a monitoring scheme and an evaluation scheme together into our daily work, if the purposes of this are explained early on to all parties in a case. Indeed, it is my experience that most clients value interim feedback on progress, both with tasks that they have agreed to pursue themselves, and in respect of those undertaken on their behalf. Here are the necessary steps:

☐ Introduce the idea early on of the need to monitor key events, whether of a positive type (which it is hoped will increase), or of a problematic type (which it is hoped will decrease), or both.

☐ Negotiate with clients as to what measures would best represent progress, and politely try to squeeze out vagueness of expression by asking for examples.

☐ Introduce the idea of record-keeping regarding both hoped-for qualitative and quantitative changes. Diaries are useful in the former case and simple graphs in the latter.

☐ At a qualitative level, standardised instruments (see Fischer & Corcoran 2007) may be used, on a pre-post basis, the validity and reliability work already having been done.

☐ Work with clients to produce estimates of the likely duration of attempts to change something. We know from the literature on task-centred case work (see Chapter 7) that this can have motivating effects.

☐ Do not be afraid to redefine goals and objectives, or to try out new approaches to problems; just restart the monitoring scheme each time.

☐ Give positive feedback to clients on any progress made. Many live lives where there is little encouragement available.

Evaluation

I have three recommendations to make regarding evaluations:

☐ Do one. Many case records inside and outside private practice contain nothing worthy of the name. In place of evaluations we tend to get summaries at the end – if the case ever reaches a proper planned, end, that is.

☐ Evaluation should be given a *much* higher profile on qualifying courses and on dedicated CBT courses than it currently has. Live case material is an excellent teaching medium in this regard. Unless staff know *how* rigorously to evaluate their own work, they become at best mere consumers of academic or agency exhortations.

☐ Pre-post-follow-up approaches probably represent the optimum level between rigour and practicability, whether qualitative comparisons are being made (e.g. handling family disputes by discussion and negotiation rather than dictation and threats) or quantitative comparisons (e.g. weight-gain, attendance at eating disorder groups). This means that we need *baseline information* before proceeding.

Conclusions

I have tried to set out what we think are the characteristics of a good assessment, and make no apology for it being an 'ideal type'. That is, we know that organisational factors, shortage of time, uncooperative clients and changing case load priorities will probably hinder the completion of stages in any neat order. The point is that if the therapist has these headings in his or her head, or better still on his or her pad, he or she will know that some information is still missing and can remedy matters when the opportunity presents.

7 Stimulus control (contingency management) techniques

We are all deeply engaged in the prediction and influencing of behaviour, or even the control of behaviour.

(Carl Rogers in discussion with B.F. Skinner 1956)

Discussions regarding the tailoring of interventions to the often complex origins and nature of problems (the 'logical fit' point made in Chapter 2) must begin with the questions raised at point 6 in Figure 7.1. One of the main problems is the weight to be given to environmental factors (reinforcement or the lack of it) where the individual has clearly acquired the capacity for certain adaptive patterns of behaviour, feelings and cognition, but current circumstances do not support these responses. Therefore, logically speaking, if we and the client have a chance to influence these contingencies or of setting them to do it, we have a chance of prompting and maintaining more appropriate reactions and ensuring that they pay off. Or, if adequate and useful responses are underdeveloped, or have simply never been learned and reinforced, then logic dictates that we need to concentrate on analysing their components, how circumstances are perceived in the first place, and then experimenting in controlled circumstances. The keyword in the diagram is *mainly*, for few cases come our way where the other challenges to more effective performance, more rational thinking, or more stable emotional reactions, are not present in the background.

Contingency management

Having decided that target behaviours are in repertoire to some degree, the therapist must look next to the factors in the environment that are failing to elicit and maintain these behaviours or that are eliciting and maintaining maladaptive responses in competition with them; that is, at the mechanics of behaviour and reinforcement. This may be just a question of coming up with a rearrangement of existing contingencies – as in a case known to me of a young man with Downs Syndrome who was a casual absconder from foster care. Given that normally there were no problems in the placement, it was suggested that staff should occasionally supply the interesting car rides he was known to enjoy, but which he currently had only when being returned by his carers or under police escort (so reinforcing his running away and 'giving himself up'). These were to be given pro rata for behaving well and (impulsivity was another of his difficulties) *not* running away. The police were also asked not to make a joke of his appearance at the station which, though good-naturedly, they often did.

Alternatively, it may be necessary to produce an entirely new set of contingencies, for instance: 'If there are three clear days without a single incident of fighting, the children will be taken to the sports centre.'

Set out below is a summary of the range of possibilities for changing behaviour by manipulation of the contingencies that surround it.

☐　Where the problem results mainly from an insufficiency of certain types of behaviour, it may be possible simply to identify and *positively reinforce* a low-level adaptive response so that it is 'amplified', performed more frequently, and its place in the individual's repertoire strengthened. In other words, we can work to improve the 'pay-off' for desirable behaviour. A good thought experiment is simply to raise the question with oneself and one's colleagues: 'What pays off for this person around here, in this setting, group, family, or organisation?' Answers based on observation often differ substantially from official views and intentions. There is also a cognitive component to all of this. In cases of attention-deficit disorders coaching young people so affected to pause and think, take a deep breath, envisage a desirable outcome thirty minutes away instead of the immediate short-term one, before stereotypical action, will only pay off if the environment is made to reward these unusual internal processes in backward, chain-like fashion. I retain interest in Homme's (1965) notion of thought patterns as 'coverants' (i.e. cognitive operants) in this regard.

☐　A performance may be *shaped* by the selective reinforcement of approximately similar behaviours, until they become progressively more like the fully fledged performance desired.

☐　Where the problem results mainly from an *excess* of certain behaviour, it may be possible to identify and positively reinforce a response which is *incompatible* with the existing (unwanted) one. That is, we may be able to encourage an alternative set of activities, which could eventually displace the existing behaviour, or which might prevent the individual from gaining reinforcement for the unwanted behaviour.

☐　Again, in respect of an excess of unwanted behaviour, it may he possible to apply *negative reinforcement*, so that whenever the individual stops this and performs some desirable alternative, an aversive stimulus is terminated. Here the contingent *removal* of the not-much-liked stimulus (e.g. being ignored) is made contingent upon the client refraining from undesirable behaviour and engaging in some more appropriate activity, which can serve to strengthen the alternative response.

☐　It may be possible to reduce the frequency of troubling behaviour by extinction; in other words, just by removing the positive reinforcement currently available for it.

☐　In certain cases, unwanted behaviour can be eliminated by *punishing* it whenever it occurs; that is, by ensuring that an aversive consequence results from its performance. More sophisticated adaptations of this principle are available, which attach different levels of punishment to different activities. These are called *response cost* schemes and involve the assignment of an agreed 'price' to each different pattern, according to its seriousness. Such programmes, mainly used with children, may be useful where there is a range of different responses which the therapist is anxious to discourage to different degrees – a sort of inverted shaping approach. However, the aim here should always be to make the consequences of different types of untoward behaviour clearer. Many of our clients already inhabit unpredictably punishing environments. Response cost schemes should aim to make controlling sanctions more predictable, contractual and rational, and eventually to shift the emphasis towards positive shaping (see pp. 201–206).

☐　Behaviour may be either encouraged or discouraged by manipulating the stimuli which *elicit* it via conditional reinforcers. Thus, it may be possible to do one or more of the following: remove or reduce the effect of the environmental cues (Sds) which signal that reinforcement is available for a particular, unwanted sequence; intensify the S^ds which trigger competing, desirable behaviours; intensify the cues which signal that no reinforcement will be forthcoming for unwanted behaviour (S^Δs); or remove the S^Δs which signal that no reinforcement will be available for desirable behaviour.

Combinations of techniques

Items in the range of possible influences on behaviour given above are presented separately so that each can be clearly identified. In a therapeutic programme it is very likely that a combination of such approaches will be used. For example, a scheme designed to extinguish troublesome behaviour by withdrawing attention from it is likely to be augmented by a programme of positive reinforcement for less controversial behaviours, the aim being to shape the individual concerned towards a more acceptable pattern of attention-getting.

Selection of reinforcers

The popular image of reinforcement is that it involves someone in authority dispensing artificial rewards for unequivocally 'good' behaviour. While each of these examples might just about serve in some circumstances with cooperative behaviour, it can be misleading to think of reinforcement in terms of someone giving some*thing* to someone else. Tharp and Wetzel (1969) once suggested the term 'reinforcing event' as more appropriate to field settings, since it is often impossible to specify exactly which part of the sequence is the potent element. Even where something tangible is being handed over conditional upon certain behaviour, it may well be the pleasant demeanour of the dispenser that is effective, or the recipient's own sense of achievement (of which the tangible reward is merely a symbol (CS), as when we earned stars or grades at school), or the fact that other people see him or her receiving preferential treatment – always providing that they have learned to care about such things. It is technically possible to conduct experiments to isolate the key factor, but this is rarely worth the effort involved, and so reinforcement often remains a 'package' of different influences. Therapists must use their common sense here and not respond mechanically to clients in the interests of accuracy.

Skinner wrote interestingly on this point in his philosophical essay *Beyond Freedom and Dignity* (we should be so lucky) (1971). He suggests that in cases of admirable behaviour the prestige accorded to an action is inversely proportional to the visibility of the forces which control it. In other words, dignity, prestige and honour are accorded approved behaviour in direct proportion to the difficulty of identifying the reinforcement which maintains it: for instance, where it appears to arise 'spontaneously'; where the individual has nothing very *obvious* to gain by performing a difficult task; and where the easiest explanation is that the behaviour is 'self-motivated' and altruistic.

My home town newspaper once carried an account of a man's heroic rescue of a drowning dog from the River Avon. Since nothing much happens around here, the following week's edition contained a follow-up story where it was recounted that this individual had saved *three* other pets from a watery grave over the past few years. Rationally speaking we should all have thought more of this canine lifeguard and recommended him for the RSPCA medal. But one's irresistible human reaction was: 'What is this man *doing* prowling the river bank? Just how do the dogs get in the river in the first place? What sort of person has the time for this?' And, quick as a flash, our evaluation of the man's behaviour has changed from 'brave' to 'a bit weird'.

The practical point here is that outside the animal laboratory, reinforcement is a *process* – a series of events with special meanings. What is given cannot be separated off from the manner or context of its giving. There is a tension here between technical specificity (making sure that reinforcers are arranged contingently and are having their intended behaviour-strengthening effects) and naturalness (taking care not to make the subject feel that he is being artificially handled and manipulated, because most of us through CS and S^d experience this as the opposite of reinforcement). The following general points about reinforcement practices arise from this discussion.

☐   Wherever possible, reinforcement for useful behaviour should arise out of the setting where it is performed and should be a natural concomitant of the performance. A set of contingencies expressed like this: 'If John helps staff and refrains from aggressive outbursts, which are distracting and time-consuming to them, then they will have time to spare to help him learn to ride his moped' is usually less resented than: 'John can have twenty minutes' supervised bike-riding if he refrains from aggressive behaviour and is helpful to staff for three hours.' In the first example a causal link is made between uncooperative and time-consuming behaviour and what happens as a result. The consequence is a fact of life; it occurs naturally, and is less of a therapeutic device. Most of us learn early in socialisation to resist over-controlling influences.

☐   Where it is not possible to link naturalistic consequences to behaviour, and some more artificial scheme is introduced as in the case of star charts displaying a record of acceptable behaviour from children, then it is important that they appreciate both the reasoning behind the scheme and that it is a special arrangement, designed to help them gain control over their behaviour. For example: 'As soon as Mark has achieved this level of school attendance, and has broken the habit of avoiding lessons he doesn't like, then the daily report cards will no longer be necessary.' This point is particularly pertinent to the design of contracts (see p. 201), but it applies to almost all work with young people. In the case of adults such schemes are usually dependent upon temporary reciprocal reinforcement schemes (if you will . . . then I agree to. . . .) (see p. 201).

☐   Artificiality and feelings of manipulation are likely to be lessened where non-material reinforcers – such as praise, approval, affection, attention and joint activities – are a main part of the programme. Where these are unlikely to be effective, material reinforcers should still always be accompanied by them. In this way acceptable, everyday rewards acquire a reinforcement value of their own, and represent a basis for the subsequent fading of the artificial (that is, socially and culturally untypical) features of schemes.

At this point it may be worth re-emphasising that reinforcers are not special in themselves. Events or commodities become reinforcers because of the particular behaviour-strengthening and positive emotional effects they happen to have on the performance of a particular individual in a particular circumstance. But note that for some, feeling angry, dominant or seeing fear in the faces of others can be positively reinforcing. This is why we need a technical term to replace reward, because some positive reinforcers look nothing like typical rewards (i.e. making a teacher lose her temper; seeing your parents argue in front of you; etc.). The only sure way to find out what reinforces a sequence of behaviour is to make an educated guess; try it, and closely observe the effects. However, there are some general guidelines to follow.

☐   We should try to observe the client's behaviour in natural or analogue settings so that the consequences which normally follow behaviour may be determined (but watch out for *post hoc ergo propter hoc* – followed by therefore caused by – mistakes). It may be possible then to reorganise these consequences (e.g. by providing more attention for useful behaviour, and removing it from unacceptable behaviour).

☐   We can make use of Premack's principle (1959) developed in the field of severe learning disabilities – but extendable to other chronic conditions. This states that a high-probability behaviour can be used to reinforce a low-probability behaviour when the performance of the former can be made contingent upon the latter. The assumption behind this approach is that if client A spends 60 per cent of his day looking out of the window, then this must be at least a lowest-common-denominator source of reward. If the same individual can he induced initially to exchange access to the dayroom couch near the window for a few minutes of rehabilitation therapy, or contact with staff, then a basis for shaping has been established. Premack's principle has had wide applications where it is difficult to discover interests through conversation – there may be none to speak of (see the case example on p. 199).

☐   Probably the commonest – and most sensible – approach to deciding what reinforcers to employ is to ask the people concerned (the client, family, friends, staff and so on) what is likely to be effective. In their work with troubled children at home, many therapists advocate the use of simple sentence-completion exercises such as: 'The person I most like to spend time with is . . .', 'The best reward costing £2 that I can think of is . . .' or 'The thing I enjoy doing most is . . .'.

☐   Reinforcement checklists are another method of giving an idea of what reinforcers to build into a programme. These cover a range of possible influences, from material rewards and objects to activities and the names of significant people.

☐   Programmes can be based on generalised reinforcers if nothing more specific seems likely to be effective. Attention, approval, free time, money, exchangeable tokens and so on are usually quite potent since they are a prerequisite for other kinds of reinforcement. Money or tokens have the advantage that they can be readily exchanged for other, more specific sources of reward, as well as taking into account the fact that appetites and interests change from day to day and from setting to setting.

The next set of factors concerns the feasibility of using particular types of reinforcement.

☐   Reinforcement needs to be powerful enough to compete with the already-present attractions of performing unwanted behaviours. It also needs to be durable over time. In addition, some thought should be given to the question of whether one type of reinforcement will affect behaviour in different settings (e.g. both inside and outside the home, where there is competition with peer group sources – which may not be entirely wholesome). There is also the problem of satiation: if the programme is based on material reinforcers, or on one type of activity, it may be that after a certain number of Pokemon cards, coloured pencils and trips to the sports centre, the child will have had enough of them. Often it is better to try to elicit *types* of activity and then to vary these systematically throughout the programme.

☐   There is little point in selecting reinforcers which will be technically difficult to present as a consequence of certain behaviour. Sometimes a signal of having earned approval will act as a conditioned reinforcer.

☐   Another consideration is whether there will be someone around to act as the therapist's mediator, to supervise and apply the new contingencies (see p. 194). Levels of co-operation, skill and understanding of the programme are important considerations here.

However, there is another awkward point to raise: professionals are always looking for someone to do 'hands-on' work for them, reserving themselves for special, expert conversations in offices with pot plants, and diplomas on the wall. Doctors and management delegate readily to nurses, which is why they are all huddled over computers so much. Psychologists have psychology assistants (who have to service psychologists so that they too can stay indoors); social workers have care assistants who do much of the work that social workers were invented to carry out. Seeing cases through in whatever place, setting, time, trouble or vulnerability kick off goes with the job in my view – as it used to do with GPs until they took the money, but outsourced the obligation for seeing their patients at home. Let's *not* do this colleagues, whatever the enticing reinforcement contingencies.

☐   The old maxim 'Start where the client is' applies in particular to cognitive-behavioural approaches. Clients will not respond to reinforcers if these are contingent upon performances (1) that they see as beyond their present capacities, or (2) where the reinforcer on offer is simply inadequate to elicit and maintain large-scale changes of behaviour – in other words, is 'not worth it' (see Figure 7.1).

Differential reinforcement programmes

These are probably the most widely used form (on the B side of CBT) of contingency management schemes and involve the setting up of a contrast between the consequences of desirable and self-defeating behaviour, always remembering that what is 'desirable' to some (car theft and joy-riding, setting fire to derelict property, using parents' credit cards to buy elicit video downloads) is undesirable to the rest of us. There are borderline cases of just about justifiable guerrilla activities where young people feel themselves to be living in oppressive circumstances, or deliberate self-harm appears to be the only means of generating concern in a fractured family, but more often 'desirable' versus 'undesirable' is a no-brainer (the

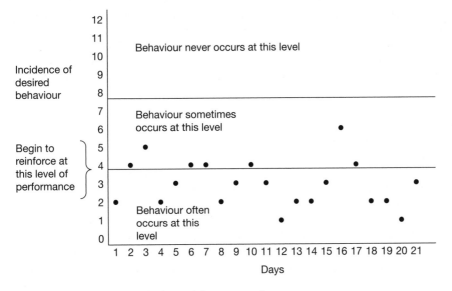

Figure 7.1 Level at which to begin a reinforcement scheme

arguments of a few leftover hip sociologists notwithstanding) because of the increasingly harmful and imprisoning (literally and figuratively) circumstances that often result.

In this approach behaviours that we want to strengthen are positively reinforced, and behaviours that we would like to weaken are placed on what is called an *operant extinction schedule* (wherein we arrange that no known reinforcement effects should follow such behaviours). To those factors may be added a third: the likelihood that in future, as a result of this clear demarcation, the client will be better able to discriminate between the two kinds of behaviour. That is, he or she will be more likely to know where, and when, each behaviour is, and is not, to be performed, as well as the likely consequences which attach to these different performances and settings. This may all sound somewhat contrived, but if you were well or even adequately brought up they are exactly the contingencies that would have been applied.

Figure 7.1 shows the daily occurrence of a behaviour which is to be reinforced. The scatter may be divided into zones labelled as above, or alternatively, 'extremely desirable range', 'desirable range' and 'extremely undesirable range'. Reinforcement should first be applied at the middle to top end of the 'frequently occurring' range, that is, it should be given for daily rates of 4 and above.

There follow some details from the case of the boy exhibiting allegedly 'disturbed behaviour' in school (hitting and pushing other children, running around the classroom, making disruptive noises, disrupting normal cooperation, behaving aggressively), which readers may recall from p. 120. The main elements of the programme are set out in the following case example:

CASE EXAMPLE 7.1

Methods used to inhibit classroom disruption:

Extinction. In practice, this meant that disruptive behaviour (as defined by teachers) was to be ignored whenever possible. If other pupils complained of Mark's behaviour (as they frequently did) they were told in a matter-of-fact way to ignore it if possible, and include him in the usual way that things were done in class.

Positive reinforcement. Any short period in which Mark's behaviour did *not* contain any of the disruptive features mentioned above (contra stereotype, these periods of peace accounted for *most* of the school day) were to be responded to by the class teacher (which is what they felt least like doing – the 'sleeping-dogs' effect) as a useful opportunity positively to reinforce behaviours incompatible with the target behaviours. This category included sitting still, working at an exercise, trying to read, neat work and so on. Where Mark joined in a group task – such as answering questions put to the whole group, or reciting an exercise – first the group would get the teacher's praise, and then Mark (and anyone else who came into this category) would receive a special mention for trying harder and for showing good progress.

The following reinforcers were used: physical proximity of the teacher and individual attention; praise and small displays of affection, such as a pat on the back (Mark would sometimes go through the motions of shrugging these off but undoubtedly looked for them each time); compliments on any work showing an improvement – whatever its absolute standard; ticks and initials on a card which was taken home to

---

show parents and could be redeemed for small monetary rewards, or trips to the swimming baths, cinema or hamburger restaurants with father. A little financial aid was given to these (not well-off) parents to establish this part of the scheme.

This classroom programme was complementary to a scheme already running at home. The daily progress card was used to link the two so that three initialled entries per day earned Mark a coloured star on his home progress chart, praise from parents, ten minutes' extra TV time per entry, plus 50p for every three entries. A bonus scheme was introduced to reinforce good weekly averages, so that initially, four stars a week resulted in an outing with father or mother. All the rates in these various parts of the programme were gradually increased (with Mark's foreknowledge) as behaviour improved.

Other procedures. An important part of the programme was an augmented remedial reading scheme implemented by teaching staff. This was sometimes carried out by a favourite second-year teacher of Mark's who did not normally have this function. This undoubtedly reduced his feelings of inadequacy and frustration in certain lessons. Mark had been seen by an educational psychologist who produced a perfect, evidence-based list of recommendations, which, unfortunately, were beyond the practical resources of the school and the Local Authority, and not to Mark's liking.

Problems. The programme's weakest point was the extinction contingency for disruptive behaviour. Some behaviour was just impossible to ignore, either because of the risk of injury to other pupils, or because of the bad example set for the rest of the class or because of other parents' complaints. Existing approaches, such as being placed outside doors, or taking notes home, had proved ineffective. Mark did not mind being put outside classroom doors as there was always plenty going on in the corridors; indeed this may have had a minor negative reinforcement effect since it put an end to what he saw as over-demanding class work. Similarly, if sent home, Mark would sometimes get a smack from his mother, but then would be free to play on his own for the rest of the day (a bargain), and mother's aversion to contact with Mark's teachers was strengthened. A further difficulty lay in persuading teachers to show interest in and affection towards Mark if his *current* behaviour justified it, and not to dwell upon either what he had recently been guilty of, or upon what he might do in the near future. Early attempts were stilted and robotic.

Time out. A time out from the reinforcement scheme was tried, and proved to be reasonably successful by at least bridging the gap until the positive reinforcement scheme influenced Mark's antisocial behaviour. A half-empty stationery storeroom was used immediately opposite the school secretary's office. A desk was placed there together with reading and writing materials. Extremely disruptive behaviour was first responded to by a pre-decided form of words, which gave Mark a clear option to sit quietly and get on with his work. If this failed he was accompanied there by his teacher, without additional comment. This occurred on eight occasions throughout the course of the programme and the periods of separation varied from five to fifteen minutes.

Changes were necessary at various stages of the programme. The extra TV time contingency, for example, did not work when there was nothing of interest being shown, and so playing out of doors for an extra fifteen minutes was substituted as a reinforcer on these occasions.

A further problem was reported by the class teacher who, in the early stages of the case, found herself having to explain to other pupils why Mark was apparently receiving 'preferential' treatment. She took advantage of time-out intervals to discuss with the class the idea that Mark needed everyone's help. An alternative approach might have been to involve other interested children in similar schemes, but geared to academic attainment or other individual considerations; however, this idea won little favour with hard-pressed staff.

Cooperation from teaching staff increased steadily as the scheme began to pay off, and staff who were involved in the scheme were increasingly free to concentrate on a home-based approach, leaving the school programme to the teachers. However, there were some early problems over defined professional 'territory' and the readily available option of 'special facilities' for this child.

Follow-up of the home and school programmes at six months revealed substantial and well-maintained gains in school, and less dramatic, but still useful gains at home. However, the main achievement in this case was that Mark continued to be taught at his ordinary school and, at the time of case closure, was seen, in the words of the headteacher, as 'still something of a challenge to discipline', rather than as a 'seriously disturbed boy' in need of 'expert help'.

This was a cost-effective exercise in multi-disciplinary cooperation resulting in a palpable degree of de-stigmatisation, showing that behavioural change influences thoughts, appraisals, attributions and prejudices, as well as the other way around.

Having discussed this case example at clinical conferences the typical reaction is that it is logically designed and did some good, but not how the services got to that point in the first place (i.e. why there was not an earlier intervention after exclusion from the first school). Why was time out necessary? Why was the mother's last-resort use of physical punishment necessary? (She thought that this worked better than the teachers' approaches which she probably largely believed would lead only to her son being referred elsewhere.) Why was a more cognitive approach not used, where Mark's perceptions of school life were redefined? It was tried throughout, and he got the message, but this did little to counter the raw behavioural/emotional contingencies in the case. Therapists presenting their clinical work often encounter such 'in the best of all possible worlds' reactions when they are bold enough to present real-world examples. It reminds one of the old nineteenth-century *Punch* cartoon of a gentleman asking the way to Dublin and being told, 'I wouldn't start from here if I was you'. However, in challenging cases, with much imminently to lose, where we are is where we are. 'Counsels of perfection' are unhelpful.

CASE EXAMPLE 7.2

In the case of the young boy (John) involved in arson (assessment data on p. 166) a wider combination of techniques was used, including the following:

☐ There was positive reinforcement of activities unconnected with periods of talk about fire and fire-related 'accidents'; self-selected activities included gardening projects supervised by John's father. (This new behaviour of his (disabled) father required considerable prompted reinforcement from his wife at first.)

☐ If 'fire talk' as it was called occurred, John's father had instructions to give one warning about it and then to come indoors at once.

☐ A diary scheme: one-hour intervals without pointed fire references earned (1) pamphlets and information about agricultural and horticultural activities from the therapist; (2) visits to a local garden centre; (3) money to take to school. This diary was reviewed by John's older brother on his visits, and outings with him (*not* to be punctuated with homilies on good behaviour) were made conditional upon a rising standard of behaviour.

☐ Extinction scheme: all talk of fire was ignored or, if it could not be ignored due to its persistence, it was responded to with a graded series of deprivations.

☐ John was instructed that if he felt himself wanting to talk about fire he was to try to think about other things instead – outings, model-making, his (largely positive) concern for his parents – and if this proved unsuccessful he was to leave the room.

☐ Targets in all schemes were gradually increased. John knew that the point of this, and understood that the purpose of the scheme was to build a happier family life and to keep him out of trouble – which, thanks to the persistence of his family, it did. This case did not, against the odds, enter the juvenile justice system, he stayed at his school, and he gave the whole thing up since his family were seen to be coming to his aid having recognised that his problems were also their concerns.

Another case example to illustrate the usefulness of a contingency management approach alongside family counselling and direct work with children. The former led to the acceptance of the latter – in most textbooks it is (somewhat romantically, I think) supposed to happen the other way around.

Case example 7.3 concerns the 9-year-old son of an army NCO referred to a Child and Family Guidance Clinic as a result of aggressive and insulting behaviour towards his now single-parent mother, his sister, occasionally towards his schoolteachers and sometimes towards passers-by in the street.

CASE EXAMPLE 7.3

The history of these problems is sad but uncomplicated. Kenneth's father was an unstable, impulsive bully to his family and there were two recorded physical assaults by him on his wife resulting in physical injury. Both incidents were witnessed by the child. A social history revealed the following stages in the development of these outrages.

The mother, herself from a deprived background, had initially found the 'macho' image of her husband to be exciting, giving her a sense of security. Their early married life was, however, punctuated by a series of disciplinary enquiries into his conduct as a soldier, and visits by the army welfare services. The charges never stuck; welfare officers were fobbed off, and a somewhat paranoid sense of triumph over 'officialdom' developed.

Kenneth's childhood consisted of (1) harsh discipline from his father; (2) exposure to grossly inappropriate magazines and videos; (3) an image of manhood based on physical prowess and domination.

Kenneth's father left the household when Kenneth was 8 – for another woman – but continued to see him fortnightly at weekends. From the age of 6 onwards Kenneth's behaviour had been a cause for concern to his mother and his teachers. He was aggressive towards other pupils and swore at his mother. On a few occasions when shopping he ran through the supermarket pushing trolleys into people. His general demeanour was aggressive and he liked to dress in combat gear and have his hair cropped in military style.

Following the departure of his father, Kenneth's mother made a determined effort to change the behaviour of her son. At the time of her son's referral to a Child Guidance Clinic she recounted that she had spoken to him at length about her embarrassment at his behaviour, tried to bribe him with expensive presents, and, as a last resort, used physical punishment, 'losing it' as she called it – all to no avail.

The approach of the therapist in this challenging case emphasised the need for consistency. Most of what had been tried before had been tried for short periods, the mother giving up and moving on to something new if an approach proved ineffective in the short term (providing negative reinforcement-effects). This also had 'immunisation-effects'. The differential reinforcement programme used in this case contained the following features:

☐ The identification of, and positive reinforcement of, low-probability behaviours somewhat incompatible with shouting, swearing and aggressive/embarrassing behaviour in the street. Those chosen were (1) improved school attendance; small-scale domestic tasks; regular attendance without incident at an 'after-school club'. The reinforcers used were stars signifying a buildup of credit towards significant purchases (e.g. his dream Nike training shoes, football kit, plus collateral reinforcement in the form of praise and small amounts of money).

☐ An ultra-reliable set of sanctions for adverse behaviour based on deprivation punishments (e.g. staying indoors; time out for fifteen-minute intervals, terminated by a believable apology (response cost); loss of television and computer privileges, and loss of credit via the star chart scheme outlined above).

☐ Basic assertion training (see p. 221) and rehearsal of typical incidents with mother (modelling – see p. 215). The most effective component.

The positive reinforcement scheme worked well from the start. A scrapbook with catalogue pictures of hoped-for purchases was used to record the necessary rates of positive behaviour to achieve these. Stars could be cancelled at agreed rates for occurrences of bad behaviour. Most effort, however, was spent on rehearsing with the mother her reactions to transgressions and stiffening her resolve to see each incident through. An attempt was made to enlist the help of the father during his fortnightly access visits. The results were mixed, with some rapid gains if he felt in the mood, some laxity resulting in setbacks in otherwise good weeks, and occasional sabotage.

Further elements in this scheme were:

- ☐ Periodic counselling appointments (in the office) with mother, which served to boost her confidence, to remind her of the agreed view of the origins of this problem, and of her plans for her own independent life – currently at risk because of the behaviour of her son.
- ☐ In-session modelling of appropriate/proportionate but determined reactions to the worst excesses of her son's behaviour.
- ☐ Periodic and unscheduled telephone contact to check on progress and to reinforce the need for consistency in Part 2 of the programme.
- ☐ The entire scheme was openly discussed in family meetings but the consequences of failing to participate in it were not glossed over. The results of his intervention were not substantially different from the mother's own attempts to deal with it. The modifications were (1) steady persistence encouraged by the therapist; (2) a move away from reliance on punishment to rewards and positive shaping.

Use of Premack's principle

Readers will recall from Chapter 2 that the definition of this approach to selective reinforcement was that a high-probability behaviour could be used to reinforce a contingent low-probability behaviour, provided that opportunities to perform the first could be made conditional upon the performance of the second. This principle is especially useful in cases where it proves difficult to find effective sources of extrinsic reinforcement – for instance, where there is nothing the client values more than the reinforcement obtained from performing a certain (high-probability) behaviour.

CASE EXAMPLE 7.4

The following case of a 4-year-old child (infantile alcoholism syndrome was suspected) with one failed foster placement behind him illustrates the principle. It was hypothesised that Ian had learned three things from his chaotic first years of life: (1) adult attention is a scarce commodity; (2) if you want it you have to make a fuss and put up with the 'impurities' when you get it, and (3) when you get it, hang on to it like grim death.

Ian was placed with carefully selected foster parents, but after a short while and despite active social work support, the placement began to break down. Foster parents complained of the following behavioural problems:

☐ 'Uncontrollable' temper tantrums, with Ian resisting all comforting or diversionary tactics.

☐ Excessive clinging to foster mother (this was seen initially as a transitory phase in the placement, but it did not go away as expected). Ian would hold on to his foster carer for most of the day, trying whenever possible to climb on to her lap. Attempts to remove him resulted in violent tantrums.

☐ Regularly entering foster parents' room at night and waking them.

☐ Breath-holding when frustrated. By the way, there was no shortage of contemporary attention and affection in this case; the deprivations came from the past, but manifested themselves in the present.

Procedure

☐ The foster-carers were advised to pay special attention to Ian's occasional bouts of solitary play and whenever he seemed to be coming to the end of such a period (before he began to 'grizzle' or seek attention) one of them would invite him to come and sit nearby and hear part of a story. It was made clear to Ian that this was a reward for playing nicely.

☐ At the end of five minutes of story-telling a 'natural break' was initiated. Ian was taken back to the scene of his earlier play activities and encouraged to resume them with the reassurance that in ten minutes or so he could come back for part two of the story. If Ian attempted to return before the time assigned, he was taken gently back to the play area. If he persisted, his foster mother would leave the room, leaving the book behind. If Ian followed and refused to be taken back, a 'time-out' scheme came into operation (sitting apart).

☐ A darkroom timer with buzzer was used in the early stages of this programme, and waiting for the signal for an interlude of close physical contact became a game in itself – otherwise time out would not have worked.

☐ Time on the foster parent's lap (high-probability behaviour) was made conditional upon increasingly long periods of play, or upon non-attention-seeking activities (low-probability behaviour).

☐ Other useful behaviours, not associated with tantrums or attention-seeking, were differentially reinforced with praise or small rewards, such as Lego pieces to add incrementally to a small model which he was being encouraged to build.

Ian eventually went to his local school – not without difficulty, but with considerably less disruption than was originally feared. His clinging behaviour reduced to easily manageable levels in thirteen weeks (due mainly to the foster carers' grasp of the general principles of the scheme and their ability to adapt it to new circumstances). Most importantly, the programme gave the foster parents a 'second wind', enabling them to continue the placement (see Macdonald & Kakavelakis (2004) for an RCT).

Contingency contracts

Contingency contracts have long been a useful procedure, and are particularly applicable to interpersonal problems. They are documents that specify behaviour which the parties would like to see performed more often, less often or not at all. They rest upon a particular interpretation of operant theory and this needs to be taken note of before describing applications.

In many cases that are referred to professionals in health and social care, it cannot be said that one person *has* the problem, or even that one person *is* the problem. Rather, difficulties lie in the conduct of relations between people. This is particularly true of family or relationship difficulties. Much of our behaviour in such settings is maintained on the basis of reciprocal reinforcement, and this process may best be thought of as an exchange, in which behaviour from person A is elicited and reinforced on the implicit understanding that behaviour from person B will be similarly treated. Different 'exchange rates' will be found within this process for certain behaviours which are differentially valued by the parties.

In most relationships there is a tendency towards a relatively enduring balance or homeostasis, maintained and controlled largely without explicit discussion. Where this balance and reciprocity breaks down, as in the case of family problems or estrangement, then four kinds of things tend to happen.

☐ Helpful behaviours, which would normally be elicited by the everyday actions of the other party, have to be specially prompted and specifically monitored. Arguments occur about relative contributions – who has done what, what the real value of such behaviour is when weighed against the behaviours performed by others, and so on. Generally speaking, people are uncomfortable in the face of this kind of greater specificity, especially since explicit prompting and control rob behaviour of much of its apparent spontaneity. The problem is that not getting what you want from another person, or getting too much of what you don't want, when left vague, often increases disputes; it *should* be a natural exchange, but what if it is not?

☐ The balance of mutual control shifts from positive reinforcement and positive shaping towards punishment, negative reinforcement and negative shaping. Respectively: 'If you do X I shall retaliate with Y', and 'Until you do A I shall keep doing B'. In other words, control of important behaviour is maintained by punishing transgressions, and by keeping 'the heat' on the other person until he or she performs actions close to those desired. This gives rise to the usual escape responses, which become increasingly sophisticated, thus requiring more powerful aversive controls, so that a negative spiral develops. I have yet to see a case of bad relations where this is not so.

☐ In such a context a well-intentioned relaxation of control is often taken advantage of by the other party, and an attempt to revert to positive reinforcement of the behaviour of the other is often seen as a ploy to be resisted. If you are now thinking of political negotiations, climate change or arms reduction treaties, you are right to do so, since these 'game theory' manoeuvres are ever-present here too, whatever the brain power of the negotiants or what is at stake.

☐ When reconciliation *is* attempted, either internally or with outside help, parties often start negotiations with an insistence that others must change their behaviour first. However, on the occasions when this happens the behaviour tends to receive little or no positive reinforcement for quite some time. Indeed, it is more often used to contrast previous behaviours (the *'about bloody time too'* syndrome, well known to anyone working with conflicted families).

These few points all add up to a view of close personal relations as a system of reciprocal reinforcement that has its own mechanisms for maintaining balance. In the same way, a gyroscope will resist small buffetings and remain stable, but a stronger force will seriously disrupt the mechanism and then equilibrium is hard to regain (see Sheldon & Macdonald 2009: ch. 8). This systemic model draws upon both operant and classical learning theories. When potentially useful, conflict-reducing actions are not reinforced (either positively or negatively) axiomatically, they are likely to recur less often. In addition, when the behaviour of another person is regularly associated with punishing effects, eventually this person's presence alone can trigger bad feelings – irrespective of what they happen to be doing at the time: the medium becomes the message (a generalisation effect through conditioned S^ds).

There is empirical evidence that relationship problems can be overcome by direct measures to reinstitute reciprocal reinforcement. A comprehensive review of recent research in this field may be found in Sexton *et al.* (2004).

The logical corollary of the views presented above is that a therapist seeking to improve interpersonal relations is unlikely to be successful if he or she works with only one part of the family system – one estranged partner or one adolescent seriously at odds with the rest of the family. The positive reinforcement potential lies in the hands of people least likely to use it, and some sort of staged reduction of hostilities (my favourite analogy for use in such families is 'SALT II', Strategic Arms Limitation Treaty negotiations), based on the exchange model outlined above. It is in this field of family and relationship problems that contingency contracts have had their widest application. They arrange for the mutually guaranteed reinforcement of adaptive behaviours, on the basis of an agreed exchange of actions which would not otherwise be performed if the reason why they are not is low expectations of reciprocity.

The design of contingency contracts

Contingency contracts are specific written agreements about future behaviour and they are based upon two major premises.

☐   That a definite, unequivocal and publicly made commitment to a future course of action is more likely to be complied with than more implicit agreements reached in more casual and reflective forms of discussion – providing that the client does not feel that he or she has been coerced into these decisions (see Festinger 1957).

☐   That with many interpersonal problems, the most powerful reinforcers available for adaptive behaviours lie with the person experiencing the other half of the problem. Therefore a prearranged and simultaneous alteration in the pattern of consequences produced by key problem-related behaviours is the best way to proceed. However, it should be noted (1) that the *withholding* of expected reinforcement, and (2) (not always accurate) attributions regarding motives and intent are often the basis for these vicious circles. None of us is exempt from such misunderstandings and, for example, a few years ago I was invited to speak at a conference (on CBT) by one of my favourite ex-students from thirty years ago, now a senior lecturer and co-author and PhD. I was pleased enough with the presentation and so was she; we got to talking about old times and most of my positive reminiscences about her seemed to come as a surprise to her – which in turn surprised me. After further discussion it turned out that she; had always thought I had a down on her, evidenced by the fact that I deliberately set her essay topics that were more demanding than those of her fellow students (just imagine this, student readers: individual tutorials, individual essay topics tailored to joint interests!). My reply was, 'Yes, because I thought you brighter than most, and that you were looking to be challenged.' Her reply was: 'But I *didn't know* that that was what you thought!' Another example of intended positive reinforcement being mis-interpreted (so this problem is not confined to an up-against-it clientele), but sadly it took me thirty years to find out.

There is considerable empirical support for the two propositions discussed above and, in the field of interpersonal problems, contingency contracts are one of cognitive-behavioural psychology's success stories.

The aims of these agreements are similar to those of most types of operant scheme. The behaviours under review must be accurately defined, and the future contingencies which are to apply must not be capable of too much misinterpretation. Where definitions of problems cannot easily be reduced to items of behaviour, then a good second best is to have an agreed list of examples to refer to, so that John's 'looking for trouble', or father's 'put-downs' can still be accurately identified when they occur. In this conciliation work there is an additional emphasis on negotiation between parties, and on identifying behaviours of approximately equal value to the participants so that in the presence of one, the other is more likely to occur. In other words, considerable effort goes into striking an equal bargain, using sequences of behaviour as the medium of exchange in the hope that re-established reciprocity will in due course infuse cognitions and feelings.

Table 7.1 (below) gives an example of a contingency contract worked out between a 14-year-old 'skinhead' boy who was referred to Social Services by the police and his parents. The three main (extant) problems were: (1) a risk of him committing further offences (property theft, damage to public property, setting fire to post-boxes with lighter fuel being a speciality); (2) his increasing estrangement from his family – his father having threatened to evict him several times; (3) a real and continuing risk of violence between father and son (the mother described their behaviour as a 'love-hate relationship' but undoubtedly rejection was in the ascendancy at the time of referral) and the father would typically wait up for his son to come home (late usually) and push and shove him to bed; often this led to violence by both father and son. To give the flavour of this hostility, the father once raised the question in front of his son as to whether there might not have been a mix-up in the maternity ward. His son was short, his father tall. His father had done well at school, his son did not; father had athletics cups on the sideboard, his son only liked fishing. His son spoke in an ersatz cockney accent to annoy his parents as a badge of gang membership though he lived in Warwickshire and his father was Deputy Town Clerk. His son was going nowhere in the father's opinion.

The provisions of this contract were suspended after eight weeks of successful operation. It did not solve every aspect of the family's problems; John's father continued to idealise his own childhood and draw unfair comparisons between the somewhat antisocial views of John and his associates and his own golden youth. Nor was it possible directly to influence John's behaviour outside the home. However, no further offences were committed over the next eighteen months and his parents thought that this was at least partly because John spent more time at home and had less interest in 'shocking' his family in retaliation for what he saw as their unreasonable treatment. This is speculative; what the contract achieved without question was an effective *truce* between the warring factions, the rules of which, as the contract was faded out, became more a part of their normal day-to-day behaviour.

Table 7.1 Contract (Skinner family)

This is an agreement between Mr and Mrs Skinner and John Skinner (aged 14). It aims to increase the level of happiness enjoyed by this family by making it clear to each member what the others expect, and what consequences follow both meeting and not meeting these terms.

Mr and Mrs Skinner	*John*
Agree that if John returns home by 10.30 p.m. on weekdays and Sundays and 11 p.m. on Saturdays, nothing will be said to him about where he has been or what he has been doing. If John is late they will ensure he forfeits time the next night.	Agrees that in exchange for being allowed out late he will: (1) Keep to time. (2) Forfeit double time for each five-minute period he is late without an acceptable excuse and twenty minutes for each five-minute period after half an hour has elapsed past the deadline – regardless of excuses. The time will be forfeited the following night.
Agree that if John stays home every Sunday evening and on one weekday, he will be allowed to attend two discos a month until 12 p.m., at which time he will be collected by his father.	Agrees that in exchange for being allowed to attend discos he will spend a specified time at home and will spend at least two hours of these days helping with household tasks; for instance, cleaning his bedroom, washing up and/or gardening; and that he will telephone home before 11 p.m. to reassure his parents.
Agree that they will give John £10 pocket money per week, £2 of which will be unconditional. Sister's pocket money will be similarly worked out and no extras given.	Agrees to forfeit money in up to £2 units if he fails to: (a) help around the house as defined; (b) telephone to reassure parents, or is spiteful to his sister (by agreed definition).
Agree to accept politely-phrased comments on their behaviour as it affects him, and to involve him more in day-to-day decisions – such as where to go out together or what TV programmes to watch.	Agrees that in exchange for being consulted, and having his views listened to, he will try harder to keep his temper, stop swearing at home and leave the room rather than shout at his parents. Failure to cooperate as defined means loss of one evening out.
Every Saturday father will spend at least three hours with John engaged in an activity acceptable to John if John meets the terms of this contract for one week. No mention will be made of past problems during these activities.	In exchange for going out alone with his father, John agrees to: (1) stop provoking his sister into rows; (2) listen to the points father makes, providing they are within the terms of this document.
Parents agree to address any worries about what company John is keeping to the social worker, and will not talk to John about them for the moment.	In exchange for the privilege of being allowed to choose his own friends, John agrees to call to see the social worker briefly once per week after school by appointment, and will be prepared to discuss his activities outside and inside the home.

There will be a fortnightly family meeting to discuss disputes and any problems arising from the use of this contract.

Signed ....   Signed ....

Date ....

Three general things may be said about contracts such as this:

☐ They work best when potential solutions to problems lie substantially within the gift of the parties directly involved. That is, where each of the protagonists genuinely possesses the power to alter things for the other(s) and satisfy them to some degree, since there is little point in trying to achieve an internal settlement to a dispute maintained largely by outside pressures. 'Hell is other people', said Jean-Paul Sartre but this is only half the truth, because happiness and a balancing of interests and security is also usually dependent upon accommodation with other people. Revenge is not in fact a dish better enjoyed cold (or hot for that matter); it is one better pushed aside.

☐ It is far better to agree relatively easily and substantially on something small, than partially and with difficulty on something major. The results of flying diplomacy may look good on paper and produce lots of photogenic handshakes, but often the shooting starts again shortly after the presidential jet (or, in this case, the departmental Citröen) has landed back at base. As with other types of behavioural schemes, the all-important early task is to provide a positive experience of rational problem-solving. A contract must prove its worth in the short term or it will not usually get a chance to prove itself in the long term. Clients rarely refuse absolutely to negotiate about behaviour, but are more concerned to establish a reasonable *level* of it, and to negotiate exchanges of positive behaviours at what they see as a reasonable 'cost', measured by the effort involved and the misgivings they hold as against the benefits received.

☐ Contracts should be focused on interpersonal 'flashpoints'; that is, upon regularly recurring 'set-piece' patterns of discord. In Table 7.1, the most important gain was in removing the nightly row (and sometimes fights) with the father and the 'may as well be hanged for a sheep as for a lamb' contingencies this set up with John.

However, if you propose an idea, or recommend a particular pattern of intervention, you never know where it will lead. Just after I wrote my first paper on contracts and relationship counselling the following headline appeared in a tabloid newspaper:

> Social workers have drawn up an amazing contract giving pretty 14-year-old Justine Carter freedom to stay out ALL NIGHT. . . . 'I begged the social worker for assistance (said Mrs Carter) and a contract is what I got . . . I signed it to keep the peace but I certainly didn't agree with it.'
>
> (*Daily Mirror* 1978)

This young girl was found by police heading home at 3 a.m. She waved a copy of the contract which did indeed cut her risks in half, and reduced these instances of her staying out and not going to school, but she had already met the requirements for that week so was on a 'contract holiday' as she saw it. The newspaper's view was that she shouldn't be behaving in this way in the first place and that Social Services were condoning the remaining 50 per cent of her errant behaviour – The Road to Dublin argument again.

In less controversial cases of this type, the best approach is to have the practical necessity for a policy of reducing problematic behaviour in stages discussed by as many of those on whom it will impinge as possible.

'The medium is the message' so far as the process of negotiating contracts is concerned. The would-be-helper, insofar as he or she has the ability to conduct open and honest negotiations and to reduce conflict by compromise, will serve as a model for the other participants. This will be so whether they are aware of the fact or not. There is, therefore, an opportunity here to go beyond negotiated truces between clients, or *détente* between the identified client and the family. The process of drawing up a contract can itself serve as a device for teaching and demonstrating the skills of non-aggressive self-assertion, or the salving, realistically achievable concessions involved in repairing damaged relationships. 'I know what: suppose we write all this stuff down and try to get rid of the flashpoints' was my opening sentence in the case described above. No one dissented.

Here is a list of further points to keep in mind when trying to produce a workable contract:

1   For a contract to be worthy of the name there must be some degree of equality between the parties to it. Legal contracts may be set aside where the relative powers held by the signatories are deemed to be grossly unequal There are similar ethical dangers with contingency contracts, where an anticipation of coercion or loss of privilege can produce the same kind of sham voluntarism.

2   If a contract is to work well, all parties must see clearly that they will get something worthwhile out of it. The benefits of keeping it must be worth the 'costs' of the changes in behaviour that it requires. It is vital, therefore, that the negotiator continually checks out the balance of real value to the respective parties.

3   The therapist must not be afraid to instigate renegotiations where the device is plainly not doing its job. In this way agreements may be adapted to changing circumstances, and clients can be given further practice in defending their points of view in a reasonable manner. Wherever possible, the contract should be couched in positive terms, or at least contain a balance of benefits and sanctions. That is, it should be clearly stated that from now on *this* pleasant consequence can be relied upon to follow *that* particular behavioural sequence; rather than arranging solely for unpleasant consequences to operate *unless* X behaves in a particular way – this can mean that the non-performance of one sequence of behaviour results in the other party having to withhold positive behaviour.

4   Once broad agreement has been reached, a draft should be produced and used as a basis for further discussion. The finished version should be logically set out, and written in plain language. Each of the signatories should have a copy. Contracts should, however, not be seen as a technique in its own right, rather as the carefully checked out set of minutes consolidating whatever can be agreed upon.

5   It is a good idea to fix in advance a regular series of meetings to review their operation. This makes it less likely that parties will withdraw unilaterally following a dispute.

6   Contracts cover most of what we do in our daily lives outside the home – in employment, and in our commercial relations. However, when they are brought in to regulate aspects of family life, they have an artificial feel. We prefer the rules by which we govern ourselves in this setting to be implicit. To some extent this is also the case with therapist/client relationships, though there are fewer definite expectations here. Given the force of this cultural norm, it is very important that the *temporary* nature of contracts should be underlined. As soon as sufficient stability has been achieved, and the main contract terms are implicitly as much as explicitly observed, the rigid terms can be phased out clause by clause. A good indicator of when to do this is provided when the clients start to apply the principle of non-acrimonious negotiation to aspects of behaviour other than those covered by the agreement.

Contingency contracts fail for three main reasons: (1) the terms are not specific enough and are interpreted differently by the various parties, leading to early disappointment; (2) new behaviour is insufficiently reinforced and/or there is too great a time lag between performance and the counter-response supposedly guaranteed; (3) there is insufficient supervision of the operation of the agreement in the early stages. They are not a panacea; nor are they always an end in themselves. Often their main function is to provide breathing space; a dependable structure within which long overdue consideration can be given to how long-standing problems achieve their daily effect through *contemporary* behaviour rather than be attempts to disinter the long-lost origins of problems.

Cognitive methods sit alongside these behavioural, exchange-theory approaches. Words from protagonists like 'never' or 'always' rarely survive rational appraisal; malintent, though frequently ascribed, rarely survives a calm discussion of what was actually in the minds of those involved at the time. In the example given in Table 7.1, to my great surprise, the young man selected time on a fishing expedition with his father, as they used to do, as his favourite activity. It brought tears to his father's eyes and, I have to admit, to mine that it came in the *truth and reconciliation* interview where the father raised the 'wrong baby brought home' hypothesis.

Contracts are the medium, not the message.

Operant extinction techniques

Extinction is a process most often used in combination with other contingency management techniques, but with unidimensional problems it can work well on its own. Figure 7.2 is an example of its use in a common problem – excessive crying in children (see p. 92 and case example on p. 95 on innate influences). Although infant crying is an everyday, or more often every night, occurrence for almost all parents, where it occurs to excess, and on top of other

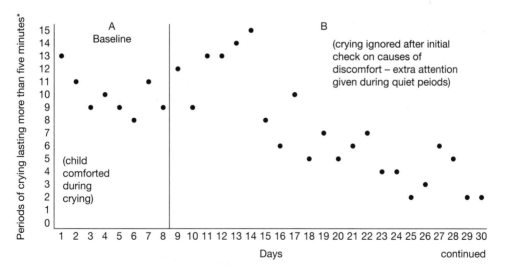

Figure 7.2 Excessive crying in a 1-year-old child (AB)

Note
* Medical examination showed no physical cause.

problems and frustrations, it can be a provocative factor in child abuse cases. (Apparently the old KGB gave up physical torture when they discovered that sleep deprivation worked better.)

Approaches based on negative reinforcement

The therapeutic application of negative reinforcement principles (see p. 110) is called *avoidance training*. Clients are taught to make responses which terminate pre-existing aversive influences. For example, in a social skills group of my experience, adolescents with a reputation for truancy and disruptiveness in the classroom were taught to reduce teacher disapproval and anxiety by admitting that they could not understand a given point, by apologising for incidents, and so on. Whether such schemes work, or descend into parody, will depend upon the willingness of adults in charge to forget what happened yesterday and seize a good opportunity when it is handed to them.

Negative reinforcement is usually just one of a number of factors in contingency management programmes. The concept itself is more useful in explaining why maladaptive behaviours are performed in the first place. Many are an easy means of escape from aversive circumstances – such as when a low achiever at school plays truant to escape criticism and the daily evidence of his ineptitude, or when someone takes a tranquilliser to 'switch off' or at least 'turn down' what appear to be the constant demands of children. In such cases the therapist has the option of trying to remove the cause of the negative reinforcement (by trying to obtain a more sympathetic approach from the teacher in the first case, or a behavioural scheme to change the behaviour of the children in the second if it is disproportionate). The 'earthing' of expected failure was a key influence in the case example above (7.2).

Shaping, fading, chaining, prompting

These procedures are grouped together partly because they have been dealt with elsewhere in this book and partly because they are all really sub-techniques rather than full-blown strategies. This means that they are more likely to be used as features of a more comprehensive programme than in their own right.

Shaping

Shaping (see p. 113) was a feature of the two main contingency management case examples used in this chapter (pp. 194 and 196), and involves the reinforcement of successive *approximations* of the desired performance. It is therefore a major feature of most contingency management programmes. In Figure 6.3 on p. 157, increasingly better approximations of non-disruptive classroom behaviour and high, then gently higher compliance rates were required before positive reinforcement occurred. These changes were linked to acknowledged *progress* in behaviour.

Fading

Fading (see p. 114) involves the standard shifting of control from stimuli occurring in one setting to those which occur in another. It is an important dimension of CBT approaches, particularly when conducted in clinical settings, where recently acquired behaviours eventually have to be performed under different, more complex circumstances. Bringing responses under the control of variables likely to be found in the outside world, by fading out 'artificial' reinforcers and introducing the more naturally occurring variety, is therefore likely to be a powerful factor in determining long-term results of any programme. In the case example on p. 194, monetary support for the outings used to reinforce adaptive behaviour was reduced by stages, as parents began to think it worthwhile to raise this for themselves – but not all can do this. Similarly, the daily report card was faded by being brought home at less frequent intervals, eventually to be replaced by a more generally phrased note of positive weekly progress.

Chaining

Chaining occurs when complex performances are broken down into their component parts and each stage in the sequence is positively reinforced. The reinforcer then becomes the discriminative stimulus that cues the next stage in the sequence. A variant of this approach, *backward chaining*, is widely used in teaching basic skills to younger clients with learning disabilities. For example, in the case of dressing, the procedure is to start with the garment already in place; one arm is removed from the sleeve, and then physically guided back in. This prompt can eventually be faded and the next stage, putting on the coat from the 'two-sleeves empty' position, can be attempted, and so on until the person has learned the whole sequence. With backward chaining the positive reinforcement of having the coat on (together with any additional praise) is immediate, becoming conditional on a longer chain as progress is made with the task.

Prompting

Prompting is a series of discriminative stimuli which indicate that a certain behaviour is now appropriate, or that if performed it will be reinforced. The example of backward chaining above includes prompting. Prompts were also used in the cases of socially unconfident clients (see pp. 160, 161 and 220), and usually took the form of gestures and facial expressions to cue verbal responses and eye-to-eye contact. Prompts can be faded as soon as the behaviour is brought under control of other, naturally occurring, situational cues.

Attention to discriminative stimuli

Behaviour can also be changed by the therapist influencing the naturally occurring discriminative stimuli which elicit it. In the case of the fractious foster child on p. 199, the carers eventually became very skilled in spotting situations that were likely to give rise to attention-seeking behaviour, and would do their best to remove these or divert the child's attention elsewhere.

Changing the environment of cues and consequences in which problematic behaviour occurs, or which blocks the emergence of adaptive sequences is an essential ingredient of CBT. Talk to reformed smokers: they are usually experts on cues.

On the cognitive side of the approach, thinking clearly about what sort of life she wanted to have, about what could reasonably be expected of a 9-year-old, and about the need to remedy a learning history for which she was in part responsible, helped the parent in the case on p. 194 to maintain control over her son's home environment and conduct when in her company. Cognitive approaches can help clients accurately to discriminate stimuli, and to try considering other possible meanings for them (e.g. is a yawn always a sign of boredom (perhaps a late night?); are some frowns due to concentration and not disapproval?).

A larger problem with all the stimulus control approaches discussed thus far lies in the ethical queasiness which some professionals have over the issue of pointed, as opposed to

Table 7.2 Summary of contingency management techniques

Techniques	Main features	Applications
Contingency management	A compendium approach using all appropriate reinforcement, extinction and punishment applications (see below). The environment is changed so as to support useful behaviours and ignore or discourage unwanted behaviours.	Used to increase the frequency, strength and so on of adaptive behaviours by providing contrasting consequences for the two. Wide range of applications: child problems, learning disability where behaviour problems block social acceptability, or any setting where some control can be gained over the consequences of behaviour.
Positive reinforcement	A consequence is provided which increases the likelihood that a given behaviour will be performed. Immediacy of reinforcement is an important factor.	Used to increase desirable behaviour. Behaviours incompatible with problematic behaviours can also be reinforced. The technique of choice in a wide range of CBT programmes, it is important that the behaviour to be reinforced should occasionally occur at reasonable strength, since this is otherwise a labour-intensive approach.
Token economy systems	Tokens (generalised reinforcers) are given for pro-social behaviours and are exchangeable for a variety of goods, privileges, access to activities and so on.	Used mainly in residential and special hospital settings (but with application in behavioural units in schools).
Use of Premack's principle	High-probability behaviours are made conditional on some performance of low-probability behaviours which are then shared.	Used where it is difficult to specify reinforcers in the usual way. Increasing levels of low-probability behaviours are usually sought in exchange for opportunities to perform high-probability behaviours.
Contingency contracts	An exchange of equally valued behaviours (which each party would like to see more of) is negotiated. The performance of one item is contingent upon the performance of an item from the other party.	Used in interpersonal difficulties – relationship work and conflicts between parents and children.
Operant extinction	Removing available reinforcement from a response.	Used for attention-seeking behaviours, usually in combination with the positive reinforcement of incompatible behaviours.

Negative reinforcement	Aversive stimulation is maintained until desired behaviour is performed, and then terminated.	Mainly used as a feature of broader contingency management programmes.
Punishment	A known aversive stimulus is presented, on contingency, or a positive one withdrawn, so reducing the frequency or intensity with which a behaviour is performed.	May be used as a suppressant of behaviours likely to interfere with programmes based on positive reinforcement. Punishment has the disadvantage that it strongly encourages escape and avoidance behaviours.
Satiation	Such an excess of negatively or positively reinforcing stimuli is provided that their reinforcing power is lost.	Used for low-level obsessions.
Shaping	Control of behaviour is shifted from one stimulus to another which resembles it fairly closely.	Used by the therapist to build on behaviours similar to those already in repertoire, and to gradually change them, so that they more closely resemble the performance required.
Fading	Therapist-supplied reinforcement is gradually withdrawn to bring new behaviour under the control of naturally occurring (non-artificial) sources of reinforcement.	An essential feature of all reinforcement programmes. Especially important in residential settings prior to discharge.
Over-learning and over-correction	This involves the intensive and over-rehearsal of an adaptive correction behaviour well beyond the level normally required. Aids clear discrimination.	Used (for example) as a special feature in programmes with enuretics. Upon the attainment of complete dryness, the client is encouraged to drink before bedtime, so that inhibiting responses are well-learned.
Attention to discriminative stimuli	The cues suspected to be eliciting behaviour are removed, or acted upon at an early stage.	Should be a feature of all behavioural programmes. Particularly useful when problematic behaviour is known to occur predictably in given settings or situations.

general background forms of taking control of problems (see Chapter 8). Yet, however well intentioned, to do nothing, or nothing much in the face of problems usually means abandoning clients to the less benign and more forceful contingencies responsible for their problems in the first place.

Looking to the environment of cues and consequences and exchanges of reinforcement as the best guide to what maintains problems in the here and now is an essential ingredient of cognitive-behavioural practice. I believe that purely cognitive approaches which seek to alter behaviour by 'remote-control', ignore these environmental influences to their detriment.

8   Response control techniques

Human beings do not simply respond to stimuli, they interpret them, and not always accurately.

(Albert Bandura)

In the previous chapter attention was drawn to techniques that exert influence through specific alterations to the client's environment, such as changing the contingencies which surround him or her – producing new cues and new consequences which affect behaviour. Now we turn to a set of approaches which focus on the nature of the *responses* produced within a given set of contingencies, rather than to the stimuli themselves. These *response control* techniques (Bandura 1969) are directed towards the production, through direct teaching, of new and more adaptive social, motor, verbal, emotional and cognitive responses. In other words, they seek to change what a person does, feels and thinks in response to the environment within which problems arise.

Let us begin, as before, by relocating ourselves on the assessment diagram (see Figure 6.1, p. 153). Response control techniques are mainly used where the answer to the question: 'Are target behaviours already in repertoire at any significant level?' is 'No'. That is, when clients have either: (1) never learned to perform the types of response which it is thought are needed to address their problems; or (2) where such responses have been learned in the past, but are now lost – as with certain psychiatric conditions and the effects of institutionalisation; or (3) where, for whatever reason, the responses occur infrequently or at a low level, and operant shaping is likely to be too labour-intensive an approach.

There are also occasions where responses are in excess, as in the case of aggressiveness, where either the therapist is unable to gain sufficient control over the contingencies supporting this behaviour, or the problem stems from behavioural deficits. These *pre-potent* responses can also be brought under control by the teaching of new behaviours which are incompatible with the old ones (see p. 193).

Sometimes problematic behaviour is under the control of variables to which the therapist does not have ready access; for instance, when the client is predominantly influenced by a peer group, or when problems occur at work. Here, although ideally it is the contingencies supporting the problem which should be modified, any help given has to concentrate on assisting the client to modify these conditions for him or herself. Although it makes sense to attack the problem of bullying at school, or exploitation at work, by trying to change the behaviour of the bullies and the exploiters, this is often very difficult, and so we are left with the option of changing the client's own responses so that bullying and exploitation become less reinforcing for those who engage in it. The aim in other cases is for an alteration to the *exchange rates* of behaviour (see Case example 8.1 overleaf).

CASE EXAMPLE 8.1

Dr P. was a single, early middle-aged physics lecturer who came to the UK from Greece. His courses were popular with students, his relations with some colleagues more complicated. He discovered that his nickname (used behind his back) was Zorba, and that his interactions were sometimes seen as 'a bit macho' – advice from a colleague. He asked one of the departmental secretaries while seated at her desk and in full view of others out on a date; she accepted, and he kissed her on the back of the head. She had second thoughts and e-mailed these to him. Other admin staff had advised her that he had overstepped the mark and should be reported. He came into the office and remonstrated with her, in front of colleagues, that she had misunderstood his (perfectly honourable) intentions (she was in a relationship, but he didn't know this, though others did). If there are stereotypes floating off the page here, these were indeed a subject of discussion, but he was frankly, and I believe, genuinely bewildered by what happened next. The secretary was persuaded under a new, rather belated 'sexual harassment and appropriate behaviour at work' code to take out a complaint against Dr P. for improper conduct. He protested his innocence through every available channel and was boiling with a sense of injustice. He was quietly advised on two occasions to just take a reprimand, apologise, and get on with his career. He replied, 'I would rather die', which he nearly did.

Probably because he approached this dispute with scientific precision, trawling through piles of policy and legal documents and presenting his arguments to departmental heads and the university inquiry as if they were courts of law, an organisational 'antibody' response developed. He was suspended for three months and refused point-blank to take a training/counselling course on 'gender relations in the workplace'. On legal advice, he attended one session but stormed out: 'These stupid people had already made up their minds that I was guilty – which I am not.' His suspension was continued; he took to drink, became very depressed, spent all day in his flat ringing colleagues for support and telling them his side of the story until they stopped taking his calls. He overdosed one night on vodka plus the Trycuclic antidepressants prescribed by his GP (quicker acting yes, but with more tolerance problems). He was taken to hospital for de-toxification, assessed for clinical depression (high on the Hamilton scale with suicidal ideation daily) and referred to me. The approach taken in this case (six sessions) was as follows:

☐   A full history of the dispute was taken; Dr P. was determined to tell it anyway, and a controlled version gave the opportunity for challenging taken-for-granted assumptions (e.g. 'This person has taken out a complaint before I have discovered.')

The approach used was as follows:

☐   The idea of 'thought experiments': i.e. 'trying on for size' another person's point of view, whatever the emotional charge carried.
☐   Prioritisation of his goals to get out of this mess, whatever its causes. He selected the ostracisation and boredom of colleagues when he tried to discuss his case with

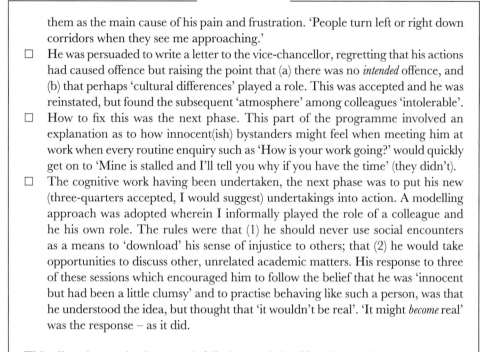

them as the main cause of his pain and frustration. 'People turn left or right down corridors when they see me approaching.'

☐ He was persuaded to write a letter to the vice-chancellor, regretting that his actions had caused offence but raising the point that (a) there was no *intended* offence, and (b) that perhaps 'cultural differences' played a role. This was accepted and he was reinstated, but found the subsequent 'atmosphere' among colleagues 'intolerable'.

☐ How to fix this was the next phase. This part of the programme involved an explanation as to how innocent(ish) bystanders might feel when meeting him at work when every routine enquiry such as 'How is your work going?' would quickly get on to 'Mine is stalled and I'll tell you why if you have the time' (they didn't).

☐ The cognitive work having been undertaken, the next phase was to put his new (three-quarters accepted, I would suggest) undertakings into action. A modelling approach was adopted wherein I informally played the role of a colleague and he his own role. The rules were that (1) he should never use social encounters as a means to 'download' his sense of injustice to others; that (2) he would take opportunities to discuss other, unrelated academic matters. His response to three of these sessions which encouraged him to follow the belief that he was 'innocent but had been a little clumsy' and to practise behaving like such a person, was that he understood the idea, but thought that 'it wouldn't be real'. 'It might *become* real' was the response – as it did.

This client is now back at work full time and the Hamilton scale measures post-treatment have fallen well into the safe zone. My own view is that he fell victim to his own cultural assumptions, to gender insensitivity, but also to the kind of 'corporate autism' that sometimes passes for staff welfare policy.

The research evidence for each of the techniques listed (see Chapter 2, p. 121 and below) has already been reviewed. Reference to this foregoing material will be made as necessary, but this chapter will concentrate mainly on practical applications of these findings.

Modelling and social skills training

Modelling is a technique that can easily be included in the therapist's repertoire of methods. Arguments have already been put forward about the dangers of relying exclusively on the interpretation of problems and verbal descriptions of what needs to be done about them, and then expecting the client to come up with the new behaviours while his environment obligingly supports these. Modelling approaches are a way of bridging the gap between an understanding of what needs to be done and developing the skills to do it.

Some authors draw a distinction between modelling and social skills training. While this is technically correct, because modelling theories attempt to explain how new responses are developed through observation alone, in most therapeutic programmes modelling is used in conjunction with rehearsal and selective feedback on performance. In addition, since therapists are mainly concerned with deficits in the problem-solving performances of clients, the distinction between the two approaches virtually disappears.

Stages in modelling

When modelling is used in the way suggested above, with feedback and appropriate reinforcement, the process normally passes through the following stages:

- ☐ Identifying specific problems resulting from gaps in the client's behavioural repertoire, and deciding what new behaviours could be developed to fill these gaps.
- ☐ Dividing the target responses into their component parts (for example, coming into a room full of people; deciding who to stand next to and what to say; introducing oneself; getting in on the conversation and so forth). Easy enough for those who have learned how to do it (but think back to adolescence); but paralysing for some.
- ☐ Identifying with clients any patterns in their thinking which may encourage over- or mis-interpretation of the motives of others and/or avoidance responses (e.g. 'People are looking at me').
- ☐ Demonstrating to the client what a competent performance looks like; repeating any problematic parts of the sequence or going through it slowly and deliberately; emphasising options and decision points. This may be done either informally during interviews – 'I'll be the neighbour, you be yourself, what do you say?' – or, in more dedicated sessions, closed-circuit TV is a very valuable tool and is usually desensitised to in a couple of sessions.
- ☐ Encouraging the client to perform simple sequences, with the therapist shaping and correcting these as required.
- ☐ Developing more complex performances by chaining together different sequences.
- ☐ Paying attention to any problems of discrimination; that is, identifying any difficulties the client may have in knowing whether a certain piece of behaviour is appropriate for a given setting.
- ☐ Gradually introducing difficulties likely to be found in real life as the client becomes more able to cope with these; for instance, not getting an immediate answer when trying to make new friends.
- ☐ Gradual fading of artificially strong or explicit prompts and reinforcements.
- ☐ Supervised practice, or practical assignments (vital, but often neglected) on which the client reports back (e.g. getting the client to initiate three short conversations or to ask for clarification from a salesperson or official).

Modelling to reduce fears

Modelling may also be used to reduce maladaptive emotional reactions (as in the case of animal or insect phobias). These, though trivial-sounding, can be crippling to people who avoid all the places where, say, spiders or dogs *might* be found; that is, just about everywhere.

The aim here is to present the client with a picture of someone coping reasonably well with the circumstances they fear and to get them to visualise themselves as coping with them. The learning components of such an approach could include any of the following. (1) Through imagining, or actually watching and experiencing the vicarious emotions, the client's fear eventually subsides, since nothing terrible happens. This is known as vicarious extinction and is a kind of exposure therapy (see below). (2) The client may learn new things about the feared objects or circumstances, or about how to handle them – in other words, that dogs do not usually bite if approached confidently, that they usually respond to affection and so on; or in the case of fears about a social performance, the client can learn that there are 'tricks of the trade'. (3) Through 'imagining-along' with the modelled performance, clients' expectations of themselves may change; they may repeatedly imagine themselves coping with such a situation, and so in future, thinking about the stimulus conditions does not trigger such powerful emotional reactions and thoughts of escape. Perceived self-efficacy is the goal.

Optimum conditions for modelling

From the foregoing discussion and the previous section on the theoretical basis of modelling, the reader will have seen that attention needs to be paid to four different components if new competency is to occur.

1   Characteristics of the modelled performance. This has to be believable but not effort-lessly competent – the equivalent of 'scales' when learning a musical instrument perhaps.
2   Cognitive components. How the client *interprets* the situations in which difficulties typically arise: talking aloud about thoughts and emotions.
3   Characteristics of the matching response: these need to be analysed stage by stage.
4   Feedback and reinforcement characteristics: positive shaping.

Taking each of these factors in turn, the ideal model is someone who can easily capture the client's attention and who has credibility in his or her eyes. This last point has little to do with formal authority. To the members of a youth offenders group, the person with the highest status may well be the toughest-sounding kid, and the convenor will be wise to make use of this fact. Credibility in rehearsals is an important consideration and staff involved in such programmes need to take precautions to ensure it. First, they can make sure that their own performances are not 'wooden', by practising beforehand and so not modelling embarrassment. Next, and again without going over the top, they can make sure that performances include appropriate emotional expression.

Particularly in the early stages of modelling, the therapist is trying to teach steadily and understandably improving *coping skills*, not mastery – which the client may conclude is beyond reach. The ideal performance is one of relaxed, growing competency.

Where complex tasks are being demonstrated, it may be useful to 'talk through' the performance so that the observers can see what features the model is attending to, and what forms the basis of his or her decision about how to behave next. If clients do the same, this may help them to remember what sequence follows the last: 'Right, here I go, the door's open so I don't bother to knock, several people are looking at me, that's fine . . . smile . . . small wave to the only person I know . . . now look expectant . . . someone's coming over . . . now for the introduction . . . is he going to shake hands or not?'

The performance characteristics of the client need only a brief comment, since the things to pay attention to here are much the same as with any type of cognitive-behavioural programme. First, the performance must be broken down into manageable stages. If the client feels more anxious as a result of participating in the programme, then a key element (lessening anxiety and engendering feelings of confidence) has been lost. Similarly, the therapist must be ready to prompt new behaviour and then to reinforce approximations of it, *as* they are performed – not just at the end – because it may not he worth the wait.

Feedback on approximate performances should always be couched in positive terms. The concept of *shaping* (see p. 113) covers what is necessary here. Clients who already associate certain kinds of social behaviour with fear and embarrassment will be very sensitive to criticism, even where this is implicit. Elaborate explanations are best avoided. Showing clients what is meant, and prompting them by a re-enactment of a similar sequence, is more effective.

The ultimate aim of any modelling programme is to bring newly developed responses under the control of naturally occurring reinforcers and of self-reinforcement. Attention and praise are often sufficient, particularly if the client accepts the need to develop new skills as likely to make life easier.

Closed-circuit television is an ideal medium for modelling new behaviours. Using portable equipment (which now costs about the same as six wasted interviews), it is possible to produce lively, believable performances, which are intrinsically interesting to observers. Sequences can be 'frozen', rerun, played without sound to concentrate attention on the non-verbal element, or run without the picture to achieve the opposite effect. Here are two examples.

CASE EXAMPLE 8.2

It was noted by nurses and social workers that patients in a psychiatric unit, due for discharge, were normally treated as individual cases, and usually held a number of fears and concerns in common. It was therefore decided to bring them together in (voluntary) groups further to define their misgivings and to rehearse with them ways of coping with these. The main problems identified in preliminary discussions were as follows:

☐   What to say to people about an unexplained period of absence.
☐   How to deal with stilted behaviour from family and friends in the know.
☐   How to approach, or try to make reparations to, family members who may have suffered as a result of the client's mental illness (schizophrenia, depression and bipolar conditions predominated; see Chapter 2).
☐   How to overcome the fear of stigmatisation at work, or by friends and neighbours.
☐   How to prevent future relapse by seeking help early on; access community-based resources.
☐   How to deal with practical and financial matters.

Assessment

Discussion of these fears or problems in the group 3 × (n = 7) suggested the following commonalities and/or deficits:

☐   Stigmatisation: beliefs that people would somehow be able to tell that they had suffered an acute psychiatric episode just by looking at them; that in varying degrees they had somehow contributed to their illnesses, and that they were something to be ashamed of. The inclusion of a previous service user in one of these groups gave it undoubted extra credibility.
☐   Trepidation regarding suggestions by staff that they might seize the initiative, be *direct* with relatives and friends, and *ask* for help and understanding during rehabilitation.
☐   A feeling of loss of control that would prevent them from seeking help to prevent relapse plus an associated view that they would not wish to waste their general

practitioners' time when they had so many 'really ill' people to see. This is a view which can still emanate as much from primary care as from clients themselves.
□ Lack of information on income support, employment-rights, housing matters and so on.

Procedure

Eight sessions in total were scheduled for each group, three within the first fortnight, then once a week, with a post-discharge meeting to review progress. The elements of the programme were as follows:

□ An informal discussion of the nature, prevalence and known causes of relevant types of mental disorder focusing on its widespread nature, and the various mixtures of biological, experiential and stress factors known to create vulnerability. A psychiatrist was present to underline lack of culpability among the patients themselves. The most interesting discussions concerned matters of cause and effect and how it is possible for us to muddle them when feeling low or anxious (e.g. that in some cases where florid symptoms had created family problems and led to temporary estrangement, this was a product of illness and fear, not of deliberate intent or incompetent behaviour on their part). Two positive factors were identified in these sessions: (1) how much better for patients to be given information about mental illness directly and systematically, rather than in ward encounters; (2) a feeling of relief that others had had similar experiences to their own – psycho-education is the posh name for this approach and in my view should be an integrated feature of all therapeutic encounters; sometimes the levels of ignorance and false belief are astonishing.
□ Role-play sessions, led by staff, based on common fears (e.g. meeting a neighbour who would say: 'Well hello, haven't seen you around for some time, hear you've had a bit of trouble?'); or, featuring a rather busy-looking GP figure who was to be induced into putting down his prescription pad and listening more carefully to the patient's fears and needs by a direct appeal or, a sticky encounter with over-solicitous relatives using the special calming voices reserved for people with psychiatric histories; or, 'earthing' a strange 'atmosphere' at work by a simple, uncluttered appeal for help while settling back in. These sessions were made palatable by staff taking the lead initially, by trying to engender a humorous, all-in-this-together-type atmosphere. The focus of these sessions was on basic assertion skills for difficult or stressful encounters: being direct but not over-forthright or aggressive; explaining feelings (the most difficult); and making specific and unequivocal requests for help and support when needed.
□ Homework or outside assignments. Towards the end of the programme clients and staff negotiated mildly challenging tasks (going in twos and threes to a local arts centre to enquire about activities and obtain leaflets); telephoning a friend or relative, or making an appointment with a doctor, the money advice centre, Social Security or a voluntary housing association. Attendance remained high throughout the programme. The evaluation cited the importance of being *shown* how to do things rather than just being spoken to, and the importance of trying to take control of potentially threatening circumstances through planning and rehearsal.

Here is another case example, dealing this time with an individual client.

CASE EXAMPLE 8.3

Paula Douglas had spent five of her twenty-six years in psychiatric units of various kinds. She was diagnosed as schizophrenic and described as 'shy', 'withdrawn', 'self-preoccupied', 'obsessive' and as being 'somewhat bizarre in her behaviour'. She avoided the centre of rooms as if they were mined; constantly hung her head; shuffled around the house; neglected dress and personal hygiene; and spent whole days in her room reading, refusing to eat or to speak to anyone. This case was referred to Social Services for 'after-care' following discharge from a psychiatric unit and her premature departure from a course of rehabilitation therapy.

Assessment

An initially grudging conversation between Paula and a social worker (with a CPN joining in from time to time concentrating on adherence to her medication regime) revealed that Paula was aware that her behaviour 'put people off', but that she was too shy to do much about it. She felt very conspicuous when confronted with new people or situations, and was ashamed of her psychiatric history.

It was decided not to delve further into the historical background of this problem (child sexual abuse and a dominating, abusive father featured in the notes), but to identify clearly one or two behavioural deficits, and to try to remedy them.

Procedure

First, the view was put to Paula that people could only think her 'mad' (her term) if her behaviour put this idea into their heads. She found the notion that 'mad is as mad does' interesting, and a series of training sessions was set up using CCTV with the explicit intention of showing her how she might behave less fearfully in the type of social circumstances she found difficult.

Two basic sequences of thinking and behaviour capable of being built on later were selected: (1) walking confidently into a room and introducing herself; (2) giving non-verbal reinforcement to other people during a conversation as a means of conveying interest and understanding, and so counteracting Paula's usually rather vacant appearance made worse by a deep fringe almost covering her eyes (she was persuaded to have it cut later since it was not a style choice but a defence).

These two classes of behaviour were broken into their component parts and modelled repeatedly by two students. They played counter-roles and also offered constructive criticism on each other's performance. The sessions became increasingly friendly and always ended in a period of conversation about novels and various other cultural pursuits known to interest the client. The length of this period (its overriding importance to Paula was only discovered later and by accident) was varied in rough proportion to the amount of effort exerted by Paula during the exercises.

After seven half-hour sessions Paula had mastered walking into rooms, and her mother was introduced into the programme. She was encouraged both to look for, and reinforce, behaviours of a similar kind throughout the rest of the day.

Believable, non-verbal signals of understanding were harder to establish. Paula's performance approximated to that of the modellers only vaguely and mechanically, and the initial programme had to be slowed down and rethought. Maintaining eye contact was discovered to be a primary problem and this was selectively reinforced with approval, initially by getting Paula to look at foreheads if she couldn't manage or hold eye-to-eye gaze. When low levels of eye contact had been established, Paula's other non-verbal behaviour improved substantially. Putting her into a room alone with a TV camera, and getting her to talk to herself (!) worked well as an adjunct. She said she thought more clearly about dealing with other people and was less fearful.

As a result, Paula acquired two new pieces of behaviour which she did not possess before; she said she thought more clearly about dealing with other people and was less fearful. She was eventually able to attend evening classes on nature conservation at a local technical college and join a cycling club, which she enjoyed. A useful amelioration of fear and loneliness.

Conclusion

Modelling is a well-researched and effective technique for developing new behaviours and reducing the anxieties that often attach to faltering, fearful social performance. One variant of it, social skills training, aims both to remedy particular deficits and to add other general-purpose skills to the client's repertoire. These techniques are being applied across a range of client groups and may be used in combination with other approaches to help with a range of different problems (see Dilk & Bond (1996) for a review).

Assertion training

Assertion training is a widely used CBT approach. It is based on a combination of cognitive restructuring (see p. 234), modelling and rehearsal, and operant reinforcement approaches. Its purpose is to teach people how proportionately to stand up for themselves without being aggressive. Since we in the helping professions tend to deal with the weakened, the powerless and the put-upon, this approach has particular relevance. However, it would be naive indeed if, as a result of our interest in psychology, we came to see these states as entirely due to internal, developmental factors. In their extreme form they are structural in origin, a corollary of the way society works. Humiliation TV, sadistic audition programmes, dominatrix headed quiz shows, and the misuse of Zimbardo's 'prisoner and guard' experiments draw in millions of viewers every week. Modelling effects are likely to occur. For anyone who doubts the effects of media images on thinking, emotions and behaviour has to account not only for the scientific research (admittedly scattered and inconclusive) but for the fact that there is a large international advertising industry with clear, bottom-line, financial outcomes. Why we like these charades is probably more to do with our own appetites and self-doubts, plus a little *schadenfreude* that others ('celebs') who deserve all they get receive their come-uppance. But then not all oppression is due to the macro-effects of the political system; a broad range of everyday misery and oppression is psychological in origin. To a considerable extent, exploitation depends on the expectations held by the exploiter (that he will be successful), and on the compliant behaviour of the 'exploitee'. Social psychology has much to tell us about the effects of these behaviourally induced factors – as demonstrated by Milgram's dramatic conformity experiments and by a legion of studies where the verbal content presented to an audience is held constant, but the style, expression and behaviour of the performers are varied to produce markedly different audience reactions (Hovland *et al.* 1953; Cohen 1964).

Assertion training can be carried out with individuals and groups and is relevant to a wide range of interpersonal problems. The approach has been well researched and a number of comparative and controlled studies exist, testifying to its effectiveness (see Craighead *et al.* 1994). However, before we proceed further we need a definition. I still like this one:

> Assertion involves direct expression of one's feelings, preferences, needs, or opinions in a manner that is neither threatening nor punishing toward another person. In addition, assertion does not involve an excessive amount of anxiety or fear. Contrary to popular opinion, assertion is not primarily a way to get what one wants, nor is it a way of controlling or subtly manipulating others. Assertion is the direct communication of one's needs, wants, and opinions without punishing, threatening, or putting down the other person.
>
> (Galassi & Galassi 1977: 3)

I hope the foregoing has convinced the reader that assertiveness is a reasonable aim: that it enables others to know better where they stand with us; that it ensures clear messages about intentions, desires and opinions; above all, that such a style of behaviour is likely to condition the behaviour of others towards us. An appropriately assertive, situation-specific style also produces important internal effects. That is, we are likely to think and feel differently about ourselves as a result of behaving less fearfully. By letting other people see, through our behaviour, that we expect to be treated as a person of worth, we are also likely to affect our own evaluation of ourselves and what we are capable of. Here, then, is an example of a cognitive-behavioural approach which follows research into the relationship between attitudes and behaviour, and suggests that the best way to improve self-esteem is to demonstrate to, and train clients in, new responses that signal a clear expectation of reasonable treatment.

Turning now to the training schemes themselves, assertion training programmes are likely to contain combinations of the following approaches.

☐ Assessment: often problems are confined to particular situations or settings (such as work or relationships) and no extra or special assessment is required. However, in cases where there is a general inadequacy – as in the case of excessively shy or withdrawn clients – an assessment schedule such as the one reproduced in Figure 6.1 (p. 153)will give a better idea of the extent of the problem. There are also standardised self-esteem scales with a wide application (see Fischer & Corcoran 2007).

☐ Discrimination training procedures: these may be used to teach the client to discriminate accurately between assertiveness, false compliance and aggression.

☐ A modelling and rehearsal component: this is usually included so that the client is *shown* in a step-by-step fashion how to behave with different degrees of assertiveness, in different kinds of situations. The client will then rehearse and attempt to perform these behaviours him or herself, receiving positively couched feedback on successive approximations.

☐ Attention needs also to be paid to the grading of tasks and assignments given, so that clients experience success rather than confirming their worst fears about themselves.

☐ A desensitisation component: as with other modelling techniques, a major aim of an assertion training scheme is progressively to remove the fear that is associated with certain behaviour. This is usually done through gradually exposing the client to such situations, but in some cases extra help with relaxation may be required (see p. 246).

☐ Generalisation: active steps must be taken to ensure that therapeutic gains generalise to the everyday experiences and problems of the client. The best way of achieving this is to vary the format of the programme and give the client experience in progressively more realistic settings.

Now let us look at each of these items in more detail.

Assessment

To start with, the client may be asked to complete a schedule, e.g. a self-esteem scale (see Fischer & Corcoran 2007). He or she does this as fully as possible, adapting the headings to particular circumstances, noting feelings and anxieties at the time of each incident, and the practical effects of a given pattern of behaviour. In addition, when it would have been appropriate to behave as suggested in Figure 6.1, but he or she did not, note may be taken of what the consequences were.

Discrimination training

Some clients have difficulty in distinguishing between suitably assertive behaviour, aggressive behaviour and falsely compliant behaviour. They may see all kinds of outspokenness as nasty, or as 'asking for trouble', and may rationalise compliancy into just a question of 'good manners'. Usually, however, people know what they would like to be able to say and do (as evidenced by the familiar internal dialogues and self-chidings that we all experience: 'Why on earth didn't I . . . why did I let . . .' after the occasion has passed by). In these cases, discrimination training is used partly to clarify the different types of behaviours, and partly to provide opportunities for occasionally helpful candour.

Modelling appropriate non-verbal behaviour

The principles of modelling and the verbal component of assertive behaviour have already been covered, and so here we should now concentrate on the non-verbal factors that make up a successful performance since these signals are often more important than the content of speech (remember the famous Nixon/Kennedy debate: Nixon won on the radio, Kennedy on the TV; and think of PM Tony Blair's famous sweaty performance – all eyes were on the perspiration and what it might mean, not on the verbal content). Sometimes right, sometimes wrong. Particular attention should be paid to the following.

☐ Stance and posture: it is difficult for clients to begin to make believably assertive response unless they face the person they are to address. If seated, leaning forward slightly demonstrates interest.

☐ Eye contact: if the client finds prolonged eye contact difficult, he or she should be persuaded to practise it at a distance first and gradually move closer. Another way of

Table 8.1 Key differences between non-assertive, aggressive and assertive behaviour

Non-assertiveness	Complying with illegitimate requests.
	Agreeing with opinions you don't really share.
	Avoiding people because they may ask you to do things and you find it difficult to say 'no'.
	Failing to express your own opinions.
	Failing to make requests of or to ask favours of others.
	Avoiding direct statements – giving mixed, vague or confused messages.
Aggressiveness	Expressing strong feelings but for your own benefit.
	Dominating conversation with threats and demands, and adopting a behavioural style that is dominating, pushy and demeaning to other people.
	Giving no consideration to the other person's rights, needs, feelings or cultural expectations.
	Possibly resorting to verbal abuse or making an attempt to humiliate the other person.
	Failing to consider, acknowledge, or act upon, the other person's point of view.
	Adopting a threatening bodily stance, with eye contact overlong and glaring, and gestures which appear to be the forerunners of physical attack.
Assertiveness	Expressing feelings directly, but without accompanying threats.
	Politely refusing unreasonable requests.
	Making reasonable requests.
	Expressing opinions, while not automatically agreeing with those of others.
	Standing up for your own rights and needs, and making clear your wants and preferences, while making no attempt to impinge upon those of others.
	Performing these behaviours without undue fear or anxiety. Being relaxed when asking for what is reasonable or legitimately due.
	Expressing anger and affection as appropriate. Maintaining appropriate eye contact.
	Matching body posture to mood.

beginning is to get the client to focus on some other part of the face and progress gradually towards eye-to-eye contact (as in the case example on p. 220). Eye contact, conveying sincerity and lack of fear, is an important characteristic of social competency and perceived honesty.

☐ Facial expression: the client can practise this alone in front of a mirror. Using this method (or closed-circuit TV) will teach clients the difference between what they feel like inside and think they might be conveying. Sometimes the difference is marked.

☐ Use of gestures: confident but not exaggerated gestures (learn to sit still, Simon Schama; otherwise we shan't hear your usually insightful opinions) do much for a social performance. These must not be aggressive – such as striking the palm of the hand – since the key point, as with facial expression, is that gestures should be congruent with other behaviour. This is a matter of practice and feedback.

☐ Voice level and tone: it is not uncommon to meet clients with loud voices who think it unlikely that they will be heard, and clients with quiet voices who think themselves perfectly audible to anyone *really* interested in listening.

Reinforcement procedures

As with the other approaches discussed in this chapter, the key principles involved in application are: simple tasks to begin with; a clearly modelled performance which is believable without being too elaborate; and reinforcement for usefully approximate matching responses, together with positive feedback to help the client improve. The programme then proceeds in step-by-step fashion to the point where first analogue and then real-life assignments are possible. Before the client undertakes complex assignments or tries out his or her new skills in situations which really matter, it may be useful to equip him or her with a range of immunised responses for dealing with rebuffs and unexpected reactions.

Desensitisation factors in assertion training

Another reason why up-against-it people feel unable to assert themselves is that they fear the emotional and behavioural consequences of so doing. Therefore, it may be useful to try to analyse with the client exactly what he or she *expects* to happen as a result of reasonable self-assertion and to point out any inconsistencies or exaggerations in these beliefs. Often clients believe that their condition of lack of social competence is inborn, or is an unalterably fixed part of their personality. While this is not so, a lifelong experience of kowtowing to other people is not easily set aside. Fear and anxiety will be partly conditioned through previous bad experiences, and via escape or avoidance responses which negatively reinforce these fears. Alternative ways of reducing anxiety must therefore be employed.

This reduction of anxiety is partly handled through the therapist's arrangement of a gradual progression from simple to demanding tasks. Such a procedure not only aids the acquisition of new responses, but also acts as a kind of desensitisation therapy (see pp. 232, 245), the client feeling increasingly relaxed as the performance improves, and a new, benign association gradually building up. However, care must be taken to ensure that clients do not get out of their depth too quickly with the result that the old vicious circle is reinstated.

Once the new assertive responses have been learned, they may be regularly reinforced in place of avoidance behaviour, since their deployment will reduce both anxiety and the often-reported sensation of having feelings 'bottled up'. These assignments are best preplanned with the client under the following headings: thoughts, fears, relaxation level, monitoring the performance and taking note of consequences.

CASE EXAMPLE 8.4

Assertion training was used with Mr Thomas. He was referred by his GP for depression (moderate on the Beck inventory), problems at work and relationship difficulties with his wife, with a suggestion of 'social phobia' in the background. He felt unable to do any of the following.

☐ Refuse unreasonable requests from his less conscientious workmates to do their work after finishing his own.
☐ Refuse overtime when he had other plans.
☐ Compliment his wife in any way.
☐ Initiate sexual intercourse.
☐ Speak up, in a meeting, or in a group of friends.

The problems that occurred at home were dealt with by a negotiated agreement based on predictable reciprocity. The work-related items (he worked in a wood yard) became the main focus of work since they caused frustration which the client was apt to bring home.

Procedure

Typical problem sequences were analysed and re-enacted with the aid of a student, with the emphasis on how to talk to the foreman when fixing which days in the week he would be available for overtime. Key phrases were written up on charts and Mr Thomas made his own notes. In the initial stages considerable praise was required for quite small gains. Mr Thomas 'psyched himself up' (as he put it) to tackle his foreman after five weeks and on his own initiative, mentioned to his younger workmates (who were apparently sitting around doing little but chatting) that he would not be free to help them later if they got behind with their work. The main positive effect of this programme was on the marital relationship, since Mr Thomas came home on time, as planned, and was a less frustrated and angry person. Self-esteem scores doubled over six sessions of CBT; depression scores fell steadily. Experimentation was the key idea.

Decisions about assertiveness training

I can think of few worse fates than being surrounded by people *constantly* and reflexively asserting their needs, wants and preferences – even if not directly at my expense – when no one is intentionally set to deprive them of anything. The important point to stress is that an assertive reaction is an *option*. Indeed, relationships can be improved by one party deliberately *refraining* from forthrightness in conditions where the other person knows full well that he or she has no right to expect an extra helping of forbearance – otherwise there would be no such thing as diplomacy. Through assertion training we are really extending the clients' *choices* of available responses, so that they know they can assert themselves when they choose and when it matters – that is, when they are too often called upon to deny their true feelings or to bear more than their fair share of the emotional costs of living in harmony with other people.

Self-management and self-control techniques

Over the past twenty years the CBT field has witnessed an upsurge of interest in self-help programmes of various kinds. Some of the theoretical reasons for this interest have already been reviewed: the development of social learning and other cognitive-mediational theories of behaviour, for example. In addition, as more people have begun to apply cognitive-behavioural principles in their work, the field has opened up to include settings far removed from clinic-based programmes. The practical problems posed by this are clearly identified in this quotation:

> How can you ensure that desired behaviours will occur at times and in places where you can neither prompt nor reinforce the behaviour? How can you get someone to do something – over there, in some other time or place – when you cannot intervene over there in that setting?
>
> (Risley 1977: 71)

An alternative to the use of mediators (for there are many settings inaccessible to them, too), and to place less optimistic reliance on generalisation effects to cover trial behaviours in natural settings, is to teach cognitive-behavioural principles to the client and enlist his or her help in administering a suitable programme. Anything which promises to extend the range of CBT methods, given the evidence for it, is an attractive proposition, but, once again, caution is necessary. A principal ingredient of 'traditional' behavioural approaches has been the attempt to manage the contingencies in the client's environment. Might not the effect of leaving this complicated task to the client be that we are led down the primrose path towards ill-designed and sloppily monitored programmes – as other disciplines have been before us? I have to confess that I am less than enamoured of computer-based self-help CBT programmes for anyone other than the 'worried well' (most NHS Direct discussions, whether online or by telephone, end with 'If you are really worried, go and see your GP'), but this might be more to do with my own learning deficits.

There are three possible safeguards against this possibility. The first is that behavioural self-control programmes tend to be monitored and evaluated rather more carefully than other kinds of self-help approaches. The second comes from a corresponding emphasis on the concreteness and specificity of the assignments given to the client, so that he or she is in no doubt as to how to respond. The third stems from the level of support given to clients in the procedures they are to apply to themselves and the amount of time given to rehearsal. It follows, then, that these are likely to be demanding programmes for clients, and so they are probably best used with people who express some desire to change, but who perhaps do not know how best to go about it, or for people who have hitherto been unwilling to pay the price of change, but may make the effort if a stage-by-stage approach is adopted.

The general aims of self-control programmes are to teach clients about the environmental factors that influence thinking, feelings and behaviour, and to widen the range of appropriate responses which they can make in the face of these. Here, in more detail, is the range of approaches that may be used in such programmes.

- ☐ Clients can be taught about eliciting stimuli (S^ds) which may 'trigger' unwanted stereotypical avoidance responses. These may be identifiable if the client fills out an ABC chart, especially if he or she is encouraged to include a record of the thoughts and feelings occurring prior to and during behaviour.
- ☐ Clients can be taught about the particular contingencies affecting them, with a view to changing these, or substituting more appropriate responses. For example, connections can be made between a client's excessive desire to please, his or her tendency to volunteer for extra work, and the hurtful criticism which he or she receives when, inevitably, he or she fails to meet the unreasonable quota.
- ☐ New associations between activities and places, which provoke fear and avoidance in the client at present, can be built up by the selective use of positive images. Some people hardly ever allow themselves pleasant reveries – 'laurelising' I call these self-congratulatory treats.
- ☐ Where external reinforcement for adaptive behaviour is weak or unavailable, clients can be taught how selectively to reinforce themselves, following agreed or pre-rehearsed procedures.
- ☐ Cognitive techniques are available, which seek to change clients' expectations about the efficacy of their own behaviour and its likely outcome (see p. 121).

CASE EXAMPLE 8.5

This is an example which relates particularly to the first three items above. The instructions set out below were used with a group of chronic night-time worriers and insomniacs who were concerned about their dependence on sleeping pills:

☐ Choose a time to experiment when you have no early morning commitments.
☐ Lie down to go to sleep *only* when you are sleepy.
☐ If alone, do not use your bed for anything except sleep or sex.
☐ If you find yourself unable to go to sleep and are 'fighting' it, get up and go into another room. Stay up as long as you wish and then return to the bedroom when sleepy. Although we do not want you to watch the clock, we want you to get out of bed if you do not fall asleep readily.
☐ If you still cannot fall asleep, repeat the step above. Do this as often as necessary throughout the night for now.
☐ Set your alarm to get up at the same time every morning, irrespective of how much sleep you get during the night. This will help your body acquire a consistent sleep rhythm.
☐ Do not sleep during the day; work or go for a walk instead.

Programmes of this type have also been used to control compulsive eating. In these cases the client may eat as often as he or she likes, but only at the table. As soon as the meal or snack is finished, the table must be cleared and everything put away. Set mealtimes must be observed, however many snacks have been taken. This sort of scheme does away with absent-minded nibbling, and with any self-deception about how much food has actually been consumed. In time it introduces a new set of discriminative stimuli (table, crockery, set mealtimes and so on), and eventually establishes a new set of associations – eating at particular times of day rather than at idle moments, and eating in particular places.

The principle used in both the previous examples is that of teaching the client how to self-re-programme the environment so that it gives maximum support for adaptive behaviours.

Cognitive components

The aim of the cognitive component of CBT is to modify the following:

☐ Negatively selective perceptions.
☐ Irrational thoughts and thinking styles.
☐ 'Catastrophic' thinking and imagery in objectively not-very-threatening circumstances.
☐ Negative self-talk and 'internal dialogues' of a self-lecturing kind.
☐ Misattribution of the causes and meaning of stimuli, particularly in social contexts, either inappropriately to the self and associated failings, or inappropriately (self-excusingly) to others.
☐ Maladaptive emotional reactions – to the extent that these are cued and/or maintained by thought patterns and thinking styles.
☐ Deficits in appropriate self-reinforcement.

The *way* in which these distortions are addressed is important. Rather than simply confronting such misreadings and negativity, cognitive-behavioural therapists tend to use 'Socratic' questioning which leaves some work to be done by the client. Gaarder, in his enchanting book, says of Socrates (470–399 BC):

> Socrates, whose mother was a midwife, used to say that his art was like the task of the midwife. She does not herself give birth to the child, but is there to help during its delivery. Similarly, Socrates saw his task as helping work to 'give birth' to the correct insight from within.
>
> (Gaarder 1995: 51)

'Up to a point', I would say again. It is better to ask questions that deliver answers in most cases: it is usually better that these questions are open-ended than closed ones indicating what the 'correct' answer is. 'Explain to me why you thought it was *inevitable* that these problems arose . . .' is better than a 'Did you think that . . .' question. However, if these approaches are overused they threaten genuineness and can seem like a psychological 'game'.

There may be occasions when cognitive events themselves are the target of modification – as in the case of obsessive thoughts and ruminations, and accompanying images of future disasters; conditions found in psychotic disorders where clients are taught to regard, for example, auditory hallucinations as internal, not external, and to experiment with ignoring them to see what actually happens (see Wykes *et al.* 1998; Thase & Jindal 2004). In addition, at a less intense level, cognitive events become the target of modification where thoughts and images about failure inhibit social performances which the client might otherwise carry out reasonably well (the Southgate penalty effect). However, in most cases we are interested to hypothesise about relations between cognitive and motor behaviour because we want to influence the latter – to change what people do; and here it must be noted that directly changing what people do often changes the accompanying thoughts and feelings.

CASE EXAMPLE 8.6

Readers are referred to p. 172 for the basic details of this case. It featured a young woman with a persistent fear of vomiting in public which in her terms was 'ruining her life'. The first stage in assessment revealed details to warm the cockles of any psychoanalyst's heart, namely a curious mixture of mollycoddling and strictness from devout Christian parents; a desire on their part that she should fulfil all the ambitions sacrificed by them for her sake and be grateful. She volunteered that she 'had had to swallow so much' in her life (!). A more prosaic version of the aetiology of this problem was that anxiety and unpredictability were a feature of her childhood and adolescence, and that her determination to 'do the right thing' carried with it psychological consequences, mediated by physiological arousal, which cued and maintained 'catastrophic thinking'.

The treatment programme was an amalgam of cognitive techniques and gentle exposure methods containing the following main elements.

☐   A plain explanation as to how anxiety (as a mild version of the fight/flight mechanism) causes drying of the mouth, constriction of the larynx and tension in the stomach – all incompatible with easy swallowing and digestion of food – plus reassurance that this problem did not make her 'a freak' (her term for herself).

☐   A concentration on the fact that her preparations to obviate a minor risk (vomiting in public) were the major part of her problem. When asked how often the feared event had occurred, she answered, shamefacedly, 'never' – an amazingly common reply.

☐   A brief introduction to the principles of relaxation therapy (see p. 246) accompanied by increasingly challenging food-swallowing exercises (iced water to begin with) in gradually more demanding circumstances (e.g. sitting near people in the canteen rather than with them) (see desensitisation, p. 245).

☐   Reality testing: singling out one or two friends and confiding in them about her problem. The client was in trepidation about this task, but contrary to expectations they were more than willing to help in the above exercises. They were seen once by me for about twenty minutes.

☐   Assertion training: learning how routinely to take control of where she sat while consuming food; in whose company; dealing with enquiries about her difficulties over food; excusing herself; briefly explaining herself on her return and so forth.

This mixed programme of cognitive reappraisal and desensitisation began to show results in three to four weeks, the client then taking it over and extending it herself. Interestingly, though originally a difficulty over swallowing food in public, the resolution of this had much wider consequences for the client's social life and sense of well-being and dispelled a fear that she was a 'latent anorexic'.

The main cognitive techniques are:

☐   Self-instructional training.
☐   Stress inoculation training.
☐   Cognitive restructuring.
☐   Covert conditioning approaches.
☐   Thought-stopping procedures.
☐   Sensitising clients to misattribution.
☐   Influencing schema and improving knowledge of how assumptions can constrict options (e.g. black and white, right/wrong thinking (see the case example on p. 236).
☐   Helping clients to understand and accurately interpret emotional responses.

These methods are discussed in more detail below, but it should be remembered that this is not a list of separate options, and routine practice usually contains *combinations* of these methods.

I am happy to report on research pertaining to these (expanding and ever more detailed) categories and titles, but I have some misgivings. That is, the research on *process* factors (see Chapter 2) is resulting in ever more complex matrices of potentially useful subtypes of intervention, but when hundreds of even blind qualitative decisions are blended together, usually with only marginally *statistically* significant concordance rates, then marginal calls as to whether a particular technique is present or not/being appropriately used or not create very weak 'signal-to-noise' ratios, which are then multiplied until the numbers (not the ratios, note) look persuasive. I believe this is why many texts on cognitive approaches read like plays, with pages and pages of dialogue (too tidy and ideographic to convince me I am afraid).

Education 'factor-analysis' research, and family therapy research took this road once; it led to nowhere in particular. I would prefer therapists to take note of particular cognitive therapy techniques; to apply them together in an integrated way against the known psycho-social origins of problems – not as if they were the equivalent of pharmaceutical preparations ('self-instructozine' versus 'cogno-restructozine'). Can't be done: different sort of field (see Orlinsky *et al.* (2004: 321, fig. 8.1) if you think I am wrong about this).

Guided self-instructional training

A major premise of self-instructional training is that what we say to ourselves – that is, the content of our 'internal dialogues' – cues, shapes and maintains our overt behaviour. The Russian psychologists Vygotsky (1962) and Luria (1961) suggested that this important relationship between language, thought and behaviour develops in three stages during socialisation. In early childhood, behaviour is controlled mainly by the speech of others (particularly adults). During the next stage, the child begins to use his own developing speech to regulate his behaviour (as in the play commentaries of young children). Remember Piaget's example of a child who asked 'How do I know what I think until I've said it?' Finally, this function is assumed by the cognitive accompaniments of speech and speech 'goes inside'. It is these sequences of cognitive cues to behaviour that we seek to influence.

In this view, behavioural excesses and deficits can result from inadequacies in cognitive controls over behaviour (lack of self-governing responses in the first case; lack of self-encouraging responses in the second). A second proposition is that it is possible to remedy these deficits by teaching clients to re-programme their responses with the aid of appropriate *self-statements.* Meichenbaum (1977) referred humorously to this approach in psychiatric care as 'teaching patients to talk to themselves'.

In problems resulting from impulsiveness, the client is instructed to interrupt the sequence of behavioural and cognitive events that leads to, say, an aggressive reaction, by deliberately thinking, or saying aloud to himself, a pre-rehearsed statement, and/or visualising a series of images which are incompatible with the behaviour he is about to embark upon. The emphasis in self-instructional training is on instigating, monitoring and maintaining coping skills and being prepared to deal with internal and external distractions, which the client brings into operation in situations which he or she finds difficult. These coping skills are maintained by cognitive cues, reinforcing images, and by covertly or overtly recited instructions, covering each step in the sequence. These techniques are, therefore, often combined with social skills training and modelling approaches (as in Case example 8.7) and incidentally, have ubiquitous applications in the field of Sports science.

CASE EXAMPLE 8.7

Here is an example of self-instructional training from a programme designed to help control paranoid ideas in a 34-year-old ex-psychiatric patient living in a hostel (see pp. 62, 161). The client (also under treatment for periodic elective mutism and chronic social withdrawal) complained initially that noises coming from other rooms seemed excessively loud, that there was more laughter to be heard than before, and that she felt that this was directed at her. She also listened intently to silences because she felt people had lowered their voices so that she could not hear the worst of their criticisms of her. This meant she could never be at peace: noise = criticism – silence = worse criticism. The hostel staff knew of nothing unusual in the behaviour of the other residents.

Procedure

These seemingly irrational beliefs (ideas of reference) were the first focus, and the inconsistencies in the client's account were gently confronted (talking in an interested but puzzled tone). These were that Laura felt people were talking about her *both* when they were behaving noisily and when they were quiet. The question was then raised: Why should other residents be so interested in her since she had nothing much to do with them? The idea that she was a person likely to excite this constant level of interest was discussed. The client was asked to think about her own interest in other individuals and whether this could ever be concentrated on one person for twenty-four hours. The client, grudgingly, thought not, and when pressed she laughed (a *very* infrequent response) and admitted that it would be boring. What then was so especially interesting about her? Her answer was that she looked strange and didn't talk to anyone – which was true. The client was then shown videotapes of herself from early on in treatment, when she looked dishevelled and had a kind of 'Old English Sheepdog' haircut, covering her eyes. These pictures were then compared with more up-to-date tapes, showing a considerable improvement. Next, the client was reminded of the effort she was making (weekly sessions, homework assignment, letter-writing and exercises in reading aloud). Wasn't she trying very hard to overcome her difficulties and become more sociable? Did all this effort count for so little? Had she not reported that other residents and staff answered her when she forced herself to say hello to them? The following self-instruction sequence was also agreed and the client was taught to review it, item by item, whenever she felt her ideas of reference returning:

- ☐ 'Steady now, deep breath.' 'It's only because I'm on my own and paying too much attention to what is going on outside my room that I am reading things into those noises that are not really there.' 'Everyone does it from time to time, I do it too much.'
- ☐ I *think* that people are talking about me because I don't have much to do with them. This may happen occasionally but definitely not all the time and among so many different people.
- ☐ I am trying very hard to overcome my shyness but I am not ready to cope with talking much to other people yet – one day I shall be.
- ☐ I look better now than before, and I intend to go on looking after myself in future. This is a problem I am getting on top of.
- ☐ Right, this is not really worth worrying about. I have better things to do – like getting something to eat or doing one of my homework exercises.

Laura first read from these typewritten instructions, and eventually memorised parts of them for use in other settings.

Use of imagery

Laura found that relaxing, and deliberately engaging in a favourite fantasy (pony trekking, or grooming a horse meticulously stage by stage), were more effective than homework exercises as an activity to follow after going through her instructions. Two further images were made use of. First, a visualisation based on videotape recordings was used, comparing her verbal skill level of nine months ago with today. This image was used whenever she felt unduly conspicuous or had thoughts about receiving derogatory comments from other people. Second, she was offered an image of the therapist praising her for the effort she was putting into her work, reminding her of the progress already made. In seven weeks (ten sessions) the ideas of reference virtually disappeared, although they occasionally reappeared when under stress (e.g. when she was asked to take a telephone call). In addition, she had abandoned a grisly self-punishing ritual of repeatedly sticking pins into her arm as atonement for whatever her neighbours were supposed to be criticizing her for (a negatively reinforced anxiety-reduction response). She later moved to a flat on her own and joined a cycling club. She has been briefly back in hospital once, now no longer avoids the CPN and receives occasional informal support from a volunteer at home. Self-esteem scores are climbing.

Stress inoculation training

This approach involves therapists in rehearsing coping skills with clients, preparatory to entering into a typically stressful situation. It is used mainly in programmes designed to combat maladaptive fears and phobias, where research is suggesting that rapid exposure to the threatening stimulus – with the client remaining in the stressful conditions using pre-rehearsed coping mechanisms – is a faster and more effective treatment approach with many clients than desensitisation (see Marks 1971, 1975; Beck *et al.* 1985) – if you can persuade clients to do it, that is. Orne (1965) introduced the concept of *immunisation* in his discussion of the importance of changing the beliefs of clients about their ability to cope with stress given appropriate rehearsal, an emphasis that should remind readers of Bandura's theories regarding the importance of modifying efficacy and outcome expectations (see Bandura 1977; Wills 2009). Table 8.2 shows a typical schedule of self-instruction, which came into operation after appropriate rehearsal with the therapist of the different elements in the process of confronting a particular stress.

A further consideration when using self-statements in this way is the voice in which clients talk to themselves. We are all familiar with the 'sound' of our parents' voices inside our heads admonishing us, and with the experience of 'hearing' ourselves praised and having our views supported by figures noted for their sanity and intelligence (I sometimes invoke the friendly ghost of Bernard Levin).

Take the a case of someone with a debilitating fear of public speaking which might seem just a worried well/lifestyle problem, except that (1) his job depended upon being able to do it; and (2) it depressed and preoccupied him (see p. 234).

In a case of mine involving a man who developed a phobia of confined spaces after being trapped in a lift (p. 107), not being able to travel in lifts might also seem a minor inconvenience, except that the patient worked on the thirteenth floor of a tower block and his files were kept centrally on the first floor. He developed a range of devices to hide his absences and his breathlessness. Fears and panicky feelings can thus affect self-concepts and a wider range of capacities that may seem distant from the original problem, but are not. For example:

> As I stand talking to the audience, I hope that my mind and voice will function properly, that I won't lose my balance, and everything else will function. But, then my heart starts to pound, I feel pressure build up in my chest as though I'm ready to explode, my tongue feels thick and heavy, my mind feels foggy and then goes blank. I can't remember what I have just said or what I am supposed to say. Then I start to choke. I can barely push the words out. My body is swaying; my hands tremble. I start to sweat and I am ready to topple off the platform. I feel terrified and I think that I will probably disgrace myself.
>
> (Beck & Emery 1985: 34)

Few academics will not have experienced such negative, emotional feedback-loop effects when confronted by a large audience of 'not *necessarily* willing to listen and take note' second-year students. We learn to cope, via raw exposure, and confess none of our fears to our colleagues.

Cognitive restructuring

The reader has already been shown an attempt to correct a disabling belief by presenting the client with arguments about its illogicality (as on p. 232). Techniques of this kind depend very much upon the pioneering work of cognitive therapists, such as Beck (1970, 1976), and on the rational-emotive approach of Albert Ellis (1979). The main theoretical assumption in this approach is that beliefs, apart from being situation-specific, cognitive and emotional accompaniments to behaviour, are themselves organised into systems, which have durable, semi-automatic effects across a *range* of settings; in other words, they operate as schemata. The logical corollary of this is that if we can influence these beliefs, or faulty thinking styles, then we can change problematic behaviour. The cognitive notion of *thinking style* is quite close to the behavioural notion of *learning history*, that is, the sum total of learning experiences which the individual is known to have undergone. It is easy to see how a particularly disjointed learning history, resulting from perverse or depressing childhood and family experiences, educational failures and so forth, can lead to a pervasively negative view of the world which, by the usual procedure of the self-fulfilling prophecy, is regularly confirmed. Ellis has noted several unnatural patterns of thinking, such as 'awfulising' – believing that it is *awful* not always to meet targets – or the belief that surrounding circumstances are always part of a mischievous conspiracy against one's legitimate aims. Readers could probably add to such a list from their own experience.

Beck has some useful advice on defining 'cognition' – a term we take for granted, but not one necessarily known to clients:

> The therapist can define cognition as 'either a thought or a visual image that you may not be very aware of until you focus your attention on it'. Characteristically, a cognition is an appraisal of events from any time perspective (past, present, or future). The typical cognitions observed in depression and other clinical disorders are often described as 'automatic thoughts', part of a habitual pattern of thinking. . . . Thus it is not uncommon

for the depressed patient to be overwhelmed by rhetorical questions (for example) 'why am I such an incompetent person?' 'Why am I so weak?' Or with unpleasant visual images (for example, 'Seeing myself looking ugly'). He takes for granted that he is weak, inept, or ugly and wonders why he has been afflicted in this way. This sequence is typical; cognitive factors maintain and sensitize beliefs; emotional factors; disturb rational appraisal. CBT depends upon breaking this vicious circle by rationally and calmly considering whether urgent emotions mean what they seem to mean, regardless of *actual* future loss or danger.

(Beck *et al.* 1979: 3)

Here is an example of what attempts to forensically unravel these patterns of thought, feeling and behaviour sounds like, this time in an anxiety disorder case:

Ruth (therapist): Now, when the anxiety got acute today, what was that like?

John (patient): Torture, extreme torture. Because I felt scared, really scared. I would equate it to a child having to go to hospital in an emergency. And you don't really know what is wrong with you and you're just really scared that something could happen, that you could die.

Ruth: Is that the thought you had, that 'I could die', when it was very bad?

John: Yeah, I was trying to repress it at the same time.

Ruth: Yeah, but you had the thought that I could die? What made you think that you could die?

John: I guess the physical sensations, you know.

Ruth: And what were they?

John: Fright. Fright was the one. It's like a paralysing feeling that comes over you.

(Scott *et al.* 1989: 33)

Self-statements were important in the severe depression case discussed on p. 236. One that worked well (she had been keen on sport) was based on the metaphor: 'You have a good idea now of what you want to achieve, but you are impatient to get there – which is good – but you are playing rugby not hockey. There may sometimes be gaps to exploit, but most of the time it is a question of gaining a useful five yards before circumstances bring you down. Then you have to look at the opportunities for *another* five yards.' The client, in conversations with herself and with her partner, condensed this into 'it's not hockey, it's rugby' as a kind of self-sustaining mantra. Table 8.2 provides some further notes on the influence of deliberate self-statements.

Marzillier, in a very useful early research review, summarised the aims and methods of the cognitive therapies as follows:

Beck and Ellis regard change in fundamental cognitive structures and beliefs as the ultimate goal of therapy. Beck (1976) describe the aims of therapy as 'to identify, reality-test and correct maladaptive, distorted conceptualizations and the dysfunctional beliefs (schemas) underlying these cognitions'; and Ellis (1979) sees therapy as needing to produce a 'profound cognitive and philosophic change in clients' basic assumptions,

Table 8.2 Self-statements

Stage	Content
Preparing for a stressor	What is it you have to do?
	You can develop a plan to deal with it.
	Just think about what you can do about it.
	That's better than getting anxious.
	No negative self-statements, just think rationally.
	Don't worry: worry won't help anything.
	Maybe what you think is anxiety is eagerness to confront the stressor.
Confronting and handling a stressor	Just psych yourself up – you can meet this challenge.
	You can convince yourself to do it. You can reason your fear away.
	One step at a time: you can handle the situation.
	Don't think about fear; just think about what you have to do. Stay relevant.
	This anxiety is what the therapist said you would feel.
	It's a reminder to do your coping exercises.
	Relax, you're in control. Take a slow deep breath and exhale.
Coping with the feeling of being overwhelmed	When fear comes, just pause.
	Keep the focus on the present; what is it you have to do?
	Label your fear from 0 to 10 and watch it change.
	Don't try to eliminate fear totally; just keep it manageable.
Reinforcing self-statements	It worked; you did it.

Source: Adapted from Meichenbaum (1974)

> especially their absolutistic, demanding, masturbatory, irrational ways of viewing themselves, others and the world'.
>
> (Marzillier 1980: 251; see Hollon & Beck (2004) for an update.)

Case example 8.8 shows predominantly cognitive techniques in use, but with some behavioural back-up.

CASE EXAMPLE 8.8

Ms M. (aged 40) was referred for CBT by her psychiatrist. Her life experience closely encapsulates the research findings discussed in Chapter 2, in that she had a series of sad and threatening life events. She was an adopted child (probably her intended role was to thaw out a frozen marriage). She was raised in a distant, arm's-length way; she later had two violent marriages herself; was raped, kidnapped, tied up in an upstairs room for three days before breaking free, her ex-husband tried to run her over as she escaped. She suffered the loss of her 18-year-old daughter in a car accident, and had to make the decision to switch off the life-support machinery. She later, understandably, had occupational difficulties, made worse by the current, 'if officially ill, stay away; if officially well, come in and perform to standard' policies.

Scores on the Hamilton Schulz & Beck Depression Inventory showed her to be in the most serious 1 per cent of cases, with suicidal ideation a daily preoccupation. Medication made her sleepy and unable to function. She was therefore likely to alternate between feeling that nothing mattered much, and occasional bursts of agitation: 'like being on your way somewhere important but "dozing off at the wheel"'; 'a dark room with nothing to do and no one to talk to is my favourite thing'.

The cognitive component of work with Ms M. concentrated on the following factors:

☐ Her brittle sense of gratitude towards her adoptive parents – 'They told me I was special because they *chose* me, but then they sent me to a boarding school three miles down the road and didn't often have me home.' She recalled going on a school nature ramble near her home and inviting her friends into the garden, where her father waved them away with the words, 'This is *not* one of your days, there is nothing in the diary about this.' She felt the loss of face and of possible close affection for twenty-five years. As an adolescent she kicked over the traces, this behaviour leading to expulsion from school. In her parents view, and, note, in *hers,* this amounted to monstrous ingratitude. Similarly, that her interest in her natural mother's fate amounted to 'a betrayal of trust'.

☐ That her early sexual experimentation ('I knew how to get boys to give me what I wanted': [therapist]: 'What was that?' Answer: 'Attention, affection') was the result of 'bad blood'. Interestingly, after years of psychiatric help, no one had ever raised with her in detail before the question of how it feels to be disposable and/or surplus to requirements as a child. She had tried to contact her natural mother but was rebuffed, and said that she had hoped to have found her 'a wreck' (which would have made her abandonment at least understandable). When she persisted and did track down her natural mother, she was married with two children, living in a nice house and 'wanting to put the past behind her'. 'But *I* am the past, I didn't ask to be' was her reaction. Would-be helpers who shy away from strong, dark emotions in the interests of 'stability' and 'looking to the future' have lost the plot regarding how bad experiences in the past stay inside us and colour every future prospect for something better.

☐ That her desire to find a 'strong man or two' who would protect her – which led to two violent relationships (the attractive macho behaviour was not supposed to be brought home) – was a result of her 'stupidity'.

☐ That she should have performed some routine checks on the state of her daughter's car (tyre pressures, brakes, etc.) before she set off on her journey, even though she had absolutely no mechanical expertise.

☐ That the person who followed her and raped her had 'had his fuse lit' by her, and that she should have known better what flirting would lead to.

☐ That getting better meant abandoning her daughter's cherished memory and 'moving on' without her, and so would constitute another betrayal. The approach used was to persuade her to take her daughter's love and the memories of her with her throughout life. She seized upon the idea.

☐ That her current, loving partner was only displaying sympathy or at best short-term love, and would leave her when he found out more about her (they are now happily married).

The behavioural components in this case were based on the idea of 'scheduling pleasant events' against a desensitisation hierarchy. The principle here is to encourage reality-testing (i.e. will the meal with friends *really* be a disaster; will the movie *really* not be enjoyable; will trips to the keep-fit club *really* not result in weight loss; will confiding more in your partner *really* distance him more than will the 'partner-management scheme' currently in place?). Does bad, manipulative sex with previous partners mean that nothing more meaningful is possible with someone quite different?

On one occasion this client and her partner came for a joint interview. He, a kindly, gentle man ('too nice for his own good' was her summation) said that he would do *anything* to help her, but that she tended to see any affection as a precursor for sex, and so rebuffed him and then felt guilty. He reasoned with her about this, and said that he only wanted intimacy when she was willing to give it freely and with no 'ghosts of the past' in the room: multiple second guessing was the problem here. He was perfectly prepared to wait and stand by her. Ms M. felt guilty about her neglect of him (both physical and emotional). 'He works late, and comes in, and I've no food to give him so he goes out for a take-away. I feel bad, but if I cooked for him he might get the wrong signals' (sex in prospect – he said *never* to that). So a little behavioural experiment was set up. Rather than 'he thinks, I think, that he thinks', tangles, it was based on the scheduling of pleasant-events principle. I suggested, since she was to be cooking, that we went to a local Italian delicatessen and bought some fresh pasta, good olive oil, parmesan cheese and pesto sauce – simple food, with a tablecloth and candle as the backdrop (it could have been beans on toast by the way). She was to telephone to say how the experiment had gone the following day, and replied, 'wonderful, a breakout' and offered 'I never expected culinary advice alongside help for depression!'. Then she laughed for about the first time I ever heard her do so. *Doing* something based on new insights is a vital ingredient in recovery.

This work led to substantial reductions in depression scale scores in eleven one-hour sessions; noteworthy experimentation (at work) and trying out a different, less pessimistic and fearful lifestyle, and to a substantial fall in preoccupations with suicide. A fluke? Not so. That this client is able to laugh again; able to work full-time; able to reconcile herself with her older, somewhat estranged child, and is willing to contemplate further developments in her recovery, is not unusual in this literature. Getting access to such help is the ongoing challenge (the government is giving some financial support) and we surely cannot leave this work to psychologists with one-year waiting lists, or to psychotherapists with a charge of £80+ per session excluding most poorer clients. So get trained if you aren't, but ask yourself why you weren't/aren't being trained (if you aren't) in the first place.

The main approach in attempts to change irrational belief systems is clearly to identify and exemplify such patterns for the client; to rehearse with him or her alternative views of reality and alternatives to negative self-statements. This can be augmented with practise in different styles of thinking, cued by pre-decided self-statements, and maintained by self-instruction schedules and appropriate self-reinforcement. There follows an example of a (famous) cognitive therapist trying, by very direct means, to render a client more aware of the automatic and illogical nature of her thoughts about the past and the future. Such a direct approach had been unusual in previous forms of psychological help owing to the status we have always accorded to the 'feelings over facts' principle of the once-dominant psychoanalytic model. This patient is clinically depressed with a history of self-harm and suicidal intent:

> *Therapist*: Why do you want to end your life?
> *Patient*: Without Raymond, I am nothing . . . I can't be happy without Raymond . . . But I can't save our marriage.
> *Therapist*: What has your marriage been like?
> *Patient*: It has been miserable from the very beginning . . . Raymond has always been unfaithful . . . I have hardly seen him in the past five years.
> *Therapist*: You say that you can't be happy without Raymond . . . . Have you found yourself happy when you are with Raymond?
> *Patient*: No, we fight all the time and I feel worse.
> *Therapist*: You say you are nothing without Raymond. Before you met Raymond, did you feel you were nothing?
> *Patient*: No, I felt I was somebody.
> *Therapist*: If you were somebody before you knew Raymond, why do you need him to be somebody now?
> *Patient*: [*Puzzled*] Hmmm . . .
>
> (Beck 1976: 289–290)

This interpretive breakthrough took ten minutes – forty to go. However, to such sequences of challenging irrationality must be added practice in alternative ways of behaving (as in Case examples 8.7 and 8.8) since, as we have seen, extrinsic reinforcement for alternative behaviours is likely to affect thinking patterns – or at least to give weight to discussions about their effects. Similarly, the evaluation of such programmes should include a behavioural indicator or two if we are to avoid working only with subjective data (see Chapter 6).

One further word of caution. Certain very well-established, and presumably functional, delusional patterns in some psychiatric cases are unlikely to yield to anything; and excessive demands in therapeutic programmes could constitute exactly the kind of 'expressed emotion' conditions known to trigger relapse. Nevertheless, with less extreme cases, good results are being recorded across a range of problems and client groups (see Ellis 1979; Wykes *et al.* 1998; Chadwick *et al.* 2000).

Covert counter-conditioning

Counter-conditioning techniques (the application of stronger, incompatible stimuli to weaken maladaptive conditioned responses) predate cognitive approaches, and their application and nature are reviewed in Chapter 4. Covert counter-conditioning (which relies upon the same principles but uses *images* rather than overt stimuli) is discussed here so that it can be seen for what it is – a cognitive technique.

Covert conditioning approaches are of two kinds. First, there are the *positive* techniques, where clients are trained to visualise themselves coping well with a particular fear-provoking circumstance but retaining control. Alternatively, clients can be trained to imagine a pre-rehearsed scene which they find unpleasant, and to relax while under stress on Wolpe's 'Can't do two incompatible things at once' theory of reciprocal inhibition (see Chapters 1 and 4). Training usually takes the form of just clarifying the image, with practice at summoning this on cue, and then visualising the circumstance that arouses the fear reaction and countering this with the positive image. Practice *in vivo* usually follows reported competence with this technique. This was an important feature of early work in the case of the agoraphobic client described on p. 104.

Second, *covert sensitisation* procedures may be employed. These techniques use punishing and negatively reinforcing images to help develop avoidance responses. They are applied to maladaptive behaviours, such as dependence on alcohol or drugs, and overeating. The client is trained first to summon up punishing images to accompany visualisation of the behaviour he or she wishes to remove.

Thought stopping

During the following discussion I want you to imagine a large, green, shiny apple. Got it? OK, now you are *not* to think of this image at all over the next two paragraphs. See how you get on.

Thought-stopping techniques have been employed by therapists of many different persuasions over the years. They may be used to control obsessive thoughts and ruminations, or as a method of controlling the self-presentation of images employed in some of the cognitive approaches reviewed above. The usual procedure is to get clients to close their eyes and summon up a clear and detailed image of what it is that is troubling or obsessively present, and then for the therapist to shout 'Stop!' The client opens his eyes immediately. He then practises this for himself, first aloud and then sub-vocally (see Hollon & Beck 2004). The aim of these devices is to interrupt the unwanted sequence of thoughts via a short, sharp environmental input. Again, the research evidence on their effectiveness is mixed. In addition, because thought-stopping techniques are usually employed in combination with other methods, it is difficult to obtain an independent measure of their potency.

Techniques for reducing anxiety and avoidance

The behavioural therapies (and now with the merger with cognitive therapy and Rational-Emotive Therapy – RET) have always been best known for the success of the work done on phobias, and on less severe, irrational fears and anxiety states (see Lambert 2004). There are a number of techniques which may be used in the face of such difficulties, and each of these is discussed in turn. (Notes on the theoretical models and research regarding these approaches are contained in Chapters 2 and 4.)

Positive counter-conditioning

By the way, how many shiny apple images have interrupted your reading? Thoughts are 'Teflon coated'; they slip through rational discourse or even pleasant emotional experience. So thought stopping is difficult to pull off and we lack controlled experiments and systematic reviews. I have had some worthwhile experiences, but then so what? Experiment and observe is the best advice.

The principle here is to 'break up' maladaptive conditioned associations (for example, fear of everyday events, objects or animals) by introducing a new response which is incompatible with, and stronger than, the existing problematic response. Again, Wolpe's principle of 'reciprocal inhibition' (Wolpe 1958) states that if we pair a response capable of *inhibiting* anxiety with the anxiety-provoking stimulus, it can be used to weaken the conditional association between that stimulus and anxiety. By pairing responses the client might, loosely speaking, 'unlearn' the association.

CASE EXAMPLE 8.9

Angela (aged 7) was brought into care after a health visitor put together a history of previous neglect punctuated by occasional physical maltreatment. The precipitating circumstances were that her father arrived home drunk one night (a regular occurrence) and found her still up and grizzling over having her hair washed before going to bed. He grabbed her and thrust her head into the sink, turning on by mistake a hot water geyser and scalding her head and neck. Following discharge from hospital to which Social Services were called, she went to live in a small group children's home prior to being fostered. Here several (understandable) problems developed which caused concern about her health and development, which in turn were regularly cited as obstacles to placement in foster care:

☐   She refused to have dressings changed without a fight.
☐   She refused to have her hair washed, or medication applied to her neck.
☐   In any situation where she was not in control (e.g. over choice of food or size of helping), she became aggressive, on one occasion threatening staff with a carving knife for spooning gravy on to her dinner when she had refused it.

The theme of control = safety here was very evident and the counter-conditioning programme used acknowledged this in general terms while focusing on specific instances of anxiety.

Procedure

☐   Circumstances or events were pre-described in respect of their purpose, and Angela was allowed to stay in charge of the speed of these (e.g. dressing changes), building in little breaks as she wished. Staff were encouraged to break down these episodes into more manageable 'chunks', and to talk out loud about what they were doing, to involve her in the task (e.g. holding dressings and bottles, carrying out similar practices on dolls to demonstrate what they were about to do). Although this was time-consuming, it resulted in far fewer episodes of distress and aggression.
☐   Angela had not had many toys in her life. Water toys were purchased, including a boat. She was left to play with these and soon found her own way to the water and gradually, washing (first hands, then face) was introduced as part of the game. The association of pleasure in the face of retention of control became incompatible with fear and anxiety, allowing scope for positive reinforcement approaches elsewhere. Her father was persuaded into treatment for his alcoholism; her mother was weaned off her anaesthetising doses of tranquillisers with the help of a GP and practice nurse; after six weeks in foster care, with planned, rising levels of parental contact and reassurance, she went home under close social services supervision and no further problems were reported.

Exposure therapy

Exposure is used in the treatment of panic and disabling fears and is derived from respondent extinction research (see p. 107). A phobia is a powerful, conditioned fear reaction to objects, animals, people, or just about any other set of environmental circumstances. Clients experience powerful physical reactions to particular stimuli, and, even if they know that their fears are illogical, they are unable to control them. Phobias are largely *learned* reactions and obey the principles of classical conditioning, though there is evidence of background temperamental influences and of genetic/biological predisposition. However, they are often maintained by negative reinforcement – maladaptive escape and avoidance responses being strengthened by the relief they bring. Phobias also generalise to circumstances which resemble the original stimulus conditions. The case described on p. 104 is one of a typical agoraphobia (fear of going out of doors); these, together with social phobias (fear of social interactions), are the types of problems most often met with in clinical practice, and can be as disabling as some psychotic conditions.

For years the established treatment for these problems was systematic desensitisation: slow, graded exposure to threatening stimuli accompanied by relaxation based on counter-conditioning principles (Wolpe 1958). This was the first of the behavioural approaches to establish itself in the therapeutic repertoire. However, later 'dismantling' research investigating the relative part played by each of the ingredients of systematic desensitisation, plus the results of increasing experimentation with rapid exposure methods, has resulted in a considerable rationalisation in this field (see the pioneering work of Marks (1975, 1978)). Instead of viewing rapid exposure and systematic desensitisation as two separate techniques, they should, on the (impressive) research evidence (see Emmelkamp 2004), for practical purposes, be thought of as a continuum from slow to rapid exposure. Although it is now reasonable to suggest that fairly rapid exposure to the feared stimulus is the treatment of choice in phobias, this is a little like suggesting that a large injection of money is the best approach to poverty. It may be a good idea but it is not always feasible. The client may be staunchly unwilling to confront his or her worst fear, however much encouragement and support is given to him or her. This leaves us having to work for an optimal solution. The problem remains: that is, getting clients to confront their worst fears as quickly as possible after due preparation, and helping them to stay there until the anxiety subsides. It is important to explain to clients that their fears and physical unrest *will* subside, however powerful the anxiety. Persuading clients to endure this is the challenge – for if they abandon the programme there is a negative reinforcement effect, and more anxiety-based defections to be got through at the next attempt.

I have usually employed a pragmatic, 'hop, skip and jump' desensitisation approach with an eye out for short cuts if there is enough stamina and motivation available. Case example 8.10 illustrates such an opportunity.

CASE EXAMPLE 8.10

M.R. was a 25-year-old, recently qualified graduate in micro-biology struggling to cope with a persistent fear of dirt and germs, who lived away from her close family. Her main fear was that she would infect them on visits home to a rather isolated and embattled

Asian community in a predominantly white, working-class area. Racial abuse was common on the streets, heightening her fears for her parents' safety and their well-being ('all they can afford so they are stuck' was the explanation for her parents remaining in the area). So the common theme of vigilant responsibility – rational or not, achievable or not – is present in this case, as was the interaction of socio-economic and psychological factors: routinely but mistakenly separated in most textbooks.

Here is where any latent Freudians who have strayed into the wrong book should prick up their ears. Her job was in a lab studying pathogens – some of which apparently had military implications(!). 'It's safer in there than anywhere; the precautions are tremendous' she replied when asked about this strange career choice for someone who disliked touching telephones, sitting on lavatories, who washed her hands relentlessly, who couldn't often drive a car because of impending disaster (no accident had even occurred). In the first of four sessions (backed by telephone counselling) M.R. produced scores of examples of infections due to failures of precautionary hygiene. The origin of these feelings lay in early teenage years but became marked during her lab work as an undergraduate. Her approach was scientific (i.e. to persuade me that her pre-occupations and fear-ridden precautions were a proportionate response to a too-little appreciated threat).

Using this mindset, M.R. was asked why she thought she didn't have an immune system like everyone else. Silence, smile: 'It's just the way I am.' 'You have no control over it then?'; 'Well, a little, now and then.' It was suggested that she keep a diary of her urges on a subjective units of anxiety scale to marry up circumstances and mood. Then using the scientific idea as the justification for her precautions, and following a little psycho-education on the nature of anxiety, the idea of experimenting with fears was introduced. She accepted that the proposal was rational.

She was invited without notice to accompany myself and a female colleague to the Ladies' toilet, where she was urged to touch the toilet seat. 'I can't!'; 'You might surprise yourself.' She did, and remained in contact for two minutes. She then headed for the wash-basins, but was persuaded away since this was an experiment. She returned to the office, and a detailed history lasting an hour was taken – the client panted and paced but stayed, answering questions. She was asked to push her hair back; refused at first, but then tried to do so, but warned that she would have to shower for at least half an hour when she got the chance, but this feeling too subsided.

(Therapist): 'What have you learned today?' (Client): 'Well, I didn't die, though I thought I might.' (Therapist): 'Have your anxiety ratings come down as we discussed?' (Client): 'Surprisingly, yes.' (Therapist): 'Then let's go to lunch.' (Client): 'I couldn't eat like this.' (Therapist): 'What is *this*?' (Client): 'I'm contaminated.' (Therapist): 'We all are but mainly it does no harm, as you have seen.' (Client): 'I'll come but I'll need to go to the toilet first' [this to wash, etc.] (Therapist): 'No, because we need to keep the experiment going if you can manage it.' (Client): 'I'll try.'

Local pub: M.R. tries to order a meal, not a sandwich like myself and my colleague. This is of course because she wants a knife and fork between her and the about-to-be-contaminated food. She is persuaded to have a sandwich and to eat some chips with her fingers.

The client is much more relaxed after the lunch and we round off the session with the need to stay with the anxiety. She is joined by a friend who is briefed to encourage her away from ablutions until bedtime. Asked again what confronting disabling fears was like she replied again: 'I didn't die after all.'

The next three sessions were dedicated to keeping this self-exposure scheme running with the help of her friend, and to reinstating her driving by taking a short course of lessons having explained her situation to the driving instructor in advance. She no longer scrubs her hands, has found a new job, and drives to and from work with increasing ease. The 'experimental' idea (admittedly with a client who well understood the term) was the predominant influence and stayed with her when she encountered new challenges.

Where the client will not cooperate with a rapid exposure approach, *slow exposure* is indicated, and to the extent that induced relaxation aids this process, we are left with a useful role for some form of systematic desensitisation.

Procedure in exposure therapy

☐   Preparation for rapid exposure is very important and may involve the therapist in using other techniques such as modelling and rehearsal. First, the causes of phobias (see Chapter 4) should be reviewed with the client. I am not suggesting here that an academic discussion should be entered into, but that some basic principles should be simply outlined. It is usually helpful for the client to grasp the ideas behind what is being proposed and to register that the method being employed is the result of considerable research and practical experimentation, not just a therapeutic style. This is not just to impress him or her, but because (as when medical procedures are necessary) stress is easier to bear when we understand the rationale behind it all and can estimate likely duration (think dentistry), can assess the limits of the effects on us, and can retain some control.

☐   The next stage involves the mapping out of a treatment rationale which is acceptable to the client. Generally speaking, the fewer the number of steps before the client confronts the stimulus conditions usually avoided, the better. Against this must be weighed the risk of premature withdrawal from a session found too overwhelming. Clients do not usually experience difficulty in describing the various stages of fear intensity and avoidance which given conditions produce, and a short hierarchy of these can be drawn up, as in Figure 8.1 on p. 246.

☐   There are many things that can be done to equip the client for coping with stress. Reassurances can be given about the relatively short-term nature of anxiety (as in the last case – it came as a surprise to M.R., never having tried it before); worst fears and irrational expectations can be underlined and analysed, clients can be encouraged to *imagine* themselves taking steps to cope with anxiety, or they can be encouraged to 'reality test' some of their lesser fears. Reassurances can also be given that the therapist will stay with them and help them to remain in contact with the feared circumstances as long as necessary until things feel better. Alternatively ('subject to availability'), relatives or friends can be trained as mediators and can help in this way. Rehearsal sessions can he started where the procedure is modelled by the therapist and then by the client.

These methods aside, programmes of this type depend greatly on a relationship of trust between client and therapist; an approach characterised by reassuring firmness in the face of fear, and by a clear commitment from clients that they will not abandon the session before the anxiety has subsided. Homework assignments can be designed to cover the period between sessions, and research rightly lays stress on the importance of these behaviour-maintenance measures.

Exposure techniques *necessarily* (deliberately) create great anxiety in clients, and without being too dramatic about it, simple precautions are needed to ensure that people with heart ailments or respiratory problems do not attempt resolutions at this pace. The best method of ensuring this is to discuss prospective cases with the GP or psychiatrist, and to enlist medical cooperation at the assessment stage. Such referrals are particularly important in the treatment of panic disorder, where clients often harbour irrational beliefs about ever-increasing heart rates, strokes or collapse into mental illness. Here, a sympathetic medical consultation can be part of the reality-testing features of the programme.

Slow exposure and systematic desensitisation

There are two kinds of systematic desensitisation: *in vivo* (live practice); and *imaginal*, a cognitive approach using the same principles but in mental form. Both approaches have the same three main therapeutic ingredients: (1) a graded hierarchy of anxiety-producing stimuli; (2) a relatively slow rate of progression through the stages of this hierarchy, the pace being dictated by a lowering of anxiety (almost boredom in some cases) before the next item is approached, and thus the idea of self-control is reinforced; (3) a counter-conditioning element in the form of relaxation. This was always an effective technique (Bandura 1969; Emmelkamp 2004), and more rapid exposure methods are only going to supersede it on the grounds that they are more efficient, more parsimonious, and also produce equally reliable results. Tests of the various elements of systematic desensitisation, to see what components are the really potent ones and which could usefully be pruned away, suggest that the relaxation element, and the idea of a smooth progression through an incremental hierarchy, are less important than was previously thought (see Cooke (1968) for the pioneering study).

This recent research leaves us having to make three separate decisions about three overlapping techniques.

☐ Will the client cooperate with the rapid exposure approach? (This decision should be based on a judgement of his or her *capabilities* as much as on expressed good intentions.)

☐ What is the optimum rate of progression towards the fear-provoking stimulus in this client's case (remembering that he or she must remain in contact with it for some time)?

☐ Will relaxation exercises serve as a coping technique to help the client through the process of exposure? Another key point is: Can clients learn to relax *outside* the consulting room, where the cues for fear and avoidance are much more evident and acute?

The first point has already been covered. Turning to the second, it is important to emphasise that the rules of slow exposure are somewhat different to those of desensitisation. In the latter approach, the idea was to slide gently up the hierarchy, keeping anxiety to a minimum and counteracting its effects in little steps. In exposure therapy, the production of some anxiety is deliberate; it is the fact that the client remains in contact with the fear-provoking stimulus until its effects subside that is the active ingredient.

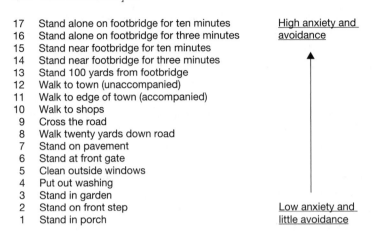

17	Stand alone on footbridge for ten minutes	High anxiety and
16	Stand alone on footbridge for three minutes	avoidance
15	Stand near footbridge for ten minutes	
14	Stand near footbridge for three minutes	
13	Stand 100 yards from footbridge	
12	Walk to town (unaccompanied)	
11	Walk to edge of town (accompanied)	
10	Walk to shops	
9	Cross the road	
8	Walk twenty yards down road	
7	Stand on pavement	
6	Stand at front gate	
5	Clean outside windows	
4	Put out washing	
3	Stand in garden	
2	Stand on front step	Low anxiety and
1	Stand in porch	little avoidance

Figure 8.1 Contact with fear-provoking stimuli (see Case example 4.4 on p. 104)

In systematic desensitisation the approach is to mollify anxiety in small steps that are not too threatening to emotional equilibrium. An illustration may help to clarify this (see Figure 8.1). In the case of the agoraphobic client (see p. 104), an extended hierarchy was constructed. It is clear that she would not have continued confronting her anxiety-provoking circumstances otherwise. She was taught the basics of progressive relaxation during these sessions, and was sometimes accompanied by the therapist, sometimes deliberately not. If the next step looked too large for her, the progression would be bridged by taking longer to complete an earlier task.

Relaxation therapy

The reasons for considering this counter-conditioning technique separately have already been given. It has specific uses for clients who have high background levels of anxiety, who suffer migraine attacks or frequent tension headaches. In addition, it may be used as a technique to cope with temporary or situation-specific stress, and has a place as an adjunct to the procedures outlined above.

Procedure

The research results of Ost and Westling (1995) show (1) clinically significant superior results for the inclusion of a relaxation element into CBT; and (2) longer-lasting gains and generalisations. Not a panacea for anxiety-based conditions, but a useful component. Here is the procedure:

☐   First, the client is taught about the nature of anxiety; that it is largely a *bodily* phenomenon developed over the eons for useful purposes, and that it can be brought under conscious control to a considerable extent, and that these conditioned warnings of impending physical damage are often just 'better safe than sorry' signals which we can analyse more rationally given that their side-effects may be worse than the benefits they convey.

☐ Next, the client is taught to distinguish clearly between muscular contraction and relaxation. The procedure is that he or she first tenses then completely relaxes each muscle, working in sequence from the toes upward to the forehead muscle, the source of most headaches.

☐ Instruction is given in deep breathing, so that a slow, deep respiration with an emphasis on sighing exhalation can be produced on cue.

☐ The client may also be encouraged to imagine pleasant, peaceful or coping scenes and with practice should be able to use these images to induce relaxation.

☐ Relaxation training is usually given with the client sitting in a comfortable chair, and practice is necessary if the client is to learn to relax while going about his or her everyday business – this is the challenge.

☐ In imaginal desensitisation, items from a pre-prepared hierarchy of threatening items are introduced one by one; while the client is in a relaxed state, he or she imagines him or herself coping with these in a step-by-step fashion.

☐ Relaxation tapes are widely available and clients can use these at home as an adjunct to treatment.

Biofeedback devices

Biofeedback instruments amplify internal organic events and levels, such as heart rate, blood pressure and Galvanic skin resistance (GSR), so that to some extent they can be brought under conscious control. Behavioural management techniques exist for heart disorders such as tachycardia; also for hypertension and migraine. The device most relevant to CBT is the GSR meter which gives an index of arousal (anxiety) by detecting small changes in the electrical resistance of the skin. Changes in GSR are part of a conditioned response, arising from the body's tendency to prepare for threat by rapid heat loss. This is a sort of 'pre-sweating' response, and part of the fight/flight reaction described in Chapter 4. Some of these machines are portable and may be worn like a hearing aid. They emit a tone, which the user attempts to reduce by whatever means he or she chooses – muscle relaxation, slower breathing, thinking of something else and so on.

Conclusions

This chapter has covered both predominantly behavioural techniques, pointing out their cognitive components, and predominantly cognitive approaches where opportunities for behavioural rehearsal and reinforcement are likely to add to their efficiency. The main line of argument taken is that the cognitive dimension and the behavioural dimension should be sensibly combined in our practice. My conclusion from a review of the outcome research is that we, the intended helpers, would be foolish to reflect the *way* in which learning history is interpreted and not just responded to; but that we would be equally foolish not to retain *in vivo* practice and support in our approaches just because it is a little stretching for us.

CBT is unsurpassed anywhere else in the applied psychology and psychotherapy literatures and, for many conditions, is now as much an ethical as a technical imperative.

Table 8.3 Summary of main response-control techniques

Technique	Main features	Application
Modelling	Demonstration of key elements in behaviours likely to prove useful to client. Usually coupled with positive feedback on successive approximations from client.	Used for learning deficits of all kinds plus vicarious extinction of fears and phobias.
Social skills training	As above, but with extra emphasis on rehearsing social and conversational skills and deciding on which occasions a given performance is appropriate.	Used for withdrawn and unconfident clients; people with learning disabilities; people with mental health problems; children, and in work with delinquents where such deficits can be implicated in offending.
Assertion training	As 'Modelling' above, but with extra emphasis on fears associated with assertiveness, and on discriminating between assertive and aggressive responses.	Used with excessively shy or withdrawn individuals. Often used in groups and as an adjunct to wider programmes.
Self-management techniques	Designed to teach coping skills. Emphasis on helping clients to re-label their experiences, change expectations of personal efficacy and the likely outcome of their behaviours. Also teaches clients to obtain environmental support for new responses by changing contingencies.	Used in a wide range of personal problems, especially with deficits and avoidance behaviours resulting from these problems.
Cognitive approaches	Means of identifying the personal constructs applied to self and to problems and making appropriate changes in these constructs. Emphasis on use of positive self-statements and self-reinforcement to maintain new responses.	Useful for wide range of performance difficulties. Particularly applicable to relatively unstructured field settings. May be used in conjunction with other behavioural programmes.
Positive counter-conditioning	The introduction of a response capable of inhibiting anxiety to weaken conditioned anxiety reactions.	Used in the treatment of specific fears and anxieties.
Exposure therapy	Controlled but rapid exposure to threatening stimuli maintained until anxiety extinguished.	May be used to control excessive fears, panic attacks and phobias in cooperative clients.
Slow exposure	Gradual exposure to hierarchy of threatening stimuli, initially to the accompaniment of muscular relaxation (systematic desensitisation).	Used to control excessive fears and phobias where clients are unable to cooperate with rapid exposure. (Muscular relaxation component may be used independently to overcome generalised stress reactions.)
Biofeedback	Use of electronic instruments to amplify and display data from bodily processes such as heart rate, galvanic skin response and blood pressure, with a view to bringing these under conscious control.	May be used in desensitisation therapy but more often employed in the treatment of stress reactions and stress-related illness.

9 Ethical considerations

First, do no harm.

(Hippocrates 400 BC)

It is a curious fact that any form of therapy with 'behaviour' or 'behavioural' in its title seems to attract more critical attention from philosophers, lawyers and journalists than any other type of psychological help in the extensive present-day repertoire – no matter how ill-conceived, and no matter what its track record in empirical research. There are two main reasons for this watchful interest: (1) With anything in which behaviour therapy is a detectable ingredient, what is done is visibly open to inspection and criticism. Its methods are not mysterious; nor are they passed on by means of long initiation ceremonies; nor do the subtleties of such approaches evaporate when exposed to the lens of a video camera. (2) Behavioural methods work well, and even better when they are combined with a cognitive element; they have practical, tangible effects, and anything that succeeds in changing people raises questions. Change for good or ill? Whose idea of change? By what right are people, and their very *thoughts*, being changed (Masson 1990)? In this sense, the critical clamour that greeted the development of the behaviour therapies, which so irritated aficionados, should really be regarded as a mark of respect. But while the use of methods with a behavioural component certainly does give rise to ethical questions, these are not, by and large, qualitatively different from those that could be raised about any type of therapeutic endeavour. It is the success of these approaches that draws the fire of critics; the fact that the target is in full view which makes it tempting.

In this chapter I would like to try to categorise, and respond to, the commonly raised objections to the use of a cognitive-behavioural approach by would-be helping professionals, as well as discuss one or two worries of my own.

The question of control

It is above all the idea of the control of human behaviour that raises the ethical hackles of critics. Partly this is a sentimental reaction made on behalf of clients who have more than enough controls in their lives as it is, but in part it may just be what Leon Festinger (1957) has called 'dissonance reduction'. Let me begin with this point. The worst accusation that can be made about professionals, in their own book, is that they are mere 'agents of social control'. This view (shouted mainly by social scientists from the touchlines) usually produces only reassurances about good intentions. A more constructive approach would be to set about discriminating between those types of social control which we might well be pleased to be identified with: the supervision of offenders as an alternative to prison; securing treatment for mentally ill people who constitute a danger to themselves and to others; protecting the rights of children by controlling those who threaten them. It will not have escaped the reader's attention that the two substantial chapters on intervention techniques in this book are called respectively 'Stimulus *control*' and 'Response *control*'. Is control what we are seeking? Not for ourselves, but for our clients. In the first case many clients (most in my practice) feel imprisoned by outside-in circumstances about which they feel they can do nothing, usually having tried, but rarely systematically. We know from psychology that loss of control and a consequent collapse of motivation (learned helplessness) is a major factor in trapping clients within their illnesses and conditions (see Seligman 1975; Gilbert 1992).

But similarly, control is involved where inside-out factors predominate, not that there are not readily available responses to personal troubles (mood, worry) or to social and familial difficulties (inappropriate external attributions – victims viewing their reactions as the *cause* of ill-temper and revenge); rather that these semi-reflexive, learned responses are self-defeating or wrong, and make things worse. Control over this repertoire of reactions via a cooler consideration of their actual effectiveness or validity, however right they might seem at an immediate emotional level, is what CBT tries to instill.

There are thus two powerful fallacies at work here.

☐   The idea that CBT (or for that matter psychological interventions in general) are such powerful media of change that, even in the face of unwillingness to cooperate, or even of determined resistance, great moral restraint is required in their application lest people be somehow 'hypnotised' or conditioned into socially convenient conformity *á la The Manchurian Candidate*, or *Clockwork Orange*.

☐   The idea that therapists introduce controls and liberty-endangering influences where none existed before. In the light of the empirical research which shows how difficult it is to produce worthwhile gains over control-group rates, and to make them stick, 'dare we use the CBT method, Dr Karloff ?' considerations (above) could be seen as a case of dubious self-flattery. Furthermore, apart from certain important exceptions (cases where substantial amounts of material aid are, or might be thought to be, dependent upon compliance, or certain residential settings where clients are literally or figuratively 'captive' and dependent upon staff for the meeting of their basic needs), the scales are heavily loaded against the would-be influencer. (The late Alan Sillitoe's play *The Loneliness of the Long Distance Runner* (1959) demonstrates this beautifully.) In reality, clients who are not persuaded of the need for help have many ways of avoiding it. Getting help when you genuinely want it is the greater ethical challenge.

Next, I would like to argue a more general point, namely that concern about the occasional unwanted side-effects of therapeutic good intent needs to be balanced by an equal concern that the 'goods' should be delivered to clients as needed, and as agreed, within reasonable time limits. I know from my own experiences as chairman of a complaints tribunal that the issue of *not* getting adequate and timely professional support constitutes the overwhelming body of concerns from service users. The following comment from Bandura still holds:

> Discussions of the moral implications of behavioral control almost always emphasize the Machiavellian role of change agents and the self-protective manoeuvers of controlees.

The fact that most people enter treatment only as a last resort, hoping to modify patterns of behavior that are seriously distressful to themselves or to others, is frequently overlooked. To the extent that therapists engage in moral agonizing, they should fret more about their own limited effectiveness in helping persons willing to undergo hardships to achieve desired changes, rather than in fantasizing about their potential powers. The tendency to exaggerate the power of behavioral control by psychological methods alone, irrespective of willing co-operation by the client, and the failure to recognize the reciprocal nature of interpersonal control, obscures both the ethical issues and the nature of social influence processes.

(Bandura 1969: 85)

Quite.

As for the second fallacy, about exercising control where none existed before, the standard defence should already be familiar: that is, that we are each bombarded daily by countless controlling influences and so to see control as a game of billiards where only one influence at a time operates is indeed to take a naive and mechanistic view of human behaviour. It is more sensible to see the therapist as entering and (if he or she is good at it) *possibly* affecting an already active field or network of contingencies, learned responses and deficits in clear thinking, feeling and behaviour. In this case, given that lots of things are *already* happening, deciding *not* to intervene (if the law allows) is as influential a decision as not intervening. The decision not to intervene, or excessive procrastination about the issues raised by intervention (as often occurs in the child abuse field) means that the behaviour of the individuals concerned is governed by forces which we have decided *not* to try to control; *not* to replace with other, hopefully more benign influences and which we have not taught the client how to exercise better control for him or herself. Sometimes it is right, or judicious, or necessary, to stay out of a case, but this should be recognised as to some extent a *potentially* mistaken abandonment of the client to *other* controls, and not as a simple decision not to seek influence. There are no real vacuums in social life and some influence or other *will* prevail. Therapeutic 'sins of commission' must therefore be weighed carefully against equally damning 'sins of omission'. The child abuse field has been reduced itself to a state of 'frozen watchfulness' by public criticism over too much or too little action. In Britain, following the death of baby Peter (2009) as a result of abuse and neglect at the hands of his mother's boyfriend and probably with his mother's complicity (they are both in gaol), the *Daily Telegraph* headline was, 'Social Workers [NB: he was also seen by a GP, a paediatrician and a health visitor] Too Slow To Bring Children Into Care'. Not much later the *Daily Telegraph* (without visible blush) opined that given the rise in admissions to care which always follow these high-profile cases, 'Are Social Workers Too Quick To Take Children Into Care?' (*Daily Telegraph*, 13 April 2010: 8). Ad hoc policy prescriptions from air-conditioned offices in Wapping, in place of an evidence-based debate about risk and its predictability (see Macdonald & MacDonald 1999; Munro 2006) just will not do as a basis for policy. They result in paralysis and a reaction which amounts to deciding that it is safer to take no active control and do nothing except worry aloud on the case record: defensive practice. It is here now, and it is a pernicious influence.

CASE EXAMPLE 9.1

Jane C. (aged 12) was referred to Social Services by a child psychiatrist. The problem was that she regularly urinated and defecated on the floor of her bedroom and sometimes spread excrement across its walls. Family interviews with the psychiatrist and with social workers had produced blank denials that anything was wrong in the family, and interviews with the child alone gave only the sense that she was equally puzzled by her behaviour but that she 'just couldn't help it'. The family tried the tactic of selective reactions to the behaviour, some based on rewards, some on punishments, but they failed to affect it much in either case. A puzzle. Interestingly for the first time, it was decided to gather information from other people who knew her (e.g. school-teachers and one or two youth groups to which she belonged). The contrast in these reports could not have been more striking. The school regarded her as a model pupil; she was a girl guide with a noteworthy interest in bringing along younger members; she attended Sunday School regularly, where the Pastor described her as a 'polite, helpful girl, mature beyond her years'. So why was she continuing to shit in her bedroom? As a protest against as yet undiscovered sexual interference – an obvious candidate theory? However, sympathetic interviews with a child specialist produced no evidence, and a strong sense of embarrassment on her part.

A medical examination having already been carried out without finding any physiological reasons for her behaviour, it was decided to abandon further forensics and to treat the behaviour. A reward-based behavioural scheme of robust design was drawn up, this in the hope that her reaction to it might at least yield more information as to causes. She agreed to the scheme with alacrity. The soiling and smearing grew worse.

Then, one day, a haunted-looking Mr C. (father) came into the office to discuss 'something' which he declared he would only talk about if he could be promised that none of it would 'go any further'. He tried hard to swear the social worker to con-fidentiality, but when informed that information that affected the rights of his daughter would have to be attributed, he still went on to tell his story.

Some eighteen months previously his wife had discovered that he had been having a long-term affair with someone at the factory where they both worked. His life had been made 'hell' since that day, and his wife, allegedly in thrall to a local Pentecostal Church, had developed the idea that 'sparing the rod was spoiling the child'. In the interview with Mr C. it became apparent that the real motivation for his wife's change in behaviour was to punish him by punishing his daughter in front of him. It also emerged that the behavioural scheme had been hijacked by the mother, and that a covert negative-image deprivation regime coexisted alongside it. Mr C. was clear that humiliation was the goal of his wife's behaviour, but it was difficult for him to think of leaving home without his daughter.

A case conference (at which the couple were present) was called, and the details which had come to light were discussed. This was an explosive affair, but the couple did agree to attend sessions with Relate counsellors while their daughter went to live temporarily with relatives. One and a half sessions were held; Mrs C. walked out during the second one.

Mr C. left home reluctantly, leaving his daughter behind. The focus of the case then moved firmly to child protection, and it was decided to seek a place at a state boarding-school for Mrs C.'s daughter, which is what she said she wanted, rather than fostering. Interestingly the reflex reaction of the Local Authority was to find a 'specialist school' for Jane, and it had to be repeatedly explained that she was a normal young girl in circumstances created by 'less normal' parents. She settled in immediately, and never soiled again. Her father went to see her on a few occasions and invited her to live with him. She always politely refused, and against the trends in child care outcomes, never went home again. She turned instead into a happy and academically able teenager.

Had Mr C.'s request for even partial confidentiality been respected in the interests of preserving a relationship which *might* have improved over time, then not only would this have transferred an injustice on to the child, but there is no guarantee that the facts would ever have emerged.

As a general principle therapists should advise clients as soon as a compromising subject is broached that while they are perfectly willing to listen to complicated stories, anything which threatens the welfare of another person, or is a serious breach of the law, cannot stay within the consulting room. In my experience, clients rarely clam up at this point, but seek help in ways to remedy matters. In this case, the revelations led at least to a controlled explosion.

It is thus vital that therapists have a clear sense as to 'who is the client?' Most cases contain multiple claims for support. In Case example 9.1, the original referral was made by the *parents* requesting 'advice'. If we look past this mere administrative category to the question of whose rights and needs were most in jeopardy; whose natural development most at risk, who was least free to speak about the problems, then the 'client' in this case was clearly Jane C. But note that her parents *lied*; they were not 'misunderstood'; nor was it the case that the 'conditions were not right for them to confide'; they lied. It happens.

Psychological techniques: their uses and abuses

Whenever therapeutic regimes, particularly residential ones, go sour, the argument is put forward that the techniques are themselves morally neutral, but are abused by the people who apply them. Such arguments may be used to justify all sorts of dubious practices – from indiscriminate arms sales to the development of germ-warfare facilities. As an argument it is technically correct (water can be used for drinking and for drowning people in), but morally unconvincing. A different ethical standard needs to be applied, that is, does a particular type of approach do anything to *encourage* wrongdoing – to make it easier, or more tempting? Our concern here is the degree to which problems are *structured* into a given approach. Are the contingencies constituted by the approach, taking into account the settings in which it is likely to be used, more likely to shape behaviour towards good rather than ill, or the reverse?

If serious problems do arise from the use of a particular approach (the example of electro-convulsive therapy springs to mind, where side-effects, class, age and ethnicity form a context around a *sometimes* apparently effective approach for some), then we need to examine the extent to which these problems are regularly accompanying factors, effects which cluster around this particular type of programme or setting. For example, if behaviour modification (e.g. token economies) schemes used in the past in juvenile detention centres were regularly to be abused across the range of such settings, and were held by the inmates to be repressive, then it would be simply naive to argue that these approaches *need not* be so applied. The key question would be: Do such measures lend themselves to abuse by giving the seal of scientific respectability to what is really crude coercion? We also need to examine to what extent the approach concentrates power without safeguard, almost as a necessary condition of its effective operation. If it does, then it may be unsafe in any hands and a regularly recurring pattern of misuse in different settings would confirm this as a serious problem.

Let us now try to measure cognitive-behavioural methods, as generally practised, against this template of moral sufficiency. Showing up clearly on the plus side is the fact that they contain their own inbuilt safeguards against hard-to-detect wrongdoing. These techniques are partly activity-based; they centre on the client doing things differently, or more or less often. It is therefore very hard to explain away either the aims or the results of CBT in obscure or euphemistic terminology. Both ends and means are open to inspection. Thus, whether a particularly objectionable 'means' is a regularly accompanying feature of programmes directed to particular problems, or to a particular client group, is open to scrutiny. Similarly, to the extent that the 'ends' being pursued are couched in behavioural terms, they will be less equivocal and less likely to be interpretable differently by the clients, the therapist and other interested parties.

The cognitive-behavioural therapies have a large and vigorously pursued literature testifying to their humane and tangibly effective application across a wide range of problems. Therefore we are permitted to raise the hypotheses as to how these approaches might be misused: transparency of aims and methods is built into the approach as in few others.

Our ethical antennae need to be particularly sensitive to the use of CBT in closed settings (e.g. secure children's homes, youth detention centres), simply because the clients are captive there, and so what looks like informed consent might not be *free* consent given the institutional and personal consequences of a lack of cooperation.

Thus, a system for discouraging aggressive behaviour among the pupils at a community school by assigning 'costs' to this behaviour (e.g. restricted privileges, loss of home visits and access to recreational facilities) is a form of coercion, albeit for a desirable purpose. The decisions about such programmes have to be made on utilitarian lines. To what extent do the rights of other people not to be abused require this sort of well-intentioned action? Journalists writing righteously about how we should never have started from here are of little help in the here and now of such cases.

Two further points may be added to those made above. First, critics should ask to what extent clients are expected to *learn* something from a therapeutic programme. Our ethical concern should increase the more the scheme is used just as a device for controlling behaviour. A good test of this issue is whether the main features of a programme are faded for individuals or for groups once unwanted behaviour is brought under its influence. In addition, critics should ask to what extent the behaviour of clients is being *positively* shaped, so that it is brought under the control of the usual socially acceptable influences. If no attempt is made to do these things, then the staff in charge must, in reality, have little confidence that their scheme is anything other than an artificial containment mechanism, the effects of which are by no means likely to generalise to more natural settings or to circumstances where different and less easily manipulated factors hold the ring.

It is possible, however, to conceive of a behavioural approach being used to 'clear the ground' for another type of therapeutic or educational emphasis – for example, by removing disruptive or interfering behaviour that is preventing new learning (see the dramatic example provided by Bucher and Lovaas (1968 with severely autistic children). However, once again, the acid test is whether obviously and continuously troublesome behaviours are eventually brought under the control of this second treatment approach, or whether positive behaviour and attitudes generated by the approach successfully displace harmful or antisocial behaviour.

A further point to be made is that the greater the emphasis on response-cost and negative reinforcement, the more closely we need to look at a programme with ethics as our main concern. At some stage, and ideally on a concurrent basis, new behaviours need to be taught, rationally justified, and potentially better, typical responses reinforced and shaped. If this stage is long delayed, or occupies only a minor role in the scheme, then, generally speaking, it is more to do with control than with therapy. Case example 9.2 shows some of the difficulties of distinguishing between these two aims.

CASE EXAMPLE 9.2

Mrs B., a widow, was only 74 years old but had rapidly advancing Alzheimer's disease which robbed her of most of her short-term memory. She had spent a year in sheltered, warden-controlled accommodation but often pressed alarm bells when she was in an agitated state and wandered off on several occasions. Medication was prescribed, but due to another slightly paranoid view of hers that people were trying to poison her, she would usually resist taking it. Many textbooks would take a rather romantic view of this troubled lady. 'Why not sit her down and explain that her husband had died four years earlier and so searching for him is in vain?' 'Why not take her to his grave in a nearby churchyard?' 'Why not get the remaining family to come in to explain matters to her, rather than just seek a solution via mood-altering pills?' Well, all of these things were done, and made only very short-term differences, because Mrs B. had no memory of what had passed between herself and these kindly would-be helpers an hour later.

An analysis of Mrs B's behaviour showed that for about 50 per cent of her day she was not agitated or upset. The reaction of staff to these quiet periods was to leave her alone. A simple reversal of these reinforcement contingencies produced useful results for two years.

Motivational issues

A frequently reported criticism of cognitive-behavioural approaches is that they only work well with 'motivated clients'. When a clinician gives examples from work with chronically ill psychiatric patients, or older people suffering from dementia, then the charge is usually amended to one of repression and mistaking the *real* needs of clients. What can sensibly be said about this issue of motivation and control?

Let us begin by analysing just what is meant by the statement 'cognitive-behavioural approaches only work with well-motivated people'. The implication here is that there are many other therapeutic approaches which work very well with 'the unmotivated' (that is to say, with people who, through fear, habit or reasoning, decide that they want little to do with therapy and therapists). This is nonsense. Whether people decide to cooperate or not depends in the last analysis on their weighing up the benefits and costs of cooperating against the benefits and costs of not opting in. Alternatively – remembering classical conditioning – it may depend on what they associate with the things on offer and the way they are being offered. For many stigmatised and oppressed groups 'help' has come to equal control because that has been their experience. Acknowledgement of this, sincerity of purpose, and the full involvement of clients in the helping process are the only factors likely to weaken this association. Potential clients may lack information on, or may misunderstand many things about what is being offered. They may overvalue the benefits of the status quo, or fear an alternative future. Attempts can be made to correct any such misapprehensions, when that is what they are. We can influence, persuade, educate, reinforce and shape clients into cooperation. But if at the end of this he or she still stands firmly against the idea of cooperation then there is little else that can or should be done. The idea that by some subtle and hard-to-write-down method of verbal 'hypnosis' clients can be 'wooed out' of their apparent recalcitrance is hard to take seriously. A much larger problem by far is that of individuals and families who are desperate for help but cannot gain access to it. My own approach with any new referral is to set up a preliminary interview: (1) to see what kinds of problems they have and whether CBT might, on the evidence, be indicated (medical referrers often have a limited grasp of the effectiveness literature); (2) to see where the approach matches their views on how they got into difficulties in the first place, and the sorts of ways out implied by these methods; and (3) whether, on early impressions, we are likely to be able to work together. Despite its informality, I regard this 'rehearsal' as the most important interview in any sequence.

It is the business of therapists and others to lay down clear views and guidelines for clients, and to enhance, within reason, the attractiveness of the solutions they are putting forward, based on evidence for them, and to work to modify any tractable environmental contingencies (often the behaviour of *other* people) which may be maintaining the status quo. When these approaches have been tried, but the attempt to build a useful relationship has failed, then the therapist has probably done all that he or she can do. If society through legislation, or the agency to which one is attached, through its regulations, insists on continuing contact, then it is important that no one should misunderstand or be able to misconstrue the nature and purpose of this enforced contact. In many cases of juvenile delinquency, where courts grant supervision orders attaching professionals to clients, what is done will be just that – the client and the people with whom he or she lives or associates will be *supervised*, looked over, watched; they will have their activities monitored and assessed. In many cases, sadly, nothing else is possible, and the wider community has its rights too. The danger lies in the distinctions between these two different kinds of intended help becoming blurred, both in the thinking and doings of would-be helpers and their clients, and in the view of a society only too willing to salve its conscience by always seeing the need for inspection as an opportunity for something 'more constructive' – in other words, therapy. Sometimes, when people decide they have nothing to lose by cooperating, there is such an opportunity, and sometimes there is not. By pretending that there almost always is (reports to courts are usually optimistic on this point), professionals are making three different mistakes.

- ☐ They are giving to the community a greatly exaggerated view of their unaided powers of influence, and the expectations to match.
- ☐ They are putting the helping professions time and again in the position of having to excuse themselves for things over which (were it not for the point made in the bullet point above) it could not reasonably be expected to have control.
- ☐ By failing to discriminate accurately those occasions when mainly inspection or containment rather than therapy is required (or is feasible), they are bringing about a considerable waste of resources. This means that staff are tied up for longer periods of

time than may be necessary, and that resources are channeled into providing quasi-therapeutic services when they could be better used to finance diversionary schemes and improvements in a decent prevention.

The above points apply mainly to those who practise CBT but whose day jobs are in the statutory Social Services and health. However, a growing source of ethical dilemmas for free-standing practitioners is becoming apparent. Self-referrals from potential clients where their employers are funding the exercise, and attempt to impose reporting duties on the therapist which threaten confidentiality and trust raises the question 'Who exactly am I working for?'

The problem here is that employment legislation requires employers to offer support (or retraining) to those they would really like to sack. This distortion of personnel services, whereby employees have either to be well and able to work to standard, or ill and therefore should not come to work at all, discriminates against people with episodic mental health problems. I have received three referrals where employers have been willing to pay fees (as a salaried academic I never charged fees in any case, except for those from the NHS under agreements). What happened next was interesting. In all three cases employers contacted me saying that (1) they *insisted* on paying, and (2) that they required weekly reports on progress, and (3) that these reports should concentrate on the issue of future employability and likely problems in the workplace. All such requests were declined on grounds of confidentiality; all three patients were treated and returned to work. This is however not the point; the employers, unless I am *very* jaded, were using CBT as a way of outsourcing their tenure decisions, which is quite different from an ethical rehabilitation policy. Watch this space for more on this problem.

In one case, bullying in the workplace was the main cause of the client's problems. It triggered and maintained the OCD condition which made the client avoid work or perform poorly. How could these clients have ever trusted me had I cooperated?

I am not arguing here for a return to the days of preciousness about therapy, when it was practised by an elite who did little else and who regarded unpaid fuel bills and bad housing as epiphenomena. I am arguing for greater discrimination about who gets it and on what ethical terms. People have a right not to be 'helped', or impelled towards 'help', and this important principle has always had a distinguished body of advocates, namely:

> The only purpose for which power can be rightfully exercised over any member of a civilized community, against his will, is to prevent harm to others. His own good, either physical or moral, is not a sufficient warrant. He cannot rightfully be compelled to do or forbear because it will be better for him to do so, because it will make him happier, because, in the opinions of others, to do so would be wise, or even right. There are good reasons for remonstrating with him, or persuading him, or entreating him, but not for compelling him, or visiting him with any evil in case he do otherwise. To justify that, the conduct from which it is desired to deter him must be calculated to produce evil to someone else. The only part of the conduct of any one, for which he is answerable to society, is that which concerns others. In the part which merely concerns himself, his independence is, of right, absolute.
>
> (Mill 1859: 73)

This is a much tougher view to hold now than in 1859. In complex industrialised societies, people are much more interconnected and interdependent, and with the arrival of the mass media the line between 'evil to oneself' and 'evil to others' is much harder to draw. Is the contemporary drug user harming only himself by his habit, or do his actions contaminate others nearby?

In any case, Mill put forward many exceptions to his rule, for instance, children, the insane, and the mentally infirm – and some of these categories demand, but at times defy, close definition. However, although this principle of not doing things to people to 'help' them if they do not themselves wish it is hedged around by all sorts of marginal cases, and has been nibbled away at the edges by bevies of philosophers, it stands nevertheless as a profound truth, a clearly visible light by which to steer ourselves. There may be all sorts of short-term justifications for changing course from it, but in the longer term I believe that we do so at our peril.

Therapy should always be on offer where we have robust knowledge and some experience to back up our expectations of a positive or ameliorative result, or where, with the client's informed consent, we are conducting a genuine experiment. But it should be something for which clients have to 'sign up'. There should always be a contractual phase to it; a period of explicit negotiation about purposes and desired outcome. Where this is not possible (as in extremes of psychological infirmity, or in the case of very young children) we must be guided by those who care for the individual, make the best judgements we can, and try to render ourselves as publicly accountable as possible. Outside this category, where no contract can be agreed, then the persons concerned are not clients in the strict sense of the word (the very notion of a compulsory client is paradoxical, as is the use of the term 'customer', or 'service user' in child protection or statutory mental health cases). They may still be people we need to see, or people that we have been put 'in charge of', and they may still (we would hope) be treated with an exemplary kindliness and concern. However, we must not delude ourselves that we can help everyone, either with cognitive-behavioural approaches or with any other method.

This said, it is a dangerous thing to see freedom and ethical purity as virtues which flourish only when there is an apparent absence of control. An absence of proper control in the case discussed on p. 252 simply allowed Mrs C. free rein to persecute her innocent daughter.

The special case of institutional and residential treatment

Any ethical concerns we have about the use of cognitive-behavioural approaches in general are likely to be multiplied when we consider their use in residential settings – particularly in closed or secure units. Much good work has been done in these settings, but together with the penal field in the US, they have, in the past, been the setting for the most disturbing examples of misuse.

My own view is that the field of residential social care offers special opportunities for intensive contact for the application of approaches combining behavioural techniques, with individual cognitive help, but that, alongside these, special safeguards are required.

However, ready access and the ability to influence local environmental dynamics have to be balanced against the particular problems and temptations, namely:

☐   As suggested above, such opportunities can be used for good or for ill. However, in line with our previous discussion about 'structured-in' problems, we need to decide whether these exist to any great extent in the application of cognitive-behavioural techniques in this type of setting. My own view is that a number of 'built-in' problems do exist, and that-while they are not insurmountable they always need to be guarded against. The first of these is the tendency of institutions to try and take short cuts with residents, to try and rub the awkward corners off them, and to socialise them into the ways of the place where they are living and its purpose. This process of institutionalisation (Goffman's (1961) *Asylums* is still well worth reading) is not usually any individual's specific intention; it occurs because of the problems thrown up by having a group of individuals, with their awkward individual needs, living in the same space. So individuality is easily sacrificed, just to keep the place ticking over. To this problem may be added our experience of what happens when the real therapeutic goals of a residential unit get subverted by the interests of administrative neatness, order, 'target-attainment', 'health and safety' and so on. Add to this covert 'risk management' (making sure, above all things and whatever the 'mission statement' says, that the agency's name stays out of the newspapers) and we have a well-prepared seedbed for therapeutically dubious practices. It need not occur; it usually doesn't; but the conditions are just right, as Zimbardo *et al.*'s Prisoners and Guards experiment (1973) demonstrated years ago, unintentionally spawning a host of TV 'reality' shows.

☐ The way out of some of these difficulties is not always as straightforward as in fieldwork settings. The obvious solution of obtaining the 'free consent' of clients who are on the receiving end of a regime needs a second look. First, what is 'free' and 'informed' consent? For any semblance of a contractual relationship between parties to exist, there has to be some semblance of equality between them. The danger is that, given the considerable disparity in actual, taken-for-granted power that exists between staff and clients, compliance can easily be mistaken for consent. Where cooperation with a therapeutic regime is – or could be thought by the client to be – linked to his or her standing or security, to the meeting of his need for comfort, human contact, affection, approval and stimulation, then a 'free choice' is virtually impossible. An unconstrained choice probably does not exist in nature anyway, and we would be fools not to make our therapeutic programmes attractive just in case anyone joined in for the wrong reasons. Perhaps the best we can do here is to argue for an absence of sanctions for not doing so. False compliance with 'anger-management' courses in prisons can lead to early parole, but, if not genuinely participated in, can lead to undiagnosed continuing risk.

It may well be that, on occasion, such precautions make programmes more attractive because entry to them is not required or automatic. Time should be spent in explaining the purposes behind the scheme and, where feasible, residents should have a hand in managing it for themselves. Worthwhile progress has been made over the past few years in handing back power to the users of services – in children's homes, homes for elderly people and hostels for the mentally ill – so that it is now more usual than not to see people, who would once have been disqualified by their client status, with seats on management committees for the facilities in which they reside or the intendedly therapeutic schemes in which they participate.

But what of those clients and patients who are ill-equipped to make any choices about participating in therapy and have no trusted relatives to act on their behalf? It may be that we sometimes underestimate the decision-making ability of our clients, whether they are children in care or psychiatric patients, and could try harder to win genuine consent and cooperation. One of the most interesting unlooked-for findings of a research project to gauge the reactions of discharged psychiatric patients to a local authority community care scheme (see Macdonald & Sheldon 1997) was the richness of opinion and testimony coming from respondents supposed to lack insight into their conditions. However, having said this, we are still faced with clients who for one reason or another cannot always be fully involved in the helping process (e.g. in dementia care). The only possible answer here is that someone has to decide for them to start with, lest the 'sins of omission' points made on pp. 250–251 are to apply. The only possible criteria for evaluating such decisions are: whether they are reasonable and evidence based; whether they are publicly made; whether they are made after due consultation with families and/or other interested parties; whether the therapist would be happy if in similar circumstances similar decisions were made about a member of his or her own family in similar circumstances (an acid test); whether they have the effect of trying to promote independence, self-sufficiency, the ability of the client to be in better control of himself or herself and his or her environment; and whether they constitute an enhancement of the range of responses the client is capable of making. Of these criteria the most important is that decisions should be clear, unambiguous and open to inspection, if necessary, by an ethics committee of the type now in routine use by clinical psychologists and in health settings, but more rarely in Social Services and private practice.

Deciding who is likely to benefit from cognitive-behavioural therapy

If the advocates of therapeutic and clinical approaches in applied psychology are guilty of anything, then it is of giving insufficient thought to their choice of targets. The reflex action of attempting to change the accessible person who happens to get referred – as if referral were always a rational and representative process – is still in place. In this way, children with educational problems, persistent truants, hospital patients, debtors and the physically disabled have all been the individual recipients of therapeutic endeavours – *services* – when in many cases the solution to their problems lay elsewhere – with the school, the hospital, the social security office, the access and dignity-denying built environment, and so on. These are all contingencies, and therapists must try to adapt them to the needs of individuals as well as individuals to their circumstances.

   The criticism that therapeutic approaches are often undertaken with the poor and the weak – people in reality suffering at the hands of others – is only partly justified. In fact it is a criticism of clinical practice as a whole rather than of any specific methods employed. The clinical model has tended to suggest that whoever comes forward should be helped, regardless of class, gender, creed and so forth, and it has thought of itself as democratic in this respect. A genuinely democratic approach would place much greater emphasis on deciding with the client what is the just, the appropriate and the propitious point for intervention. In its concentration on environmental factors (usually the behaviour of other people), it should be part of CBT courses to actively counteract the tendency to see the problem as belonging primarily to the person complaining of it, or referred for it.

Feelings about the imposition of techniques

There is a certain arrogance about intervening in the life of another person, never better expounded than by Barbara Wootton (1959), who argued tartly that if psycho-social case work could really do the things claimed for it in textbooks then such skills were perhaps being squandered on the poor and troubled, and should be applied immediately to the UN, politicians and world leaders for the prevention of war, famine and pestilence. Basic CBT principles are what I always shout back at the radio, whenever I hear of another twist in the Palestine/Israel conflict, but I have never been contacted for advice. P.G. Wodehouse, after seeing *Othello* for the first time and enjoying the drama, observed: 'But I couldn't help but think that the whole thing could have been settled with a bit of give and take on both sides.'

But then professional helpers have always been well aware of this sort of thing, arguably too well aware, and not well enough aware of the charges of procrastination. The literature positively oozes with cautionary phrases about 'starting where the client is', noting carefully his or her version of events, never offering advice except as a last resort, however much clients clamour for it. As discussed in Chapter 1, this overreaction and hedging around what professionals are supposed actually to *do* about someone's problem can leave us with the impression that psychological therapists are meant to serve the same function as a warm bath – good for all sorts of aches and pains, so long as they amount to nothing very serious or specific; otherwise refer to a specialist (the results are as good if front-line staff take on these functions themselves (see Lambert 2004)).

Conclusions

1   There *is* an ethical threat present in current health and social care practice. It is that all but *very* high-risk cases are often handled with brief, containing encounters. It is almost as if a group of professionals and their managers had been converted to the psycho-social equivalent of homeopathy, implying by their behaviour that a *very* small molecule dose of contact will be somehow remembered in the minds and circumstances of ill and troubled people and make them better. This is a strange turn of events, since early experiments in task-centred case-work and brief psychotherapy were (despite the positive evidence) derided on the grounds that long-established problems, which nearly always rested in childhood for the psychoanalysts, could not possibly deliver meaningful and lasting change (they do, as we have seen in Chapter 2). But now we find ourselves fighting to maintain even the 8–10–15 session protocols recommended by CBT research. This is a technical requirement – a *course* of treatment is required on technical grounds, but also on *ethical* grounds. Imagine a situation where GPs, knowing the need to prescribe full courses of antibiotics or antidepressants, were routinely required to give just one or two pills for now.

2   Learning and cognitive theory teaches us that blame, culpability and the prospects of reform need to be taken in the full understanding that 'the environment' – both yesterday's and today's – gets inside us through conditioning. These influences play a key part in influencing behaviour, thinking, emotions and their wider consequences. There is nothing in the nature of the procedures discussed in this book to suggest that they need to be applied in an excessively clinical or mechanical way. Indeed, the principles themselves suggest that this would be self-defeating. Cognitive-behavioural approaches do suggest specific remedies for specifically defined problems, but *how* these remedies are applied is also very important (see p. 69).

3   Knowledge of basic research and of the procedures themselves has been available for some time, but has until comparatively recently produced only a patchy response from the professions equipped to use them. Other preoccupations aside, one reason for this may be that the effective use of cognitive-behavioural techniques effectively requires a *detailed* and a *specific* knowledge of the various reports, theories and procedures. This discipline cannot be approached in the same way as so much else is on our overcrowded training curricula – as general, background or contextual knowledge – where the method of application is left almost entirely to the professional. Staff are not always well equipped by training in all settings where these methods have a place. Indeed, in certain cases (e.g. depression with an appreciable risk of self-harm), knowing the limits of one's own skills, the scope of treatments, and when to refer on is the most important ethical consideration.

4   'Tribal' differences and empire-building are also an ethical concern. There is more than enough work here for us all, and, given basic professional competence, clients will benefit more from interdisciplinary cooperation than demarcation disputes. The most reassuring thing to repeat is that against demanding protocols of modern systematic reviews (see Lambert 2004; Littell 2008) the ubiquitous entry in the 'harms reported' category in CBT research is 'none'. Few if any other approaches can claim this: not pharmacotherapy, certainly not psychoanalysis, not family therapy. There has been a long struggle to establish the level of disinterested appraisal in research reviews that we have today. The Cochrane Collaboration (see www.cochrane.org) led the way, where, under the determined leadership of Professor Geraldine Macdonald (Queen's University, Belfast) as coordinator for reviews, the same essential principles have now been spread to psychosocial interventions – a cause for celebration.

Sins of omission rather than of commission should now be our main ethical concern. If you are mentally ill and/or black and/or elderly, your chances of obtaining this, or other psychosocial, evidence-based help is four times lower. If you are a child in trouble, your chances of seeing a cognitive-behavioural therapist are three times lower than seeing a counsellor (technique unspecified) than a supervising social worker, a nurse-therapist, a psychotherapist or a psychotherapist skilled in CBT. *These* are the concerns which should exercise us alongside a wariness over requests to help adjust individuals cognitively and/or emotionally to unfair, unjust, unsupportive or illogical circumstances rather than focusing on changing these circumstances:

> Thus, the idea of Reason and Feeling as distinct forces battling for control of our lives is always a distorted one. Yet it has been a powerful pattern in the European tradition and, in spite of various attacks on it, it is still with us today. The name of 'reason' is often given not to thought itself but to a certain set of rather bourgeois motives centring on prudence and social harmony.
>
> (Midgley 2005: 164)

Bibliography

Abramowitz, J.S. (1997) Effectiveness of psychological and pharmacological treatments for obsessive-compulsive disorder: a quantitative review. *Journal of Consulting and Clinical Psychology* 65(1): 44–52.

Acheson, D. (1998) *Independent Inquiry into Inequalities in Health*, London: HMSO.

Allport, G. (1937) *Personality: A Psychological Interpretation*, New York: Holt.

Alsobrook, J.P. and Pauls, D.L. (1998) The genetics of obsessive-compulsive disorder, in Jenike, M.A., Baer, L. and Mirchello, W.E. (eds) *Obsessive-Compulsive Disorders*, St. Louis, MO: Mosby.

Appleby, L. (1997) *National Confidential Inquiry: Progress Report into Suicide and Homicide by People with a Mental Illness*, London: Department of Health.

Auden, W.H. (1976) *Collected Poems*, London: Faber and Faber.

Auden, W.H. (1977) *The English Auden. Poems, Essays and Dramatic Writings*, ed. Edward Mendelson, London: Faber and Faber.

Ayer, A.J. (1973/1991) *The Central Questions of Philosophy*, Harmondsworth: Penguin.

Bacon, F. (1605) *The Advancement of Learning*, ed. G.W. Kitchen (1965), London: Dent.

Bagley, C. and Ramsay, R. (1997) *Suicidal Behaviour in Adolescents and Adults: Research, Taxonomy and Prevention*, Aldershot: Ashgate.

Bandura, A. (1965) Influence of models' reinforcement contingencies on the acquisition of imitative responses. *Journal of Personality and Social Psychology* 1: 589–595.

Bandura, A. (1969) *Principles of Behavior Modification*, New York: Holt, Rinehart & Winston.

Bandura, A. (1977) *Social Learning Theory*, Englewood Cliffs, NJ: Prentice-Hall.

Barlingame, G.M., Mackenzie, K.R. and Strauss, B. (2004) Small group treatment: evidence for effectiveness and mechanisms for change, in Lambert, M.J. (ed.) *Bergin and Garfield's Handbook of Psychotherapy and Behavior Change* (5th edn), New York: John Wiley.

Barlow, D.H. and Letiman, C.L. (1996) Advances in the psychosocial treatment of anxiety disorders. *Archives of General Psychiatry* 53: 727, 735.

Bateson, G., Jackson, D.P., Haley, J. and Weatland, J. (1956) Towards a theory of schizophrenia. *Behavioural Science* 1: 251–264.

BBC Horizon Publications (1993) *Wot U Looking At?* London BBC Broadcasting Support Services 24.5.

Bebbington, P.E. (1998) Epidemiology of obsessive-compulsive disorder. *British Journal of Psychiatry* 35 (suppl.): 2–6.

Beck, A.T. (1964) Thinking and depression, 2: Theory and therapy. *Archives of General Psychiatry* 10: 501–571.

Beck, A.T. (1970) Cognitive therapy: nature and relationship to behaviour therapy. *Behavior Therapy* 1: 184–200.

Beck, A.T. (1976) *Cognitive Therapy and the Emotional Disorders*, New York: International Universities Press.

Beck, A.T. (1999) Cognitive aspects of personality disorders and their relation to syndromal disorders: a psycho-evolutionary approach, in Cloninger, C.R. (ed.) *Personality and Psychopathology*, Washington DC: American Psychiatric Press.

Beck, A.T. and Emery, G. (1985) *Anxiety Disorders and Phobias; A Cognitive Perspective*, New York: Basic Books.

Beck, A.T., Steer, R.A. and Garbin, M.G. (1988) Psychometric properties of the Beck Depression Intervention: treatments five years later. *Clinical Psychology Review* 8: 77–100.

Beck, A.T., Rush, A.J., Shaw, B.F. and Emery, G. (1979) *Cognitive Therapy of Depression*, New York: Guilford Press.

Beck, A., Wright, F.D., Newman, C.F. and Liese, B. (1993) *Cognitive Therapy of Substance Abuse*, New York: Guilford Press.

Beck, A.T., Hollon, S.D., Young, J.E., Bedrosian, R.C. and Badenz, D. (1985) Treatment of depression with cognitive therapy and amitryptine. *Archives of General Psychiatry* 42: 142–148.

Beck, A.T., Ward, C.H., Mendelson, M., Mock, J. and Erbaugh, J. (1961) An inventory for measuring depression. *Archives of General Psychiatry* 4: 561–571.

Bem, D.J. (1967) Self perception: an alternative interpretation of cognitive dissonance phenomena. *Psychological Review* 74: 183–200.

Bem, D.J. (1972) Self-perception theory, in Berkowitz, R. (ed.) *Advances in Experimental Social Psychology*, Vol. 6, New York: Academic Press.

Bem, D.J. and Alan, A. (1974) On predicting some of the people some of the time: the search for cross-situational theories in behaviour. *Psychology Review* 81: 506–520.

Bennett-Levy, J., McManns, F., Westling, B.E. and Fennell, M. (2009) Acquiring and refining CBT skills and competencies. Which training methods are perceived to be most effective? *Behavioural and Cognitive Psychotherapy* 37(5): 571–583.

Berger, M. (1985) Temperament and individual differences, in Rutter, M. and Hersov, L. (eds) *Childhood and Adolescent Psychiatry: Modern Approaches*, London: Blackwell Scientific.

Bergin, A.E. and Garfield, S. (1971, 1978, 1986, 1994) *Handbook of Psychotherapy and Behavior Change* (1st to 4th edns), Chichester: John Wiley.

Berk, L.E. (ed.) (2005) *Child Development*, London: Allyn & Bacon.

Berlin, I. (1996) *The Sense of Reality: Studies in Ideas and their History*, London: Chatto & Windus.

Birchwood, M. and Tarrier, N. (eds) (1992) *Innovations in the Psychological Management of Schizophrenia: Assessment, Treatment and Services*, Chichester: John Wiley.

Birchwood, M., Hallett, S. and Preston, M. (1988) *Schizophrenia: An Integrated Approach to Research and Treatment*, Harlow: Longman.

Black, D., Morris, J., Smith, C. and Townsend, P. (1980) *Black Report: Inequalities in Health*, London: BMJ Publishing Group.

Blakemore, C. (1977) *Mechanisms of the Mind*, Cambridge: Cambridge University Press.

Blanchard, E.B. (1994) Behavioral medicine and health psychology, in Bergin, A.E. and Garfield, S.L. (eds) *Handbook of Psychotherapy and Behavior Change* (4th edn), New York: John Wiley.

Bolton, D. and Hill, J. (1996) *Mind, Meaning and Mental Disorder*, Oxford: Oxford University Press.

Boswell, J. (1740) *Life of Johnson*, Oxford: Oxford University Press.

Boyle, M. (1993) *Schizophrenia, A Scientific Delusion?* London: Routledge.

Braithwaite, R. (2001) *Managing Aggression*, London: Routledge.

Brewer, C. and Lait, J.C. (1980) *Can Social Work Survive?* London: Temple Smith.

British Medical Journal (BMJ) (2002) *Trials for Tomorrow*, London: BMJ Publishing Group.

British Medical Journal (BMJ) (2006) *Clinical Evidence: Mental Health*, London: BMJ Publishing Group.

Brooks, M. (2009) *Thirteen Things That Don't Make Sense*, London: Profile Books.

Brown, G.W. and Birley, J. (1968) Crises and life changes and the onset of schizophrenia. *Journal of Health and Social Behaviour* 9: 269–312.

Brown, G.W. and Harris, T. (1979) *Social Origins of Depression*, London: Tavistock Publications.

Brown, G.W., Birley, J.L.T. and Wing, J.T. (1972) Influence of family life on the course of schizophrenia disorders: a replication. *British Journal of Psychiatry* 121: 241–258.

Bucher, B. and Lovaas, O.I. (1968) Use of aversive stimulation in behaviour modification, in Jones, M.R. (ed.) *Miami Symposium on the Prediction of Behaviour: Aversive Stimulation*, Miami, FL: University of Miami Press.

Cannon, W.B. (1927) The James–Lange theory of emotions: an analytical examination and an alternative theory. *American Journal of Psychology* 39: 100–105.

Carr, A. (ed.) (2000) *What Works with Children and Adolescents?* London: Brunner Routledge

Carroll, L. (1865, 1872) *Alice's Adventures in Wonderland*, London: The Bodley Head.

Caspi, A., Harrington, H., Milne, B., Amell, J.W. and Theodore, R.F. (2003) Children's behavioural styles at age 3 are limited to their adult personality traits at age 26. *Journal of Personality*, 71(4): 495–513.

Cattell, R.B. (1965) *The Scientific Analysis of Personality*, Baltimore, MD: Penguin.

Centre for Reviews and Dissemination, University of York.

Chadwick, P., Birchwood, M. and Trower, P. (1996) *Cognitive Therapy for Delusions, Voices and Paranoia*, Chichester: John Wiley.

Cigno, K. and Bourn, D. (eds) (1998) *Cognitive-Behavioural Social Work in Practice*, Aldershot: Ashgate/Arena.

Clare, J. (1821) *John Clare; Selected Poems*, ed. J.W. Tibble and A. Tibble (1964) London: Dent

Claridge, G. (1985) *Origins of Mental Illness*, Oxford: Blackwell.

Clark, D.M. and Salkovskis, P. (1991) *Cognitive Therapy with Panic and Hypochondriasis*, New York: Pergamon Press.

Clark, D.M., Salkovskis, P., Hackmann, A., Middleton, H., Anastasides, P. and Gelder, M. (1994) A comparison of cognitive therapy, applied relaxation and Imipramine in the treatment of panic disorder. *British Journal of Psychiatry* 164: 759–769.

Clark, D.M., Salkovskis, P., Hackmann, A., Wells, A, Fennell, M., Ludgate, J., Ahmad, S., Richards, H.C. and Gelder, M. (1998) The psychological treatment of hypochondriasis: a randomized controlled trial. *British Journal of Psychiatry* 173: 218–225.

Cobb, R. (1997) *The End of the Line*, London: John Murray.

Cochrane Database of Systematic Review (www.cochrane.org) The York Database of Reviews of Effectiveness (DARE) The Cochrane Library, London: BMJ Publishing Group.

Cohen, A.R. (1964) *Attitude Change and Social Influence*, New York: Basic Books.

Cooke, G. (1968) Evaluation of the efficiency of the components of reciprocal inhibitions psychotherapy. *Journal of Abnormal Psychology* 73: 44–51.

Craighead, W.E., Craighead, L.W. and Lilardi, S. (1998) Psycho-social treatments for major depressive disorder, in Nathan, P.E. and Gorman, J.M. (eds) *Treatments that Work*, Oxford: Oxford University Press.

Craighead, L.W., Craighead, E.W., Kazdin, A.E. and Mahoney, M.J. (1994) *Cognitive and Behavioural Interventions: An Empirical Approach to Mental Health Problems*, Massachusetts: Allyn and Bacon.

Creer, T.L., Holroyd, K.A., Glasgow, R. and Smith, T.W. (2004) Health psychology, in Lambert, M.J. (ed.) *Bergin and Garfield's Handbook of Psychotherapy and Behavior Change* (5th edn), New York: John Wiley.

Crisp, A.H., Norton, K., Gowers, S., Haleck, C., Bowyer, C., Yeldham, D., Levett, G. and Bart, H. (1991) A controlled study of the effects of therapies aimed at adolescent and family psychopathology in anorexia nervosa. *British Journal of Psychiatry* 159: 325–333.

Dalrymple, J. (1994) Devils Island: what really happened on the Orkneys. London: *Sunday Times*, 27 February.

Damassio, A.R. (1994) *Descartes' Error*, London: Macmillan.

Darley, J.M. and Batson, C.D. (1973) 'From Jerusalem to Jericho': a study of situational and dispositional variables in helping behaviour. *Journal of Personality and Social Psychology* 27(1): 100–108.

Darwin, C.J. (1871) *The Descent of Man*, Cambridge: Cambridge University Press.

Dennett, D. (1991) *Consciousness Explained*, London: Allen Lane.

Dennett, D. (2003) *Freedom Evolves*, London: Allen Lane.

Dennett, D. (2006*) Breaking the Spell: Religion as a National Phenomenon*, London: Allen Lane.

DeRubeis, R.J. and Crits-Christoph, P. (1998) Empirically supported individual and group psychological treatments for adult mental disorders. *Journal of Consulting and Clinical Psychology* 66: 33–52.

Descartes, R. (1637) *The Philosophical Works of Descartes*, trans. E.S. Haldane and G.R. Ross (Vol. II), New York: Cambridge Minority Press.

Descartes, R. (1664) *Traité de l'homme*, trans. and ed. T.S. Holt, Cambridge: Cambridge University Press; see also: Descartes, R. (1667) *The Passions of the Soul*, Cambridge: Cambridge University Press.

Dilk, M.N. and Bond, G. (1996) Meta-analytic evaluation of skills training research for individuals with severe mental illness. *Journal of Consulting and Clinical Psychology* 64: 1337–1346.

Dixon, N. (1976) *On the Psychology of Military Incompetence*, London: Jonathan Cape.

Dixon, N. (1981) *Preconscious Processing*, Chichester: John Wiley.

Dobson, K.S. (1989) A meta-analysis of the efficacy of cognitive therapy for depression. *Journal of Consulting and Clinical Psychology* 57: 414–419.

Donaldson, M. (1978) *Children's Minds*, London: Fontana Press.

Dowson, J.H. and Grounds, A.T. (1995) *Personality Disorders: Recognition and Clinical Management*, Cambridge: Cambridge University Press.

DSM IV^{TR} *The Diagnostic and Statistical Manual of the American Psychiatric Association* (4th ed), Text Revision. Washington, DC: American Psychiatric Association.

Ecclestone, C., Williams, A.C. and Morley, S. (2009) Psychological therapies for the management of chronic pain (excluding headache). *Cochrane Database of Systematic Reviews*, Issue 2, Art. no. CD007407.

Edelman, G. (1987) *Neural Darwinism*, New York: Basic Books.

Elkin, I. (1994) The NIHM treatment of depression program: where we began and where we are. In Bergin, A.E. and Garfield, S.L. (eds) *Handbook of Psychotherapy and Behavior Change* (4th edn), New York: John Wiley.

Ellis, A. (1979) *The Basic Clinical Theory of Rational Emotive Therapy*, New York: Van Nostrand Reinhold.

Emmelkamp, P.M. (2004) Behaviour therapy with adults, in Lambert, M.J. (ed.) *Bergin and Garfield's Handbook of Psychotherapy and Behavior Change* (5th edn), New York: John Wiley.

Eysenck, H.J. (1960) *Fact and Fiction in Psychology*, Harmondsworth: Penguin.

Eysenck, H.J. (1965) *Sense and Nonsense in Psychology* Harmondsworth, Penguin.

Eysenck, H.J. (1978) Expectations as control elements in behavioural change'. *Advances in Behaviour Research and Therapy* 1(4): 7–15.

Eysenck, H.J. (1985) *The Decline and Fall of the Freudian Empire*, Harmondsworth: Viking.

Eysenck, H.J. and Kamin, L. (1981) *Intelligence: The Battle for the Mind*, London: Pan Books.

Eysenck, M. and Keane, M.T. (1990) *Cognitive Psychology*, London: Lawrence Erlbaum.

Falloon, I.R.H., Boyd, J.L. and McGill, C.W. (1984) *Family Care of Schizophrenia*, New York: Guilford Press.

Falloon, I.R.H., Kretorian, H., Shanaham, W.J., Laporta, M. and McLees, S. (1990) The Buckingham Project: a comprehensive mental health service based upon behavioural psychotherapy. *Behaviour Change* 7: 51–57.

Fava, G.A., Bartolucci, G., Rajanelli, C. and Mangelli, L. (2001) Cognitive-behavioural management of patients with bipolar disorder who relapsed while on lithium prophylaxis. *Journal of Clinical Psychiatry* 62: 556–559.

Ferster, C.B. and Skinner, B.F. (1957) *Schedules of Reinforcement*, New York: Appleton-Century Crofts.

Festinger, L. (1957) *A Theory of Cognitive Dissonance*, Evanston, IL: Row Peterson.

Fischer, J. (1973) Is casework effective? A review. *Social Work* 1: 107–110.

Fischer, J. (1976) *The Effectiveness of Social Casework*, Springfield, IL: Charles C. Thomas.

Fischer, J. and Corcoran, K. (2007) *Measures for Clinical Practice (Vol. I. – Children; Vol. II – Adults)*, London: Free Press.

Fisher, M., Newton, C. and Sainsbury, E. (1984) *Mental Health Social Work Observed*, London: George Allen & Unwin.

Foucault, M. (1965) *Madness and Civilization*, New York: Pantheon.

Foucault, M. (1967) *Madness and Civilization: A History of Insanity in the Age of Reason*, London: Tavistock.

Foucault, M. (1987) *Mental Illness and Psychology*, Berkeley: University of California Press.

Frank, E., Swartz, H.A. and Kapfer, D.J. (2000) Interpersonal and social rhythm therapy: managing the chaos of bipolar disorder. *Biological Psychiatry* 48: 593–604.

Franklin, M.E.E, Abramowitz, J.S., Foa, E.B., Kozak, M.J. and Levitt, J.T. (1998). Effectiveness of exposure and ritual prevention for obsessive compulsive disorder: randomized compound with non-randomized samples. *Journal of Consulting and Clinical Psychology* 68: 594–602.

Gaarder, J. (1995) *Sophie's World*, London: Phoenix House.

Gallasi, M.D. and Gallasi, T.P. (1977) *Assert Yourself!*, New York: Human Sciences Press.

Gambrill, E.D. (1997) *Social Work Practice: A Critical Thinker's Guide*, Oxford: Oxford University Press.

Gambrill, E.D. (2010) *Propaganda in the Human Services*, New York: Oxford University Press.

Gambrill, E.D. and Schlonsky, A. (2001) The need for comprehensive risk management systems in child welfare. *Children and Youth Services Review* 23: 79–107.

Gardner, H. (1987) *The Mind's New Science: A History of the Cognitive Revolutions*, New York: Basic Books.

Garland, J.E. (2004) Facing the evidence: antidepressant treatment in children and adolescents. *Canadian Medical Journal:* 489–491.

Gibbs, L.E. (1991) *Scientific Reasoning for Social Workers: Bridging the Gap between Research and Practice*, New York: Macmillan.

Gigerenzer, G. (2007) *Gut Feelings: The Intelligence of the Unconscious*, London: Allen Lane

Gilbert, P. (1992) *Depression: The Evolution of Powerlessness*, London: Lawrence Erlbaum.

Gleick, J. (1988) *Chaos: Making a New Science*, London: Heinemann.

Goffman, E. (1961) *Asylums*, New York: Doubleday Anchor.

Goldberg, D. and Huxley, P. (1992) *Common Mental Disorders: A Bio-Social Model*, London: Routledge.

Goodwin, F.K. and Redfield-Jamison, K. (2004) *Manic Depressive Illness*, Oxford: Oxford University Press.

Gottesman, I.I. (1982) *Schizophrenia: The Epigenetic Puzzle*, Cambridge: Cambridge University Press.

Gottesman, I.I. (1991) *Schizophrenia Genesis: The Origins Of Madness*, New York: Freeman.

Gray, J.A. (1975) *Elements of a Two Process Theory of Learning*, London: Academic Press.

Gregory, R. (1970) *Odd Perceptions*, London: Routledge.

Halsey, A.H. and Webb, J. (eds) (2000) *Twentieth-century British Social Trends* (3rd edn), Basingstoke: Macmillan.

Hamilton, M. (1960) A rating scale for depression. *Journal of Neurology, Neuro-surgery and Psychiatry* 32: 50–55.

Harris, P. (1972) Perception and cognition in infancy, in Connolly, K. (ed.) *Psychology Survey, no 2*. London: George Allen and Unwin.

Hašek J. (1923) *The Good Soldier Schweik*, Synek Publishers.

Hays, V. and Waddell, K. (1976) A self reinforcing procedure for thought stopping. *Behaviour Therapy* 1: 12–24.

Hebb, D.O. (1972) *Textbook of Psychology* (3rd edn), Philadelphia, PA: Saunders.

Heider, F. (1958) *The Psychology of Interpersonal Relations*, New York: John Wiley.

Heinssen, R., Liberman, R.P. and Kopelowicz, A. (2000) Psycho-social skills training for schizophrenia: lessons from the laboratory. *Schizophrenia Bulletin* 26: 21–45.

Henggeler, S.W., Schoenwald, S.K., Borduin, C.M., Rowland, M.D. and Cunningham, P.B. (1998) *Multisystemic Treatment of Anti-social Behavior in Children and Adolescents*, New York: Guilford Press.

Herbert, J.D., Gaudiano, B.A., Rheingold, A.A., Myers, V.H., Dalrymple, K. and Nolan, E.M. (2005) Social skills training augments the effectiveness of cognitive-behavioural group therapy for social anxiety disorder. *Behaviour Therapy* 36: 125–138.

Herbert, M. (1978) *Conduct Disorders of Childhood and Adolescence*, Chichester: John Wiley.

Hetherington, E.M. and Parke, R.D. (1986) *Child Psychology*, London: McGraw Hill.

Hilgard, E.R. (1948) *Theories of Learning*, New York: Appleton-Century Crofts.

Hilgard, E.R., Atkinson, R.C. and Atkinson, R.L. (1979) *An Introduction to Psychology* (7th edn), New York: Harcourt, Brace, Jovanovich.

Hill, C.A. and Lambert, M.J. (2004) Methodological issues in studying psychotherapy processes and outcomes, in Lambert, M.J. (ed.) *Bergin and Garfield's Handbook of Psychology and Behavior Change* (5th edn), New York: John Wiley.

Hillner, K.P. (1979) *Conditioning in Contemporary Perspective*, New York: Springer.

Hollon, S.D. and Beck, A.T. (1994) Cognitive and cognitive-behavioral therapy, in Bergin, A.E. and Garfield, S.L. (eds) *Handbook of Psychotherapy and Behavior Change* (4th edn), Chichester: John Wiley.

Hollon, S.D. and Beck, A.T. (2004) Cognitive and cognitive-behavioral therapies, in Lambert, M.J. (ed.) *Bergin and Garfield's Handbook of Psychotherapy and Behavior Change* (5th edn), New York: John Wiley.

Homme, L.E. (1965) Perspectives in psychology 24: control of coverants, the operants of the mind. *Psychological Record* 15: 501–511.

Hovland, C., Janis, I. and Kelly, H.H. (1953) *Communication and Persuasion*, New Haven, CT: Yale University Press.

Howard, H.I., Kopta, S.M., Krause, M.S. and Orlinsky, D.E. (1986) The dose–effect relationship in psychotherapy. *American Psychologist* 41: 159–164.

ICD 10 (1992) *International Classification of Disease*, World Health Organisation.

Isaacs, W., Thomas, J. and Golddiamond, I. (1966) Application of operant conditioning to reinstate verbal behaviour in psychotics, in Ulrich, R., Stachnic, T. and Mabry, J. (eds) *Control of Human Behavior*, vol. 1, Glenville, IL: Scott Foreman.

James Lind Library, Oxford. www.jameslindlibrary.org.

James, W. (1890) *The Principles of Psychology*, New York: Dover Press.

Jones, C., Cormac, I., Silveira da Mota Neto, J.I. and Campbell, C. (2004) Cognitive behaviour therapy for schizophrenia. *Cochrane Database of Systematic Reviews*, Issue 4, Art. no. CD000524.

Kazdin, A.E. (2004) Pschotherapy for children and adolescents, in Lambert, M.J. (ed.) *Bergin and Garfield's Handbook of Psychotherapy and Behavior Change* (5th edn), New York: John Wiley.

Kazdin, A.E., and Weisz, J.R. (1998) Identifying and developing empirically supported child and adolescent treatments. *Journal of Consulting and Clinical Psychology* 60: 576–585.

Kazdin A.E. and Wilson, G.T. (1978) Criteria for evaluating psychotherapy. *Archives of General Psychiatry* 35: 407–418.

Keats, J. *John Keats's Poems*, ed. G. Bullett (1964) London: Everyman Library.

Kendler, K.S. and Evans, L.J. (1986) Models for the joint effect of genotype and environment on liability to psychiatric illness. *American Journal of Psychiatry* 143: 279–289.

Kick, P.E. and McElroy, S.L. (1998) Pharmacological treatment of bipolar disorder, in Nathan, P.E. and Gorman J.M. (eds) *Treatments that Work*, Oxford: Oxford University Press.

Knight, S.H. (1921) *Uncertainty and Profit*, New York: Essential Reprints.

Kohlberg, L. (1981) *The Philosophy of Moral Development*, New York: Harper Row.

Kornor, H., Winje, D., Ekeberg, O., Weisaeth, L., Kirkenhel, I., Johansen, K. and Steiro, A. (2008) Early trauma-focussed cognitive-behavioural therapy to prevent chronic post-traumatic stress disorder and related symptoms: a systematic review and meta-analysis. *BMC Psychiatry*, 8 September, arH. D.81.

Kuhn, T. (1970) *The Structure of Scientific Revolution* (2nd edn), Chicago, IL: University of Chicago Press.

Laing, R.D. (1960) *The Divided Self*, Harmondsworth: Penguin.

Lambert, M.J. (ed.) (2004) *Bergin and Garfield's Handbook of Psychotherapy and Behavior Change* (5th edn), New York: John Wiley.

Lambert, M.J. and Ogles, B.M. (2004) The efficacy and effectiveness of psychotherapy, in Lambert, M.J. (ed.) *Bergin and Garfield's Handbook of Psychotherapy and Behavior Change* (5th edn), New York: John Wiley.

Lambert, M.J., Bergin, A.E. and Garfield, S.L. (2004) Historical overview, in Lambert, M.J. (ed.) *Bergin and Garfield's Handbook of Psychotherapy and Behavior Change* (5th edn), New York: John Wiley.

Le Doux, J. (2003) *The Emotional Brain*, London: Phoenix.

Leff, J. (ed.) (1997) *Care in the Community: Illusion or Reality?* Chichester: John Wiley.

Leff, J., Knipers, L., Berkowitz, R., Erberleinen, R., Vries, R. and Sturgeon, D. (1982) A controlled trial of social intervention with schizophrenia patients. *British Journal of Psychiatry* 141: 121–134.

Lewinsohn, P.M., Steinmetz, J.L., Larson, D.W. and Franklin, J.L (1981) Depression-related cognitions: antecedent or consequence? *Journal of Abnormal Psychology* 90: 213–219.

Libet, B. (1999) 'Do we have free will?, in Freeman, A. and Sutherland, V. (eds) *The Volitional Brain*, Exeter: Imprint Academic.

Liese, B. and Franz, R.A. (1996) Treating substance use disorders with cognitive therapy: lessons learned and implications for the future, in Salkovskis, P. (ed.) *Frontiers of Cognitive Therapy*, New York: Guilford Press.

Littell, J.H. (2008) Evidence-based or biased? The quality of published reviews of evidence-based practices. *Children and Youth Services Review* 6: 1299–1317.

Lopata, C., Thomeer, M.L., Volker, M.A. and Nida, R.A. (2007) Effectiveness of cognitive-behavioural treatment on the social behaviours of children with Asperger's Disorder. *Focus on Autism and Other Developmental Disabilities* 21: 237–244.

Lovaas, O.I. (1967) A programme for the establishment of speech in psychotic children, in Wind, J.K. (ed.) *Early Childhood Autism*, Oxford: Pergamon Press.

Lovaas, O.I. (1987) Behavioural treatment and normal educational/intellectual functioning in young autistic children. *Journal of Consulting and Clinical Psychology* 55: 3–9.

Luborsky, L., Singer, B. and Luborsky, L. (1975) Comparative studies of psychotherapies: is it true that 'everyone has one and all must have prizes?' *Archive on General Psychiatry* 32: 995–1008.

Luria, A. (1961) *The Role of Speech in the Regulation of Normal and Abnormal Behaviour*, New York: Liveright.

McCrae, R., Costa, P.T., Ostendorf, F., Angleitnes, A., Hrebickova, M., Avia, M.D., Sanz, J., Sauchez-Bernardos, M.L., Kusdil, M.E., Woodfield, R., Saunders, P.R. and Smith, P.B. (1997) Nature over nurture: temperament, personality and life span development. *Journal of Personality and Social Psychology* 78: 173–186.

Macdonald, G.M. (2001) *Effective Interventions for Child Abuse and Neglect, An Evidence-Based Approach to Assessment, Planning and Evaluation*, Chichester: John Wiley.

Macdonald, G.M. and Kakavelakis, I. (2004) *Helping Foster Carers to Manage Challenging Behaviour. Evaluation of a Cognitive-Behavioural Training Programme for Foster Carers*, University of Exeter: Centre for Evidence-based Social Services.

Macdonald, G.M. and MacDonald, K.I. (1999) Perceptions of risk, in Parsloe, P. (ed.) *Risk Assessment in Social Care and Social Work*, London: Jessica Kingsley.

Macdonald, G.M. and Roberts, H. (1995) *What Works in the Early Years*, Barbados: Barkingside.

Macdonald, G.M. and Sheldon, B. (1992) Contemporary studies of the effectiveness of social work. *British Journal of Social Work* 22: 615–643.

Macdonald, G.M. and Sheldon, B. (1997) Community services for the mentally ill, consumers views. *International Journal of Social Psychiatry* 43: 35–55.

McGuffin, P., Owen, M.J. and Gottesman, I.I. (2005) *Psychiatric Genetics and Genomics*, Oxford: Oxford University Press.

Malcolm, J.L. (1984) *In the Freud Archives*, London: Jonathan Cape.

Malik, N., Kingdon, D., Pelton, J., Mehta, R.M. and Turkington, D. (2009) Effectiveness of brief cognitive-behavioural therapy for schizophrenia, delivered by mental health nurses: relapse and recovery at 24 months. *Journal of Clinical Psychiatry* 70: 201–207.

Maranon, G. (1924) Contribution a l'étude de l'action émotive de l'adrenolin. *Revue française d'endocrin* 21: 301–325.

Marshall, M., Gray, A., Lockwood, A. and Green, R. (1998) Case management for people with severe mental disorders. *Cochrane Database of Systematic Reviews*, Issue 2, Art. no. CD000050. DOI:10.1002/14651858.CD000050.

Marks, I.M. (1975) Behavioural treatments of phobic and obsessive-compulsive disorders: a critical appraisal, in Hersen, R. *et al.* (eds) *Progress in Behaviour Therapy*, London: Academic Press.

Marks, I.M. (1978) Behavioural psychotherapy of neurotic disorders, in Bergin, A.E. and Garfield, S.L. (eds) *Handbook of Psychotherapy and Behavior Change* (2nd edn), Chichester: John Wiley.

Marzillier, J.S. (1980) Cognitive therapy and behavioural practice. *Behaviour Research and Therapy* 18: 17–28.

Masserman, J. (1943) *Behaviour and Neurosis*, Chicago, IL: University of Chicago Press.

Masson, J. (1990) *Against Therapy*, London: Fontana.

Matt, G.E. and Navarro, A.W. (1997) What meta-analyses have and have not taught us about psychotherapy effects: a review and future directions. *Clinical Psychology Review* 17: 1–32.

Mayer, J.E. and Timms, N. (1970) *The Client Speaks: Working Class Impressions of Casework*. London: Routledge & Kegan Paul.

Medical Research Council (MRC) (2003) *Clinical Trials for Tomorrow*, London: BMJ Publishing.

Meichenbaum, D. (1974) *Cognitive Behaviour Modification*, Morristown, NJ: General Learning Press.

Meichenbaum, D. (1977) *Cognitive Behaviour Modification: An Integrative Approach*, New York: Plenum.

Midgley, M. (2003) *The Myths We Live By*, London: Routledge.

Midgley, M. (2005) *The Owl of Minerva*, London: Routledge.

Milgram, S. (1974) *Obedience to Authority*, London: Tavistock.

Milkowitz, D.J., Somonean, T.C., Sachs-Erikson, N., Warner, R. and Suddarth, R. (1996) Family risk indicators in the course of bipolar affected disorder, in Mundt, C., Goldstein, K., Hahlweg, P. and Fielder, P. (eds) *Interpersonal factors in the Origin and Course of Affective Disorders*, London: Gaskell Books.

Mill, J.S. (1859) *On Liberty*, London: Dent.

Müller, O., Berghöfr, A. and Baner, M. (2002) Bi-polar disorder. *The Lancet* 359: 19.

Munro, E. (2006) *Effective Child Protection*, London: Sage.

National Institute for Clinical Excellence (NICE) (2004) *Depression (Amended) Management of Depression in Primary and Secondary Care*, London: NHS.

National Institute of Health and Clinical Excellence (NIHCE) (2005a) *Obsessive-compulsive Disorder: Core Interventions in the Treatment of Obsessive-compulsive Disorder and Body Dysmorphic Disorder*, Clinical Guideline 31, London: National Collaborating Centre for Mental Health.

National Institute of Health and Clinical Excellence (NIHCE) (2005b) *Post Traumatic Stress Disorder (PTSD): The Management of PTSD in Adults and Children in Primary and Secondary Care*, Clinical Guideline 26, London: National Collaborating Centre for Mental Health.

National Institute of Health and Clinical Excellence (NIHCE) (2006) *Eating Disorders*, Clinical Guideline a., London: National Collaborating Centre for Mental Health.

National Institute of Health and Clinical Excellence (NIHCE) (2007a) *Depression (Amended)*, Clinical Guideline 23, London: National Collaborating Centre for Mental Health.

National Institute of Health and Clinical Excellence (NIHCE) (2007b) *Anxiety (Amended)*, Clinical Guideline 22, London: National Collaborating Centre for Mental Health.

National Institute of Health and Clinical Excellence (NIHCE) (2007c) *Clinical Guideline, Schizophrenia*, London: National Collaborating Centre for Mental Health.

Nida, R.E., Lopata, C., Thomeer, M.L. and Volker, M.A. (2006) Effectiveness of a cognitive-behavioural treatment and the social behaviours of children with Aspergers disorder. *Focus on Autism and other Developmental Disabilities* 21: 237–244.

O'Neill, O. (2002) *A Question of Trust: 2002 BBC Reith Lectures*, Cambridge: Cambridge University Press.

Oakley, A. (2000) *Experiments in Knowing: Gender and Method in the Social Sciences*, Cambridge: Polity Press.

Olds, J. (1956) Pleasure center of the brain. *Scientific American* 195: 105–116.

Olsen, M.R. (ed.) (1984) *Social Work and Mental Health*, London: Tavistock.

Orlinsky, D.E. and Parks, B.K. (1994) Process and outcome in psychotherapy: *Noch einmal*, in Bergin, A.E. and Garfield, S.L. (eds) *Handbook of Psychotherapy and Behavior Change* (4th edn), New York: John Wiley.

Orlinsky, D.E., Ronnestad, M.H. and Willntski, N. (2004) Fifty years of psychotherapy process – outcome research: continuity and change, in Lambert, M.J. (ed.) *Bergin and Garfields Handbook of Psychotherapy and Behavior Change* (5th edn), New York: John Wiley.

Orne, M. (1965) Psychological factors maintaining resistance to stress, in Krauser, S. (ed.) *The Quest For Self-Control*, New York: Free Press.

Ost, L.G. and Westling, B.E. (1995) Applied relaxation vs cognitive therapy in the treatment of panic disorder. *Behaviour Research and Therapy* 33: 145–158.

Parsloe, P. (ed.) (1999) *Risk Assessment in Social Work and Social Care*, Research Highlights, 36. London: Jessica Kingsley.

Pavlov, I.P. (1897) *Lectures on Conditional Reflexes,* trans. W.H. Gannt (1928), Oxford: Oxford University Press.

Pavlov, I.P. (1927) *Conditional Reflexes*, New York: Dover Press.

Persons, J.B. (2009) *The Case Formulation Approach to Cognitive-Behaviour Therapy*, New York: Guilford Press.

Peters, W. (1987) *A Class Divided, Then and Now,* London: Yale University Press.

Pharoah, F., Mari, J., Rathbone, J. and Wong, W. (2006) Family intervention for schizophrenia. *Cochrane Database of Systematic Reviews*, Issue 4, Art. no. CD0000, 88. DOI: 1002114651858. pub.2.

Piaget, J. (1929) T*he Child's Conception of the World,* London: Routledge & Kegan Paul.

Piaget, J. (1958) *The Child's Construction of Reality*, London: Routledge & Kegan Paul.

Pinker, S. (1996) *The Language Instinct*, London: Allen Lane.

Pinker, S. (1999) *Words and Rules: The Ingredients of Language*, London: Weidenfeld & Nicolson.

Pinker, S. (2004) *The Blank Slate*, London: Allen Lane.

Pinker, S. (2007) *The Stuff of Thought*, London: Allen Lane.

Plomin, R., Defries, J.C. and Lochlin, J.C. (1977) Genotype–environment interaction and correlation in the analysis of human behaviour. *Psychological Bulletin* 85: 309–322.

Plomin, R., Owen, M.J. and McGuffin, P. (1999) The genetic basis of complex human behaviours, in Slater, A. and Muir, D. (eds) *Developmental Psychology*, Oxford: Blackwell.

Popper, K.R. (1963) *Conjectures and Refutations*, London: Routledge & Kegan Paul.

Popper, K.R. (1982) *The Open Universe: An Argument for Indeterminism*, London: Hutchinson.

Popper, K.R. and Eccles, J.C. (1977) *The Self and its Brain*, New York: Springer.

Porter, P. (1983) *The Rest on the Flight*, London: Picador.

Premack, D. (1959) Towards empirical behaviour laws, 1, Positive reinforcement. *Psychological Review* 66: 11–17.

Prideaux, S. (2005) *Edward Munch, Behind the Scream*, London: Yale University Press.

Rachman, S.J. and Wilson, G.T. (1980) *The Effects of Psychological Therapy*, Oxford: Pergamon Press.

Rajecki, D.W. (1982) *Attitudes: Theories and Advances*, Sunderland, MA: Sinauer Associates.

Redfield-Jamison, K. (1995) *An Unquiet Mind: A Memoir of Moods and Madness*, London: Picador.

Rees, M. (Astronomer Royal) (2010) *Reith Lectures, 2010*, London: BBC.

Reid, W.J. and Hanrahan, P. (1980) The effectiveness of social work, recent evidence, in Goldberg, E.W. and Connolly, N. (eds) *Evaluative Research in Social Care*, London: Heinemann Educational Books.

Reid, W.J. and Shyne, A.W. (1969) *Brief and Extended Casework*, New York: Columbia University Press.

Richard Phillips Inquiry (1995) London: Westminster City Council.

Richmond, M. (1917) *Social Diagnosis*, New York: Russell Sage Foundation.

Risley, T.L. (1977) The social context of self-control, in Stuart, R.B. (ed.) *Behavioral Self-Control*, New York: Brunner-Mazel.

Rivers, W.H. (1922) *Conflict and Dreams*, London: Chatto and Windus.

Rogers, C.R. (1951) *Client-centred Therapy: Its Current Practice, Implications and Theory*, Boston, MA: Houghton Mifflin.

Rogers, C.R. and Skinner, B.F. (1956) Some issues concerning the control of human behaviour: a symposium. *Science* 124: 3231, 1050–1066.

Rosa-Alcazar, A.I., Sanchez-Meca, J., Gomez-Conesa, A. and Mariv-Martinez, F. (2008). Psychological treatment of obsessive-compulsive disorder; a meta-analysis. *Clinical Psychology Review* 28: 1310–1325.

Roth, A.D. and Pilling, S. (2008) Using an evidence-based methodology to identify the competencies required to deliver effective cognitive and behavioural treatment for depression and anxiety disorders. *Behavioural and Cognitive Psychology* 36: 129–147.

Rutter, M. (2006) Is a 'Sure Start' to an effective preventative intervention? *Child and Adolescent Mental Health* 11: 135–141.

Rutter, M. (2007) Gene–environment interdependence. *Redeveloped Science* 10: 12–18.

Rutter, M. and Hersov, L. (eds) (1987) *Child and Adolescent Psychiatry: Modern Approaches*, Oxford: Blackwell Science.

Ryle, G. (1949) *The Concept of Mind*, London: Hutchinson.

Ryle, G. (1979) *On thinking*, Oxford: Blackwell.

Sackett, D.L., Rosenberg, W.M., Gray, J.H.M., Haynes, R.B. and Richardson, W.S. (1996) Evidence-based practice: what it is and what it isn't. *British Medical Journal* 312: 71–72.

Sacks, O. (1985) *The Man Who Mistook His Wife for a Hat and Other Clinical Tales*, New York: Summit.

Salzberger-Wittenberg, I. (1970) *Psychoanalytical Insights and Relationships*, London: Routledge & Kegan Paul.

Scarr, S. and McCartney, K. (1983) How people make their own environments: a theory of genotype–environment effects. *Child Development* 4: 424–435.

Schacter, S. (1964) The interaction of cognitive and physiological determinants of emotional state, in Berkowitz, L. (ed.) *Advances in Experimental Social Psychology*, New York: Academic Press.

Schacter, S. and Singer, J.E. (1962) Cognitive, social and physiological determinants of emotional states. *Psychological Review* 69: 378–399.

Schlick, M. (1936) *Philosophical Papers*, trans. Reidal, 1979, vol. 2.

Schulz, K. (2010) *Being Wrong: Adventures in the Margin of Error*, London: Portobello Books.

Scott, J., Williams, J.M. and Beck, A.T. (1989) *Cognitive Therapy in Clinical Practice; An Illustrative Casebook*, London: Routledge.

Scull, A. (1993) *The Most Solitary of Afflictions: Madness and Society in Britain, 1700–1900*, London: Yale University Press.

Seligman, M.E.P. (1975) *Helplessness*, San Francisco, CA: Freeman.

Serfaty, M.A., Turkington, D., Heap, M., Ledsham, L. and Jolley, E. (1999) Cognitive therapy versus dietary counselling in the out patient treatment of anorexia nervosa: effects of the treatment phase. *European Eating Disorder Review* 7: 334–350.

Sexton, T.L., Alexander, J.F. and Leigh Mease, A. (2004) Levels of evidence for the models and mechanisms of therapeutic change in family and couple therapy, in Lambert, M.J. (ed.) *Bergin and Garfield's Handbook of Psychotherapy and Behavior Change* (5th edn), New York: John Wiley.

Sheldon, B. (1977) Goal analysis, do you know where you are going? *Social Work Today* 1: 4.

Sheldon, B. (1978) Theory and practice in social work; a re-examination of a tenuous relationship. *British Journal of Social Work* 8: 1–22.

Sheldon, B. (1982) *Behaviour Modification*, London: Tavistock.

Sheldon, B. (1985) Evaluation-oriented case-recording, in *Managing Information in Practice*, Edinburgh: Scottish Education Department/Social Work Services Group.

Sheldon, B. (1986) Social work effectiveness experiments: review and implications. *British Journal of Social Work* 16: 223–242.

Sheldon, B. (1987) The psychology of incompetence, in Drewry, G., Martin, B. and Sheldon, B. (eds) *After Beckford? Essays on Child Abuse*, Egham: Royal Holloway College.

Sheldon, B. (1994) Biological and social factors in mental disorders: implications for services. *International Journal of Social Psychiatry* 40: 87–105.

Sheldon, B. (1995) *Cognitive-Behavioural Therapy: Research, Practice and Philosophy*, London: Routledge.

Sheldon, B. (2001) The validity of evidence-based practice in social work: a reply to Stephen Webb. *British Journal of Social Work* 31: 801–809.

Sheldon, B. and Baird, P. (1982) The use of closed circuit television in training social workers. *Social Work Today* 13: 2.

Sheldon, B. and Chilvers, R. (2000) *Evidence-based Social Care*, Lyme Regis: Russell House Publishing.

Sheldon, B. and Macdonald, G.M. (2009) *A Textbook of Social Work*, London: Routledge.

Shenger-Kristovnikova, N.R. (1921) Contributions to the question of differentiation of visual stimuli and the limits of differentiation by the visual analyses of the dog. *Bulletin of the Institute of Science*.

Shields, J. and Slater, E. (1967) Genetic aspects of schizophrenia. *Hospital Medicine*: 579–584.

Skinner, B.F. (1953) *Science and Human Behavior*, London: Collier Macmillan.

Skinner, B.F. (1971) *Beyond Freedom and Dignity*, Harmondsworth: Penguin.

Skinner, B.F. (1974) *About Behaviourism*, London: Jonathan Cape.

Skoog, G. and Scoog, I. (1999) A forty year follow-up of patients with obsessive-compulsive disorder. *Archives of General Psychiatry* 56: 121–127.

Slater, E. and Cowie, V. (1971) *The Genetics of Mental Disorders*, London: Oxford University Press.

Slater, A. and Muir, D. (eds) (1999) *Developmental Psychology*, Oxford: Blackwell.

Sloane, R.B., Stantes, F.R., Cristol, A.H., Yorkston, N.J. and Whipple, K. (1975) *Psychotherapy vs Behavior Therapy*, Cambridge, MA: Harvard University Press.

Smith, M.L. and Glass, G.V. (1977) Meta analysis of psychotherapy outcomes. *American Psychologist* 32: 752–740.

Strongman, K.T. (1987) *The Psychology of Emotion* (3rd edn), Chichester: John Wiley.

Strupp, H.H., Hadley, S.W. and Gomes-Schwartz, B. (1977) *Psychotherapy for Better or Worse: The Problem of Negative Effect*, New York: Aronson.

Sutherland, S. (1992) *Irrationality: The Enemy Within*, London: Constable.

Szasz, T. (1961) *The Myth of Mental Illness*, New York: Harper and Row.

Taylor, T. and Montgomery, P. (2007) Can cognitive-behavioural therapy increase self-esteem among depressed adolescents? A systematic review. *Children and Youth Services Review* 29: 823–839.

Tharp, R.G. and Wetzel, R. J. (1969) *Behaviour Modification in the Natural Environment*, London: Academic Press.

Thase, M.E. and Jindal, R.D. (2004) Combining psychotherapy and psychopharmacology in the treatment of mental disorders, in Lambert, M.J. (ed.) *Bergin and Garfield's Handbook of Psychotherapy and Behavior Change* (5th edn) New York: John Wiley.

Thase, M.E. Greenhouse, J.B., Frank, E., Reynolds, C.F., Pilkonis, P.A., Hunnley, K., Grochocinski, V. and Kunfer, D.J. (2004) Treatment of major depression with psychotherapy or psychotherapy-pharmacotherapy combinations. *Archives of General Psychiatry* 54: 1009–1013.

Thiele, L.P. (2006) *The Heat of Judgement: Practical Wisdom, Neuroscience and Narrative*, Cambridge: Cambridge University Press.

Thomas, A., Chess, S. and Birch, H.G. (1968) *Temperament and Behavior Disorders in Children*, New York: New York University Press.

Thorndike, E.L. (1898) Animal intelligence: an experimental study of the associative process in animals. *Psychological Review*. Monograph 2.

Thwaite, R. and Bennett-Levy, J. (2007) Conceptualizing empathy in cognitive behaviour therapy. Making the implicit explicit. *Behavioural and Cognitive Psychotherapy* 35: 591–612.

Tierney, S. (2004) *A Study of the Effectiveness of Interventions for Eating Disorder*, CEBSS, University of Exeter.

Tolman, E.C. (1932) *Collected Papers in Psychology*, Berkeley, CA: University of California Press.

Treasure, J., Claudino, A.M. and Zuckers, N. (2010) Eating disorders. *Lancet Seminar*. 583–593.

Trower, P., Bryant, B. and Argyle, M. (1978) *Social Skills and Mental Health*, London: Methuen.

Truax, C. and Carkhuff, R. (1967) *Towards Effective Counselling and Psychotherapy*, Chicago, IL: Aldine.

Tsuang, M.T. and Vandermey, R. (1980) *Genes and the Mind: Inheritance of Mental Illness*, Oxford: Oxford University Press.

Vaughn, C.E. and Leff, J.P. (1976) The measurement of expressed emotion in families of psychiatric patients. *British Journal of Social and Clinical Psychology* 15: 159–165.

Verworn, M. (1916) *Irritability*, New Haven, CT: Yale University Press.

Vittengh, J.R., Clarke, L.A., Dunn, T.W. and Jarrett, R.B. (2007) Reducing relapse and recurrence in unipolar depression: a comparative meta-analysis of cognitive-behavioural therapy's effects. *Journal of Consulting and Clinical Psychology* 75: 474–488.

Vlaeyen, P.E. and Gorman, J.M. (1998) *A Guide to Treatments That Work*, Oxford: Oxford University Press.

Vygotsky, L. (1962) *Thought and Language*, New York: John Wiley.

Wanless, D. (2006) *Securing Good Care for Older People: Taking a Long Term View*, London: Kings Fund.

Watson, J.B. and Raynor, R. (1920) Conditioned emotional reactions. *Journal of Experimental Psychology* 3: 1–14.

Webb, S.A. (2001) Some considerations on the validity of evidence-based practice in social work. *Bristol Journal of Social Work* B: 1–14.

Weisz, J.R., Huey, J. and Weevsing, V.R. (1998) Psychotherapy outcome research with children and adolescents, in Ollendick, T.H. and Prinz, R.J. (eds) *Advances in Clinical Psychology* (vol. 20), New York: Plenum Press.

Weisz, J.R., Sonthan-Gerrow, M.A., Gordis, E.N., Connor-Smith, J.K., Langer, B.C., McLeod, B.D., Amanda, J-D., Updegraff, A. and Weiss, B. (2009) Cognitive-behavioral therapy versus usual clinical care for youth depression: an initial test of transportability to community clinics and clinicians. *Journal of Consulting and Clinical Psychology* 77: 383–394.

Westbrook, D. and Kirk, J. (2007) The clinical effectiveness of cognitive behaviour therapy: outcome for a large sample of adults treated in routine practice. *Behaviour Research and Therapy* 43(10): 1243–1261.

Westbrook, P., Kennedy, H. and Kirk. J. (2007) *An Introduction to Cognitive Behaviour Therapy; Skills and Applications*, London: Sage.

Westbrook, D., Sedgwick-Taylor, A., Bennet-Levy, J., Butler, G. and McManus, F. (2008) A pilot evaluation of a brief CBT training course. Impact on trainee's satisfaction, clinical skills and patient outcomes. *Behavioural and Cognitive Psychotherapy* 36.

Wills, F. (2009) *Becks Cognitive Therapy Distinctive Features*, London: Routledge.

Wilson, T. and Fairburn, C (1998) Treatments for eating disorders, in Nathan, P. and Gorman, J. (eds) *A Guide to Treatments that Work*, New York: Oxford University Press.

Winokur, G., Coryell, W. and Keller, M. (1995) A family study of manic-depression (bipolar I.) disease. Is it a distinct illness separable from primary unipolar depression? *Archives of General Psychiatry* 52: 367–373.

Wodarski, J.S. and Thyer, B.H. (eds) (1998) *Handbook of Empirical Social Work Practice*, Chichester: John Wiley.

Wolpe, L. (1958) *Psychotherapy by Reciprocal Inhibition*, Stanford, CA: Stanford University Press.

Wolpert, L. (1999) *Malignant Sadness*, London: Faber and Faber.

Woodcock, A. and Davis, M. (1978) *Catastrophe Theory*, Harmondsworth: Penguin.

Woolf, V. (1927) *The Essays of Virginia Woolf*, vol. 5, ed. S.N. Clarke (2009), London: The Hogarth Press.

Wootton, B. (1959) *Social Science and Social Pathology*, London: Allen & Unwin.

Wundt, W. (1907) *Outlines of Psychology*, trans. C.H. Judd, Leipzig: Englemann.

www.babcp.org, British Association for Behavioural and Cognitive Psychotherapies.

Wykes, T., Tarrier, N. and Lewis, S. (1998) *Outcome and Innovation in Psychological Treatment of Schizophrenia*, Chichester: John Wiley.

Zerbin–Rüdin, E. (1967) Endogene Psychosen, in Becker, P.E. (ed.) *Human Genetik; em kurzes Handbuch*, vol. 2, Stuttgart.

Zimbardo, P.G. (1992) *Psychology and Life* (13th edn), New York: HarperCollins.

Zimbardo, P. (2003) *Psychology and Life* (14th edn), New York: HarperCollins.

Zimbardo, P.G., Hanney, C., Brooks, W.C. and Jaffe, D.C. (1973) The psychology of imprisonment. Privation, power and pathology, in Rosenham, D. and London, P. (eds) *Theory and Research in Abnormal Psychology* (2nd edn), New York: Holt, Rinehart Winston.

Zung, W.K. (1965) A self-rating depression scale. *Archives of General Psychiatry* 12: 63–70.

Index

Page numbers in **bold** refer to figures, page numbers in *italic* refer to tables.

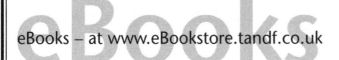